BEYOND THE 120-YEAR DIET

p44   b50 markers

BEYOND

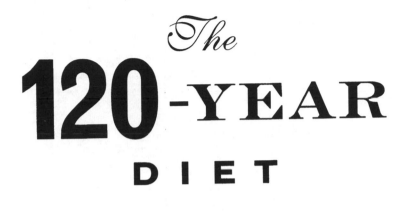

The
120-YEAR
DIET

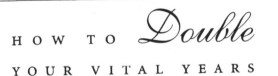

HOW TO *Double*
YOUR VITAL YEARS

ROY L. WALFORD, M.D.

FOUR WALLS EIGHT WINDOWS

New York · London

ACKNOWLEDGEMENT

I am grateful to my administrative assistants, Peri Doslu and Helga Bradish, for expert support including library research, bibliographic work, and careful perusal of the manuscript; to my daughter, Lisa Walford, for writing a portion of Chapter 8 and for her coverage of the menu items in the Appendix; again to Lisa Walford, and to Karen McMann, for their respective roles (Karen as programmer) for the software development so important in the genesis of *Beyond the 120-Year Diet*; and to my editor, Kathryn Belden, at Four Walls Eight Windows, for useful suggestions and careful editing. Finally, I acknowledge a debt to the useful and interesting postings of the Internet Calorie Restriction Society (see Readings and Resources, Internet Information Sources).

CONTENTS

CHAPTER 5

CHAPTER 6

CHAPTER 7

CHAPTER 10

FOODS AND TIPS FOR A CRON-DIET CUISINE

PREFACE

TO THE SECOND EDITION

====

THE PUBLIC ATTITUDE TOWARDS RETARDING AGING AND greatly extending life span has undergone a remarkable change since the first edition of this book, in 1986. Beginning a book tour for that edition, my first encounter was with Charles Gibson, cohost of *Good Morning America*. As I awaited my turn in the anteroom, I watched Gibson interviewing Shirley MacLaine about her recently published account of her travels into the spirit world. Gibson accepted all of her assertions about the reality of spirits without batting an eye. So I thought I would have an easy interview. But when I faced him for my four minutes of time, he began waving *The 120 Year Diet* in the air like a madman, and declared, "Your publisher must have insisted on this title."

"No, it's a title I chose," I replied, somewhat startled.

"That can't be. It's absurd to think we can extend the human life span that much!" he insisted (and kept on insisting for the whole four minutes).

The misled Mr. Gibson's attitude was typical of the time. Until the past two to four years, significant life extension has been regarded with about as much credulity as believing in ghosts. It has furthermore been a curiously taboo subject, even among biologists, as discussed at length in my earlier book, *Maximum Life Span*. [1]

It's not taboo any longer! For his January 1, year 2000 essay in the *New York Times*, feature columnist William Safire chose as a title, "Why Die?" and went on to discuss briefly not only the probability of life extension but its social ramifications.

Today, few informed people doubt that life extension by means of

xi

molecular genetics or other (simple) manipulation lies on the horizon. The question now is, how far away is it? The answer of course is that we don't quite know when the work with stem cells, telomerase, free radical scavengers. . . or whatever, will fructify with a human application, and begin leading to life spans of 150 years, 200 years, and progressively longer as gerontology advances.

One sure thing: laypersons tend to anticipate advances sooner than they happen, i.e., they overpredict, whereas experts underpredict. In the last part of the nineteenth century and first part of the twentieth, lay pundits were predicting that by the year 2000 we would have colonies through much of the solar system.[2] That was overprediction. In 1935 the three greatest physicists of the first half of the century (Einstein, Bohr, and Lord Rutherford) all predicted that we would never get power from the atom. About ten years later, with Hiroshima, the atomic (nuclear) age was born. And at the dawn of the information age, Mr. Bill Gates made his famous underprediction, "Nobody will ever need more than 64K of memory."

Since we cannot predict when there will be human applications for certain life extension techniques, what can we do in the meantime to enhance our chances of still being alive and vital when the more sophisticated techniques arrive? The answer to that question forms the subject of the present book. Calorie restriction with optimal nutrition, which I call the "CRON diet," will retard your rate of aging, extend life span (up to perhaps 150 to 160 years, depending on when you start and how thoroughly you hold to it), and markedly decrease susceptibility to most major diseases. If you want to hang around longer than you otherwise would, all the while leading an active healthy life, this is currently the only proven way to go. It's an interim solution, and may be difficult for the first six to twelve months, but it works!

There have been a number of significant developments in research since the first edition of this book. The CRON-diet principles have now tested positive in three separate monkey colonies, and I myself performed the first closely monitored human experiment (in Biosphere 2). The overall results strongly reinforce the evidence that the diet will do everything I claim for it. Also, we know much more now than in 1986 as to what constitutes "optimal nutrition" within a low-calorie regimen. The breakdown of the fatty acids (the omega-3 and omega-6 fatty acids), the glycemic index, the health enhancement attributed to the phytochemicals . . . are all new (and will be explained later in the book). They are certainly not substitutes for calorie restriction, but they may enhance your health over the years of life you will gain on a CRON diet.

CHAPTER 1

BETTER HEALTH
AND
GREATER LONGEVITY

LET'S GET ORIENTED

NOT MANY YEARS AGO, ABOUT ALL A PHYSICIAN ASKED himself when he saw a new patient was, What disease does this patient have? How can I *cure* it? Today's physicians are beginning to add the questions, What diseases is this patient susceptible to? How can I prevent them? In early Chinese medicine, the patient paid the doctor only as long as he (or she) stayed well. When the patient got sick, the doctor paid. Imagine how different American medicine would be today if such a system prevailed!

Whomever you are, reading this book, I can tell you with more than 75 percent accuracy that you will die of heart attack, hypertension, stroke, cancer, diabetes, kidney failure, or complications arising from osteoporosis. It's sad but safe to make this prediction because three out of four Americans do indeed succumb to these major killer diseases. Fortunately, you can do a great deal to cut your chances of being struck down by any of them. But avoiding them is just part of what you must do to live longer and better.

Even if you avoid all of the killer diseases, still you will grow old, and at about the same rate. Your skin will dry out and wrinkle, your hair grow thin and turn gray, your sight will dim, your hearing capacity will decline. You'll get heavier and a bit shorter. Your muscles will shrink, your joints stiffen. Your heart will pump blood less well... your lungs will take in less oxygen, and your tissues will use the oxygen less efficiently. Your kidney function will diminish and your endocrine glands will secrete a lower level of hormones. Your breasts will sag or your erection flag. Your resistance to infection will be less than a fourth what it was in youth. There will be slowing of your reaction time to a stimulus, such as the sight of a car hurtling toward you. Some phases of your learning process may slow down, with a lapse in memory for recent events, such as what movie you saw three nights ago. You may not come down with a major disease, but your vulnerability to changes in your environment, the weather, and in your personal life will markedly increase with age. Finally you will die from what for a young person might not be a serious problem at all: a mild attack of the flu will become the big sleep, or you won't manage to jump out of the way of that speeding red Pontiac.

> It's like a lion at the door,
> And when the door begins to crack,
> It's like a stick across your back,
> And when your back begins to smart,
> It's like a penknife in your heart,
> And when your heart begins to bleed,
> You're dead, and dead, and dead indeed.
>
> —NURSERY RHYME

Even if we avoid disease, we age just about as I've described, because aging is not itself a disease but the last stage of development. I am going to tell you how this unpleasant process of aging can be slowed down and even postponed to a much later time in life than it would otherwise occur. The method mainly involves losing weight gradually on a carefully selected diet that is high in nutrition but low in calories, or what I shall refer to henceforth as the CRON diet, where CRON stands for calorie restriction with optimal nutrition.[1]* (Note: An asterisk after a reference number indicates a discussion in the References and Notes section at the back of this book. The notes may comprise more detail than the average reader wishes to bother with. Suit yourself.)

In conservative scientific circles, what I recommend may be regarded as "controversial." That's another way of saying "not completely verified." Whether one should recommend measures to prevent disease and retard aging for which there is strong evidence that they do indeed work, but which are not 100 percent verified, will evoke different and sometimes (in fact, usually) heated opinions from biologists and medical doctors. Nevertheless, it is safe to say that far less skepticism exists today about the age retardation promised by a CRON regime in humans than in 1986 when the first edition of this book was published. Continuing research is proving me right, as we shall see.

PROOF AND PROBABILITY

For many years, firm but not conclusive evidence suggested that lowering the amount of cholesterol in the blood would help prevent heart disease.

Populations with high blood cholesterol levels experienced more heart attacks than those with low levels. But this neat correlation was not considered absolute "proof," and rightly not, because other differences between the populations might show a similar correlation but have nothing to do with susceptibility to heart attacks. The population with more attacks might be mostly blue eyed, and the other one brown eyed, but it wouldn't necessarily mean that to be blue eyed was to carry a time bomb in your chest. Correlation is not the same as proof of causation! It tells you where to look, but you have to be careful about drawing conclusions.

Despite population data and other "correlation" evidence, the only way to obtain scientifically acceptable proof of the association between blood cholesterol and heart disease would be to take a large number of persons from *the same population,* put half of them on a cholesterol-lowering regimen, and see if that half develops less heart disease than the rest. This critical test was performed in a seven-to-ten-year, $150-million study conducted by the National Institute of Health. It provided formal evidence that lowering blood cholesterol will substantially decrease the chance of a heart attack. There have been further refinements of this yardstick in that the cholesterol/HDL ratio in the blood, and more recently the triglyceride/HDL ratio yield even better predictions, and possibly (most recently) the level of blood homocysteine.

Years before the proof of the importance of the blood lipid levels in heart disease was published, many very creditable physicians, including professors at major medical schools, recommended measures aimed at lowering blood cholesterol. They did so on the basis of inferential, or "probable," evidence gained from observations in humans and experiments in animals. Other equally prestigious doctors didn't agree that the evidence was enough to act upon. Until formal proof is established, matters like this remain legitimate questions of judgment, which varies from one physician to another, and even between panels of experts. In 1980, for example, the Food and Nutrition Board of the National Research Council was unwilling on the basis of available data to recommend much at all in the way of nutritional change in the American diet, whereas in the same year and *on the same body* of data a committee of the American Heart Association advised lifelong adoption of a considerably altered diet. This illustrates our situation concerning many aspects of preventive medicine, including ways to slow down the aging process. Should we wait for "conclusive" evidence, which may be years away and too late for some of us? Can we, in some instances, accept probable evidence?

Physicians, patients, and bodies of experts alike should realize that not taking a stand, insisting on waiting until all the evidence is in, is itself a position and a recommendation. Not taking a stand is not really the neutral position it is made out to be.

We cannot easily run a $150-million seven-to-ten-year conclusive study on every promising assembly of probable evidence about preventing disease and retarding aging, so we must either stay neutral and do nothing or take a stand on the basis of imperfect evidence. Physicians like to pretend, and many have kidded themselves into believing, that whatever they espouse has been "scientifically proved." Nonsense! A great deal of what established medicine recommends with good conscience is not formally "proved." The health benefits of exercise, for example: the *formal* proof on that is not yet in, yet practically all physicians recommend it. And they are right to do so, because the probable evidence is excellent.

Recommendations about disease prevention and life extension are only as good as the ability of the recommending person to analyze and judge a wide assortment of important but inconclusive evidence. In this book I undertake to explain and rate the evidence, analyze it, judge it, and make specific recommendations. My credentials in relation to age retardation are among the best in the world. In the matter of disease prevention, they are less, but they reflect extensive reading on the subject, plus my experience as a teacher and practitioner at the University of California School of Medicine.

By *rating the evidence* I mean stating whether any case in point can be considered to display a very high order of probability (almost certain), a high order of probability, a moderate order, or less.

I judged it highly probable 14 years ago (for the first edition of this book) that a diet super high in nutritive quality but low in calories (the CRON diet as described herein) would retard the basic rate of aging in humans, greatly extending the period of youth and middle age; postpone the onset of such late-life diseases as heart disease, diabetes, and cancer; and even lower the overall susceptibility to disease at any age. In the intervening time, much additional evidence has accumulated, not only from further rodent investigations but also now from monkey and human studies, to support all of these assertions.

PRINCIPLES OF THE CRON DIET

The CRON diet is based upon many years of animal experimentation in my own laboratory at the UCLA Medical School, and in other laboratories in other major universities in the United States and Europe; in more recent studies of calorie-restricted monkey colonies at the Universities of Wisconsin and Maryland; at the National Institute on Aging; and my own studies on humans inside Biosphere 2 for two years.

There is no doubt at all that the life span of animals can be extended by up to 50 percent by dietary means, corresponding to humans living to be 150 or 160 years old. I don't actually expect to achieve quite this much life extension in humans. The necessary regimen would be too tough; but a less rigorous regimen will still add many years to your life, as well as life to your years. The former without the latter would not be so good, but the CRON dietary program promises both.

The CRON diet emphasizes food combinations and menus arrived at by computer techniques so that the Recommended Daily Allowances of all important nutrients are approximated with *minimal caloric intake.* The program calls for *gradual* weight loss over six months to a year or so, until you reach and remain at a new weight point substantially below your "set point." Your set point is the weight toward which you naturally gravitate if you neither over- nor under-eat. Your new weight point, if you are on the proper nutritive program, is your point of maximum metabolic efficiency, maximum health, and maximum life span.

(The CRON diet would also serve superbly well as a quick-weight-loss regimen, but I do not recommend such an undertaking, as it would be counterproductive in terms of good health and longevity, and, as I will show later, might even temporarily raise the levels of certain fat-soluble pesticide residues in your blood.)

I will also tell you how to determine fairly soon after beginning the diet whether markers of your health status have been improved, and to estimate (over a longer period) your individual aging rate, as well as can be done with present techniques. You can then determine how well the program is working for you. And you will soon observe, if you stick to the program, that you simply feel better. You will need less sleep, have more energy, enhanced vitality, and a clearer head than before.

The CRON diet is well founded scientifically. But evidence that taking fairly large amounts of certain vitamins, drugs, and chemicals will give an added boost to health and longevity varies from very good (for increasing health and *average life span*) to less than moderate (for increasing *maximum life span*—see below for definition of this important term). It does exist, however, and we must at least consider supplementation as a part of our program. The proper types (more than one) and amounts of exercise may yield additional advantages.

We shall thus be discussing evidence at every order of probability. In consultation with your personal physician, you must finally decide which recommendations you want to adopt.

INTERACTING WITH YOUR CHOSEN PHYSICIAN

Don't use this book just to strike out on your own, regulating your diet, testing your progress, and swallowing a lot of chemicals and pills. My recommendations may apply to an average across-the-board person but still not be appropriate for a particular individual like yourself. You should discuss the book with a physician qualified to establish your current health status and supervise your longevity and health program. Such qualifications are more easily asked for than found, although the situation has greatly improved in the last dozen years as experimental gerontology and geriatrics have become important medical disciplines. Nevertheless, modern medical training, while strong in disease treatment, remains weak in disease prevention. Nutrition, for example is still a woefully small part of the medical-school curriculum. The average physician may be vaguely familiar with much of the evidence I cite in this book, but will recognize that *some* of my recommendations are not in line with what establishment medicine preaches. He (or she) is apt to feel safe in hiding his ignorance of the subject behind his doctoral authority. That's not what you need.

Establishment medicine is in general excellent, but as pointed out by medical historian P. Starr,[2] it maintains its status and authority by two maneuvers: consensus, and the assumption of complexity. By *consensus* is meant that biologists and doctors may squabble among themselves, but they try to present a unified front to the public. *Assumption of complexity* means they behave as though arguments about health care were too complicated for even a reasonably educated layperson to understand. The acceptance of doctors as all-wise authority figures (which, believe it or not, dates only from about 1920) signifies "a surrender of private judgment" on the part of patients.[3] In considering what I say in this book, I ask you not to surrender your private judgment.

Warped into the habit of consensus viewing, your physician may not be willing even to consider evidence and recommendations contained in a popular book such as this one. In that case, he or she will find the hard-core scientific evidence for much of what I say here more extensively and rigorously documented in a book my former UCLA colleague Dr. Richard Weindruch (now at the University of Wisconsin) and I have written, *The Retardation of Aging by Dietary Restriction*, published by Charles C. Thomas in 1988, plus other, rigorous scientific monographs (see Readings and Resources, at the end of the book). What I say here may well be debatable, but it is based upon sound scientific investigations carried out at numerous recognized universities by many different investigators. All this will become apparent as we go along, in particular if you read the References and Notes section, also at the end of the book.

The National Institute on Aging and the National Center for Toxicological Research have maintained colonies of more than 30,000 rats and mice, about half of which are on an animal version of the CRON diet and the other half on a traditional diet. These colonies were established so that investigators throughout the country could test the hallmarks of this life span-prolonging, age-retarding regimen without the enormous trouble of setting up their own animal groups, as nutritional scientists have had to do until recently. The regulation of aging by diet, an area in which I and my associates have done some of the pioneering work, has become a major field of investigation into the aging process. If your doctor does not know about it, he or she should do some reading.

To establish the best interplay between yourself and your physician, you must take an active participatory interest. Anyone—either layperson or physician—can easily see from his two fine books *Anatomy of an Illness* and *The Healing Heart*, that Norman Cousins mastered the technique of the patient/physician interplay. Because of that, he received more careful, informed care from his doctors than if he had blindly followed their authoritarian advice. His books portray a new kind of patient/doctor relationship. Be guided by their example.

Of course you should seek advice from your personal physician. Still, in preventive medicine you must assume a large measure of responsibility for your own health. This means knowing or learning how to evaluate evidence. Even respectable medical journals contain a great deal of hogwash, lay journals a lot more, and television commercials almost nothing but. But hogwash is not hard to recognize, wherever it occurs, if you have the key concepts of what constitutes good evidence.

Finally, to hold up your side of the patient/physician interplay, you must acquire a basic knowledge about the major killer diseases of late life, and about certain critical aspects of the biology of aging. This knowledge is provided by the book you have in your hand.

AVERAGE AND MAXIMUM LIFE SPANS

To begin to understand aging and how to retard it, you must understand survival curves, in particular the significance of the average and maximum life-span points on those curves. Figure 1.1 shows four curves, A, B, C, and D. Curves A, B, and C are from actual populations; D is hypothetical. The vertical axis on the left indicates the percentage of the population that is alive at any age.

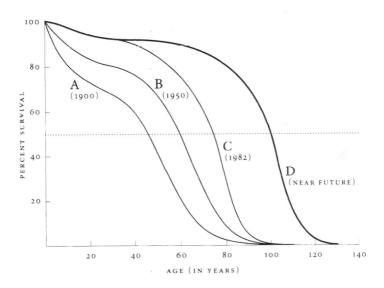

FIGURE 1.1 *Survival curves for the United States in 1900 (curve A), 1950 (curve B), and 1982 (curve C) and for a near-future subpopulation (people on the CRON diet) whose aging rate has been slowed (curve D)*

At birth all these population members were alive, so we start with 100 percent. In population A, half the people were dead by the age of 44; in population B, by 60; in population C, by 74; in hypothetical population D, by 100 years of age. All these 50 percent survival points express *average life spans* (also known as *life expectancies at birth*) for the four populations. Curves A, B, and C are the survival curves for the United States in 1900, 1950, and 1982. The average life span has been increasing since the turn of the century.

This largely reflects our conquest of many infectious diseases and to some extent other diseases in First World societies. But it can be shown mathematically that if *all* known diseases were cured—no heart disease, no stroke, no cancer, no diabetes—the average life span would move up to 85 years of age, but no further, unless the aging process itself were brought under control. The remarkable increase in average life span since 1900 does not reflect any retardation of the basic aging process!

Notice in Figure 1.1 that the maximum life spans are the same for curves A, B, and C. Maximum life span reflects the genetically determined longevity potential for our species. [4*] At the same time, it's a good measure of the basic aging process. It has remained at about 110 years not only since 1900, but even since the time of ancient Rome—and even before that. (There are of course a few outliers: two persons have lived to 113, one to 119, and the recently deceased French woman, Jeanne Calment, to 122). According to Genesis 6:3, "man also is flesh: yet his days shall be an hundred and twenty years." That's close enough to the observed 110-year maximum! No matter how off base His devotees have portrayed Him with respect to evolution, God shines through, at least in this passage, as an excellent gerontologist.

The survival curves A, B, and C teach us that we cannot influence maximum life span just by curing diseases. Even if all the major diseases were eliminated, the disease-free, older-growing population would simply become vulnerable to smaller and smaller environmental assaults, and still die off by 110 years. Only measures that truly retard biologic aging and stretch out the periods of youth and middle age will budge the shoulder of this maximal survival point and create a long-living society like the one represented in curve D. That's what the CRON diet will do.

I shall tell you not only how you can jump from curve A onto B or C, or from B onto C—thus increasing your average survival potential—but how you can jump onto curve D itself, becoming a member of the longest-living society that has ever existed. There is already an Internet-connected group of long-livers on this regime.... Many of them will be around to celebrate the twenty-second century.

So we have two goals in this book. They are related, but not quite the same. We want to learn how to improve our survival chances in terms of average life span. That means preventing as much as possible those diseases most of us would otherwise die of. Second, we want to learn how to slow down the rate of aging, so that while we avoid the diseases, we also do not age so rapidly. In other words, we will not only *live* longer we will stay *younger* longer. We will neither sag nor flag nor forget where we are or where we have been or where we are going in this fast-moving and exciting world.

QUESTIONS AND ANSWERS

I expect by now you have a lot of questions. I have encountered many of them in connection with the first edition of this book, my other books, lectures, and various events. The more specific and practical questions will be answered as we go along, but it will help if I answer some of the more common general ones right here.

QUESTION 1: Who wants to live to be 120 years old (or older) anyway?

ANSWER: I find I can evoke an "I do" or a "not me" answer from most people, depending on how this question is phrased. The very fact that it is often asked reflects the negative attitude about aging so common today. This attitude prevents people from properly imagining what a long-living society will be like when it arrives.

Do you ever hear a positive joke about the elderly? Most jokes about aging are nasty or condescending, like "Her face is so wrinkled, when she wears long earrings she looks like a venetian blind." That tasteless quip brings a terrible image to mind. With such an image, people don't think rationally. Of course they say, "No, I don't want to live to be 120."

Who can blame them? But this image of decrepitude is not the true picture at all. The 120-year (or even much longer) survival curve cannot be produced by addition of old years to old years, but only by stretching out the period of youth and middle age. In the new society I envision, an 80-year-old person will look and act and feel like a 40-year-old person of today. That allows us to ask the question differently. Who wants to be younger longer and middle aged longer, and in full possession of his or her faculties over that extended period? The person who doesn't say "I do" to that one is simply not having a good time in life. Alas, for these people I have no remedy.

In thinking about a 120- to 140-year society, we must not be overly influenced by the mentality and outlook of the 110-year society we live in now. In a long-living society, for example, people will have multiple careers. How many times have you heard a friend exclaim, "If I could just do it over again with what I know now?" But we become old, worn out, and even one career is exhausting enough.

Intensely creative people sometimes die soon after their one career reaches its end. James Joyce succumbed two years after finishing *Finnegans Wake*, Marcel Proust not long after completing *Remembrance of Things Past*, and poet Robert Lowell did not outlive his muse. Novelist Romain Gary wrote in his final note that the reason for his suicide was "I have explained myself fully."

These abrupt terminations would be less likely to happen if the persons involved were *functionally* only 35 to 45 years old, and ready for a new career. They would just roll over and arise from the other sides of their lifestyle beds, in a sense reborn, as I did at the age of 67 when I entered upon the experience of being a crew member inside Biosphere 2. Young people don't realize at gut level that they'll ever become old. Older people forget the energy, tirelessness, and vitality of youth; that wonderful sustaining feeling of physical well-being. But keep that energized vitality and you'll want to reach 120 or 140, want to go from one career to another, be able to "do it again with what I know now."

Of course some people will get stuck. They're the ones to feel sorry for. How would you like the elegantly boring job of being Queen Elizabeth II for 120 years?

I don't believe one grows older. I think that what happens early in life is that at a certain age one stands still and stagnates.

—T. S. Eliot [5]

QUESTION 2: The search to retard aging is an old one. After thousands of years of fruitless effort in the life-extension game, why do you think we've arrived now, or at least are close to some major breakthroughs?

ANSWER: For the following four good reasons:

ONE: We can with an order of probability bordering on certainty extend maximum human life span by means of the CRON diet right now, so at least one breakthrough has already taken place.

TWO: Like the Red Army in 1945, biology is advancing rapidly on a broad front. This is not only the day of the "information revolution", with computers going full blast around the country, but also the day of the "biological revolution." An enormous fallout cascades into the sphere of gerontology, the science of aging. And we know that science sometimes advances faster than many of its own experts have predicted.[6] We seem to be in such a period now.

THREE: For a long time people looked upon major extension of maximum life span as a pipe dream, and life-extensionists as impractical visionaries. Starting sometime in the late '70s or early '80s, however, this view began to change. In 1983 I was invited to testify before the U.S. Senate Finance Committee.[7] It seemed that government statisticians had been underestimating the numbers of old people accumulating in the population, making it difficult for the Finance Committee to anticipate Social Security requirements. My task was not to discuss these statistics but to portray the possibility of a true retardation of aging, and its socioeconomic effects. I noticed that when I spoke of the prospect that a long-living society, or at least a long-living subpopulation, might evolve in the near future, I got no skeptical feedback from the senators, or even the assembled statisticians. They did not think I was merely indulging in a science-fiction fantasy. The prospects were accepted as serious possibilities. If I had said the same thing five or ten years earlier, everyone would have thought: "Dr. Walford may have impressive credentials, but the poor man has obviously gone over the hill."

About this same time the Population Reference Bureau in Washington, D.C., predicted that eliminating cancer and heart disease would prolong millions of lives but add burdensome costs to society in caring for the elderly, whose average life spans have been extended into the period of being "functionally old." The Bureau urged the government to focus research on slowing the aging process *because a chronologically old but "functionally young" elderly population would not be a burden but a great social asset* .[8]

This change in public consciousness has accelerated remarkably during the '90s, and acceptance of the possibility of progress in any area greatly facilitates actual progress. If people still thought going to the Moon and Mars mere pipe dreams, the rockets would not be streaking up off their launch pads in Florida, even if the technology were available. Belief, hope, and confidence foreshadow practical action. In terms of life extension, there is not much doubt today in either the scientific community or the public that it's coming. The question is, when? Other methods are still in the future, but the CRON diet is now. If you want to still be around in good functional health when newer methods arrive, so you can take full advantage of their promise, this is what to do now.

FOUR: My fourth reason for optimism is fanciful and romantic, I admit. Throughout its long history, mankind has dreamed three classic dreams: to go to the Moon and other planets; to change one element into another, like lead into gold (the old alchemical dream of the philosopher's stone); and to be immortal, or at least to live a lot longer than we do. Of these three great dreams, the first two not only have been realized, but in our own lifetimes. We have already been to the Moon. No one doubts we are bound for the planets. With the techniques of modern physics we can change one element into another. Is it too fantastic to believe we shall also realize the third dream, the longevity dream, within the lifetimes of many of us now alive?

QUESTION 3: Dr. Walford, a lot of the research you cite as "evidence" for the life-extending benefits of the CRON diet was done in rodents. How do you know it applies to humans?

ANSWER: We won't know absolutely until a cohort of CRON dieters lives to be over 120, but the order of probability is now close to being overwhelming, that the CRON diet will extend maximum life span in humans just as it does in all animal species so far tested. And since this book's first edition 14 years ago, studies in monkeys and humans have been done. Life span has not yet been measured, as primates live a very long time; but there is no doubt the same extensive physiologic changes, including immunologic, biochemical, neurological, and hormonal changes, occur in monkeys and humans on a CRON diet as in rodents. And the CRON monkeys look younger than the control monkeys, and have not yet developed any of the diseases of aging, whereas the controls are becoming diabetic, one of the major diseases of aging in monkeys.

We are dealing with the question of "translatability." What is the probability that a phenomenon observed in animals can be translated to humans? Well, it depends on the phenomenon. Fertilization, growth, development, and aging are basically much the same across large species differences. There may be an occasional uniqueness in the mechanism of aging. Salmon and octopuses, for example, age almost overnight as the result of a programmed hormonal outpouring. And a few animals, lobsters for example, don't show any features of aging; [9] they simply outgrow their ecological niche. But these are easily recognized exceptions. Nobody doubts that most animals—for example, mice, rats, horses, chimpanzees, and humans—age by similar mechanisms. Any general process that retards aging in one such species ought to do so in another. The CRON-dietary regimen is such a process. [10]*The fact that it induces the same physiologic changes in all mammalian species so far tested further reinforces the likelihood of life extension for humans.

Most gerontologists, although perhaps not quite all, agree that calorie restriction will extend maximum human life span. I am aware, however, that some scientists have adopted a "wait and see" attitude. Of course, if they wait that long and don't do it themselves, they will not be alive to see.

QUESTION 4: But suppose that despite that extremely high order of probability you are so fond of talking about, the animal work on extending maximum life span turns out in fact not to apply to humans? What then?

ANSWER: In that unlikely case, all I can promise you is that your susceptibility to cancer, heart disease, stroke, diabetes, autoimmune disease, and probably even osteoporosis will be less than half that of the other people in your car pool. Your expected years of average survival will be better even than those of the people represented by curve C, and certainly far better than those of A or B if you happen to belong genetically to one of those less fortunate curves (Figure 1.1), even if your maximum survival chances are not improved. Nontranslatability of maximum life span still adds about ten or more years to your life, and healthier years at that, as a "worst case" estimate.

QUESTION 5: Do I have to give up all that good food?

ANSWER: If you are currently on the typical Western-style American diet, you do have to change your attitude towards, and your built-in social programming about, food. But you didn't write your own attitudes or programs anyway. They have been written into you by the experiences of childhood and a lifelong daily barrage of slick advertising, which tries to make you believe you are somehow deprived if you are not eating junk food, or that it's deliciously decadent and chic to be dining on the precursors of arteriosclerotic plaques. Indulge! they tell you. Have a fabulous time! Die young!

Of course, this notion of dire deprivation is simply a prejudice.

People who don't smoke do not feel deprived; they just don't smoke. Vegetarians (not that I particularly advocate vegetarianism) don't feel they are leading lives of deprivation; they just don't eat meat. But even scientists aren't immune to these notions. In commenting on the potential role of high-fat diets in causing arteriosclerosis, Rockefeller University's Dr. Edward Ahrens was quoted by *Time* magazine [11] as saying, "To deny everyone red meat could mean taking away the joy of life unnecessarily"—thereby denying joy to millions of Hindus, Jains, Seventh-day Adventists, and at least 3 million American vegetarians, few of whom feel deprived by not eating meat. And Dr. Suzanne Oparel, a scientist at the University of Alabama Medical Center studying the role of salt in causing high blood pressure, was quoted as saying, "Not being able to eat [a lot of] salt is losing one of the pleasures of life."

It's not that hard to reprogram yourself, and it's worth it. Besides lowering your disease susceptibility, the CRON diet will give you better eyesight and hearing at every age; a sharper, more alert problem-solving mind; an increased feeling of well-being; enhanced sexuality and fertility at a more advanced age. True, you may have to give up angel food cake, but to those for whom sight, alert senses, well-being, and sexuality are less important than angel food cake, I have nothing to offer. "Let them eat cake!"

You might also remember that there are seven deadly sins: pride, greed, lust, envy, gluttony, anger, and sloth. If you must have a certain measure of sin, I suggest you give up gluttony and accentuate one of the others: lust, for example. Indeed no less an authority than Dante informs us in both the *Inferno* and the *Purgatorio* that lust is the *least* of the seven deadly sins. In short, God ranks gluttony as worse than lust. Edward Ahrens, Suzanne Oparel, and all you other belly-oriented sinners, give up gluttony and double your lust! You'll live longer, healthier, jollier lives, and have a better chance of making it to Heaven.

QUESTION 6: What do you think about the Pritikin program, and the Ornish program?

ANSWER: On the positive side, I believe the Pritikin program is excellent, and with a fairly high order of probability will live up to most of its promises. The program has been disparaged by establishment medicine because Pritikin was not a trained health professional and the documentation in published articles from his center (although appearing in reputable biological journals) sometimes lacks good control data; but his evidence is nevertheless quite impressive. The Pritikin program knowledgeably addresses itself to general health problems and to prevention of the killer diseases. The strongest aspect of the program is that it *reprograms* those who go through it, into a more healthful lifestyle. I give it high marks on most counts.

On the questionable side, Pritikin was quite naive on the subject of life extension. He mixed up ideas about disease susceptibility and the basic biology of aging. Also, he was totally against supplementation, which seems to me too severe. Finally, he based his program on what he thought primitive man consumed, since that would be supposedly what humans are genetically "programmed" to eat, digest, and metabolize. But he erroneously considered primitive man to be represented by the early agricultural societies, or their modern equivalents like the Tarahumara indians. In fact primitive man was not agricultural man, who has existed for only about 10,000 years, but hunter/gatherer man, who existed for 1½ million years (*Homo erectus* and early *Homosapiens*). [12] Cereals and grains, which form a high proportion of the Pritikin diet, were not a large part of the diet of Paleolithic hunter/gatherer man. Early man subsisted largely on meat, vegetables, nuts, roots (tubers), and fruits, with not much grain or cereals and virtually no dairy products.[13] Despite his naivete, however, Pritikin lucked in: the wild animals eaten by a hunter/gatherer were only about 5 percent fat, compared with the 35 to 40 percent body fat of modern cattle. So the low-fat recommendations of Pritikin may be less inconsistent with the intake of the earliest humans than what modern Westerners customarily eat, or what certain current fad diets recommend.

The Ornish program resembles Pritikin's in that it is low fat and with a strong emphasis on wholesome foods, and with both exercise and educational counselling components. The results are well documented in top journals in the scientific literature, including the demonstration that arteriosclerotic clogging of arteries can sometimes be reversed. [14] I heartily agree with Ornish [15] that in most cases heart-disease patients should be offered dietary therapy before being subjected to bypass cardiac surgery. Only if they cannot or will not follow an appropriate dietary/exercise program should invasive techniques be turned to.

QUESTION 7: What do you think of the so-called "Zone" diet as promulgated in the various books of Barry Sears, in particular his latest one, *The Anti-Aging Zone*?

ANSWER: Certainly Sears and his assistants get high marks for marketing, beginning with the title of the first book. *Enter the Zone* has all the thrilling innuendo of a *Star Trek* episode or a theme-park ride. And in *The Anti-Aging Zone* you will find repeated over and over again that the Zone diet *reverses aging*. Now reversing disease is possible (see Ornish, above), and slowing down the rate of aging is also possible; but reversing basic aging itself—no one has ever done this, or seriously claimed it except alchemists and magicians. Sears presents no evidence whatsoever for this claim, but its constant repetition throughout the book reminds me of the technique of the TV commercial: repeat it often enough and people will come to believe it, regardless of the evidence, or lack thereof. Sears' first book does not include a bibliography or reference list, although you can obtain one if you send off a request; the latest book, *The Anti-Aging Zone*, does contain a lengthy list. However, there are no reference *numbers* in the text of either directing the reader to relevant references. Sears' reference lists are impressively long but essentially useless. So, for a starter, we have *proof* by repetition and merely the *pretense* of a helpful reference list.

If you look up Sears in Medline (National Library of Medicine) on the Internet, which gives exhaustive coverage of the medical-biological literature, you will find that he published about half a dozen solid experimental scientific papers in top journals in the '70s, one review paper in 1982, and one diet paper in the state dental journal in 1993. That's about it. According to his own account, most of the '80s he was off trying to corner the market on an ethnobotanical plant, borage. That didn't work out. His diet books have done much better. I find them all slickly written but unconvincing on numerous issues.[16]* I will limit further comments to his recent book on diet and aging.

Sears proposes a new theory of aging, dealing largely with eicosanoids. The evidence for this theory is at best marginal, compared to that amassed for any of the various theories of aging being considered by modern gerontology, for example the free radical theory,[17] DNA-repair theory, immunologic theory, glycemic theory, telomere theory, to name a few. But without subjecting his ideas to the critical review of publication in a scientific journal, which he does know how to accomplish, judging from his 1970s publications, Sears tries to shuffle all these into his own theory as though his were the gerontological equivalent of Einstein's long-sought unified field theory. One doesn't quite know whether to shout "bravo" (for performance) or "baloney" (for content), but I am inclined towards the latter.

Accepting that calorie restriction gives the best hope for age retardation and life extension, Sears then attempts a takeover of the area (One is reminded of his borage period!) by seeking to persuade us that only the Zone diet, with its relatively high fat content, will allow one to follow a calorie-restricted regime and be satisfied. Here he is on slippery ground as evidence also suggests that bulk of material eaten per calorie is more important than fat content, in leading to satiety.[18] I may also point out that all the changes Sears attributes to a Zone diet, e.g. low blood glucose, low insulin, low glycolsylated hemoglobin, were produced by the Biospherian diet[19] in which I participated, and which in its ratios of calories derived from protein, fat, and carbohydrate (roughly 12 percent, 12 percent, and 76 percent respectively[20]) were about as un-Zone-like as one could possibly get. Yet Sears quotes the Biospherian experience as supporting his theories. It certainly does not.

I do confess I find Sears entertaining. On pages 186 to 187 of *The Anti-Aging Zone* he lists a number of signs or, if you will, "biomarkers," to inform you whether you are "in the Zone" or not, i.e., whether you are following the Zone diet properly. These include how you feel generally, whether you are groggy in the morning, are fatigued, have headaches, and ten other markers of similar sophistication.[21]* One of these biomarker signs is the following, and I quote Sears exactly,

"When the stool is isodense with water (i.e., it floats), that becomes a very good indicator of optimal eicosanoid balance." In other words, if your shit floats, you are "in the Zone." To this I have but one question, "Where are you when it hits the fan?"

QUESTION 8: What do you think of the books of Durk Pearson and Sandy Shaw, including their best-selling book *Life Extension: A Practical Scientific Approach?*

ANSWER: In my book *Maximum Life Span* I gave examples showing that gerontology has always been the happy hunting ground for faddists, charlatans, pseudoscientific fringe characters, and just misinformed enthusiasts with "ready cures" for aging. Self-proclaimed "experts" spring up on all sides. Pearson and Shaw are among this long line of opportunists. The fact that they wrote a best-seller means nothing. Judy Mazel's *The Beverly Hills Diet* was a best-seller and it's probably the most ignorant diet book ever written. The only worse health advice I know of is that of Pearson and Shaw themselves. They argue that it's quite all right to lead a sedentary life and eat a high-fat, sugar-rich diet as long as you consume their formulation of vitamins, chemicals, drugs, and nutrient supplements. This is simply nonsense.

Pearson and Shaw are colorful television performers, but scientifically they are a joke. While presenting themselves in person and in writing as "scientists," so far as I know they have never done any regular biological research; never published an article in any reputable biological journal; never been on the faculty of any college, university, or biological research institution. As Dr. Ed Schneider, deputy director of the National Institute on Aging, has remarked of the fabulous twosome, "They're fun, but I wish they weren't in aging."

Okay, I can hear you ask: so they have no credentials and misrepresent themselves—but are they totally wrong? After all, they've been *reading* about the field of life extension for years, and they are basically intelligent people. They must know *something*.

True enough, but remember that in preventive medicine and life extension we are often obliged to deal with inferential evidence. Absolute answers are few. The best we can do is assess the degree of probability that different procedures will be effective. Every year several hundred articles are published in the world's scientific literature about, for example, vitamin E. You can shuffle that many articles together and come up with any answer that suits your prejudice. Pearson and Shaw lack the training and experience in science, the constant intimate contact with actual working scientists, the firsthand experience of having even one's own seemingly proved experiments explode into error, to *judge* and *analyze* the validity of the enormous body of constantly outpouring literature of biology. What they say is therefore a mixture of fact, fantasy, and fallacy. They are wishful thinkers and self-propagandists who do not really understand the nature of evidence.

THE NATURE OF EVIDENCE

If you get nothing out of this book except what I say in this section, you're way ahead. I'll be focusing on the biology of aging, but what I say will have general applicability to how you should evaluate any scientific or material claim, whether it be about your body, your automobile, your rose garden, or whatever—but not necessarily ethical, aesthetic, or religious claims, which are of course separate areas.

Throughout much of this book I'll be presenting you with evidence followed by recommendations. I want you to be informed and then to make up your own mind, remembering that you should seek guidance from your own doctor but not be dominated by his or her assumption of authority. The frequent bamboozling of the public by health faddists is partly the fault of medicine itself, which has taught people to rely on someone else's judgment, rather than teaching them how to examine evidence.

Evidence falls into four categories: testimonial, argumentative ("make the case for"), correlational, and experimental. *Testimonial* evidence is the principal type coming from the faddists, charlatans, and know-nothings. They will give you a list of people who took the treatment and say it did them good. If the list includes movie stars and professional athletes, or Olympic athletes, so much the better.

Testimonial evidence (related closely to "anecdotal" evidence) is highly unreliable. The list rarely includes people who took the treatment and did not receive any benefit. It almost never includes people who did not take the treatment but got better anyway, spontaneously. And testimonial evidence is abundantly available for almost every claim, from the benefits of Christian Science to experience with spiritualism, herbalism, black magic, faith healing, ghosts, Scientology, UFOs, Bigfoot . . . you name it. If you accept testimonial evidence, you will end up believing just about anything and everything. Testimonial evidence isn't necessarily and inherently wrong, but it's almost impossible to evaluate.

Interestingly enough, establishment medicine is also sometimes guilty of too much reliance on testimonial evidence, but it gives it another name: the "clinical anecdote." Dr. X has seen 35 patients with a certain malady and on the basis of his experience thinks that treating them with compound Z has been beneficial. He has no controls. His opinion represents a subjective guess. He will usually say, "My impression is …" or "My clinical experience is …" and then give the guess. This medical version of testimonial evidence is often wrong.

Argumentative evidence consists in marshaling known facts or experimental results and reasoning from them that something else ought to be so. Exercise, for instance, increases the level of high-density lipoproteins (HDL) in the blood, and these are usually associated with a lower degree of arteriosclerosis, so exercise *ought* to increase resistance to heart attacks. That's a logical argument. But do people who exercise actually experience fewer heart attacks? Maybe so, but you cannot stop with a plausibility argument! You have to test your hypothesis in the real world of what is happening.

Examples of argumentative evidence in gerontology concern the antioxidants: substances like vitamin E and the mineral selenium. These, it is argued, neutralize the damaging so-called "free radicals" that are by-products of normal metabolism. You can make an excellent case for the idea that free radicals cause aging, and that including antioxidants in the diet ought to retard it. But sad to say, including antioxidants in the diet, while it may to a certain degree indeed be health enhancing, has not so far been shown to extend the maximum life span of any species. Antioxidants so far have failed this critical test. Making a plausible case for something is not enough! Most of the Pearson/Shaw book relies upon this lower-order category of evidence, and upon the testimonial posturing of Pearson and Shaw themselves.

Sandy Shaw takes antioxidants and bends horseshoes on television, thus proving that antioxidants retard aging! Bah!

The two final types of scientific evidence, and the only really solid ones, are correlational and experimental. *Correlation* implies that when two things occur together all or most of the time, there may be a direct causal relationship between them, or that perhaps both are caused by some third (not necessarily apparent) phenomenon. Correlation can be seductive, but it's not actual proof. Nations whose citizens eat a high-fat diet generally display a higher incidence of heart disease than nations with low-fat diets. That sounds reasonable, but it's not proof. When the Santa Ana wind blows in California, a lot of people develop hay fever. The wind also causes an elevation in barometric pressure. Does elevated barometric pressure, then, cause hay fever? Of course not. The wind blows pollens around; that's what leads to the hay fever. Barometric pressure is irrelevant. Yet the correlation exists.

In this book we shall be concerned a great deal with correlational evidence. In fact it can be very useful, but one has to be careful. It was observed on examination of the data from a large number of insurance companies that people who are slightly overweight seem to enjoy a better average survival. This data might well be accurate, but the true biological interpretation may be quite different from what the data *seem* to indicate—that is, that it's intrinsically healthy to be slightly overweight. More on this later, but here's another interpretation, just to illustrate possibilities: perhaps the modern U.S. processed-food and junk-food diet is so poor that the average eater must consume excess calories just to get enough vitamins and essential nutriments to remain healthy and not be *mal*nourished.

The only kind of scientific evidence acceptable as genuine "proof" of a hypothesis is that of repeatable experiments, usually accompanied by what are called "control" data. Under appropriate conditions you do something, and that changes something else. And this something/something else always happens! When another investigator repeats the experiment on the other side of town or in Uttar Pradesh, the same result is obtained. The experiment, if done well, establishes the causal nature of a relationship between two phenomena. It constitutes *experimental evidence.*

Repeatedly confirmed experiments in my laboratory and in many other university laboratories have proved that cutting down calories, plus increasing the quality of the diet, produces very lean, extremely healthy animals, greatly extends their maximum life spans, markedly lowers their susceptibility to disease, and keeps them young in outward appearance, in their physiology and biochemistry, and in their physical and intellectual performance.

Correlation, if extensive enough, and experiment, if well conceived and carried out, constitute good evidence. Argument, or plausibility-constructs, are the building blocks of hypotheses. They are good for pointing the investigator in what he hopes is the right direction and for suggesting how to proceed in testing his hypothesis, but if acted on directly, because they "sound reasonable," they can lead you astray. Jumping on the latest supplement bandwagon might be a case in point. Testimonial evidence is the least reliable of all, but the most frequently used in advertising.

Having categorized the evidence, you have to *interpret* it. What does it mean biologically? American insurance company statistics seemed at one time to indicate that it's better to be slightly overweight; experiments in animals, that it's better to be underweight. The correlational evidence in one instance and experimental evidence in the other were both correct, but they seemed contradictory. Why? I've just given you one hint, and we'll be discussing these matters at some length in a later chapter. But when two sets of data both seem valid in fact but directly opposed in meaning, it often turns out in science that both are correct, and you have just not found the right interpretation.

I cannot teach you the fine points of interpretation of scientific evidence. That takes years of training and lots of experience. But you should be able to recognize the *category* of the evidence being presented to you: by me, in discussions with your friends, by other writers or lecturers, by popular health magazines, by newspapers, and of course by the 30-second flash-ad media blitzes. If your barber, hairdresser, or favorite celebrity tells you, "I went to Mexico and they shot me up with XYZ and I feel great. My cancer melted away, my arches rose, my bunions decamped, and lights went on in my head," you can recognize the statement as testimonial evidence.

I hope you will look just as critically at all the evidence in this book. That's your first step toward a super-healthy and extended life.

CHAPTER 2

GAUGING AGING AND MEASURING SUCCESS:

WHAT IS YOUR BIOLOGIC AGE?
IS THE CRON DIET WORKING FOR YOU?

═══════

THE CONCEPT OF BIOMARKERS

A BIOMARKER IS A TEST OR INDICATOR THAT SUGGESTS some event is happening or that some situation, be it normal or abnormal, exists in the body. For example, if you experience a sudden severe chest pain, you might be having a heart attack. The chest pain is a biomarker. By itself, however, it merely suggests the possibility of a heart attack. It doesn't prove you are actually having one. Maybe you've just swallowed a chicken bone and it's stuck in your esophagus. Or you are having gastric regurgitation (so-called "heart burn"). On the other hand, if your chest pain radiates to the left shoulder and down your arm (another biomarker for heart attack), you break out in a cold sweat (another biomarker), and your pulse becomes rapid and faint (another), then you probably are in fact having a heart attack. The biomarkers add up! Better get to a hospital right away!

In this chapter I'll be discussing two categories of biomarker:

ONE: The biomarkers of aging. A number of physiologic values, for example blood pressure, show average changes with age in a population. In general, blood pressure increases gradually with age in Western societies. Compared to the average person born the same year as you, you may be 50 years old by birthday age, but only 40 by the *functional* test of your blood pressure. By itself that doesn't mean you are functionally only 40 years old. But if your visual accomodation, hearing acuity, and lung volume match up to those of a 40-year-old (the biomarkers add up!), then you are *functionally* ten years younger than your birthday age. The reason you want to know this, outside of mere curiosity, is that if you adopt a regime that purports to retard aging, you want to know if it is really doing so. If you stick to the regime for six years, have you *functionally* aged only three years?

TWO: The biomarkers of success. By this I mean success in following a CRON diet. Are you really doing what it takes to retard aging or are you just playing around? You don't have to wait six years to find the answer to this important question. Six months is time enough. Your doctor can do a number of tests before you start and then six months later, tests which show rapid changes if you are on track with the program, tests including levels of blood sugar, cholesterol, blood pressure, and a number of other parameters. I did not include these as biomarkers in the first edition of this book because 13 years ago there were no hard data on primates (humans and monkeys) on suitably reduced calorie/ optimally nourishing regimes. Now, however, there is substantial data, as we shall see.

Some biomarkers belong to both of the above categories, but I'll start with those dealing primarily with aging itself .

THE BIOMARKERS OF AGING

We can place animals or people on the CRON diet or some other regimen we believe may slow their rates of aging and/or increase their resistance to cancer, heart attack, and other diseases, but how can we tell if it is working? If you take a pill for a headache, you know soon enough. The headache goes away or it doesn't. But if you take six packages of cholestyramine a day to lower your chance of having a heart attack, how do you know if it's working? Are you just going to a lot of trouble—every time you're in a restaurant asking for a glass of water without ice, pouring the packet of orange cholestyramine into the water, and drinking it up like some hypochondriac fool in a movie? How does one know if preventive medicine is working, since the indication that it works is that something does not happen?

Finding whether an anti-aging regimen works is much easier in short-lived species than in man. A mouse or a rat lives on *average* for about 24 months. Its *maximum* life span is 38 to 39 months. Put 50 of the animals on an experimental regimen and if the average reaches 40 months and the *maximum* 48 months, the regimen is a success. Aging has been retarded. And by performing autopsies on all that die, and sacrificing some of the population at various times before natural death, you can perceive how the frequency of disease has been influenced.

Are there fewer lung cancers among animals on the regimen? Are cancers that do occur postponed until a later time in life? This kind of information is hard to get in long-lived species. The maximum authenticated life span of rabbits is 15 years; of dogs, 20; cats, 25; horses, 40; chimpanzees, 50; and man, 122 years. If we put 50 six-year-old spaniels on what we hope is an anti-aging program, we must wait more than 14 years to see if any exceed the maximum life span for dogs. In humans, the time required would be almost totally prohibitive. Not many investigators are willing to initiate a 50-to 75-year experiment.

Who could blame them, in their "publish or perish" academic community? True, they might live longer (if they were part of the test group), but academically they'd be dead, and better things would almost certainly be coming along to render their dedication a waste of time, as in the science fiction story in which the young fellows take off in the primitive slow rocket, heroically resigned to growing old and gray in their cramped craft as it plows through infinite boring space, carrying the legends of man. Finally, just as they—now old men—are heading into the far star system of their youthful dreams, along comes a *new* and infinitely faster starship built 50 years after they had left Earth on their old workhorse. It hurtles by full of blond young ladies and gentlemen tinkling glasses of iced champagne as they come *as tourists* to visit the star system the old fellows have given their lives to reach.

No, thank you—formal lifetime experiments are not attractive.

Then how do we determine in a long-lived species like man, but in a reasonably short stretch of time, whether our program is working to retard the rate of aging? For that we need biomarkers that determine functional age, ways of measuring age besides just how many years our subjects have been alive. To calculate functional age, we can use a battery of different tests whose average values change with age in the population. This battery provides a checkpoint against which to measure an individual relative to the expectation for his years. We can assess his reaction time and vision and lung capacity and a range of other easily measured functions, combine the results, and provide a measure of his functional age. Though he is 60, his biomarker "score" may be that of a 45-year-old man, if he has taken care of himself, or of a 70-year-old man if he has not.

Functional age is not the same as chronologic age. Since 1850, for example, only one British prime minister has died before the age of 70. Seven passed the age of 80. Churchill was over 90 when he died. The prime ministers would probably have tested younger on a "functional" age battery than, say, construction workers of the same chronologic ages. In men, a younger functional age and longer life are associated with a longer period of education, higher income, and more interesting work; for women, the important factors seem to be longer education and physically active leisure time.

What criteria must a useful biomarker satisfy? What should we measure? It's not good enough simply to choose anything that changes substantially with age. The biomarker must make biological sense. For example, people eat fewer calories as they grow older, but obviously it would not make good sense to use caloric intake as a measure of a person's "functional" age. Old gluttons would score young on such a test.

Nor is blood cholesterol a good marker for basic aging! True, it increases with aging in the U.S. population, but in many societies it does not. A good biomarker for aging ought to reflect a universal species characteristic. Even in the United States, the increase in blood cholesterol with age is much greater among the rich, who eat richer food. Blood cholesterol may be a reasonably good marker of susceptibility to arteriosclerotic heart disease, but disease susceptibility, as our study of average survival from 1900 to 1982 has taught us (see Figure 1.1), is not the same as intrinsic aging.

The very best biomarkers of aging will reflect changes that are not susceptible to major influence by environmental factors. Exercise enhances cardiovascular fitness and increases average life span, but it has not, perhaps surprisingly, been shown to have much influence on maximum life span in either humans or long-lived strains of animals. Rats or mice allowed to exercise but given free access to food do not exceed the characteristic maximum survival time of 38 to 39 months.

Markers that change with age but are greatly influenced by exercise, physical fitness, occupation, or economic class may confuse the issue. On the other hand, they may, like cholesterol and the other blood lipids, be good markers for disease susceptibility. We shall want to employ them because the CRON diet influences both the aging rate and disease susceptibility.

In Table 2.1 I have listed a number of human biomarkers, dividing them into those that in part reflect true, intrinsic "functional" age; those that may have predictive value for how long you have left to live, whatever your cause of death; and those that reflect either susceptibility to a particular disease or perhaps accelerated aging of one or several organ systems.[1]*

Predictive value is important but difficult to achieve. It refers to the ability of the biomarker to indicate on the average how much longer you are likely to live, barring accidents. Having antibodies in your blood that react with your own tissues (autoantibodies) predicts a shorter average survival.[2] Many tests correlate well with chronologic age but have no predictive value at all. For example, graying of hair shows a high correlation with age, but premature graying does not indicate accelerated aging, except perhaps of the hair. Gray hair is not, however, an indication that your functional age is higher than someone whose hair isn't gray.

Remember that in *Alice in Wonderland* the White Queen says, "It's a poor sort of memory that only works backward." In the same vein, biomarkers that tell you only how old you are, when of course you know that already, and not how long you may expect to live might be considered of limited practical use. But in fact this is not quite the case. In laboratory animals the CRON diet both extends maximum life span and postpones graying of hair. If you decelerate aging in the whole body, the hair goes along. Retarding aging will postpone the graying relative to whatever your individual graying rate is.

TABLE 2.1 *Three categories of human biomarkers*

1. "FUNCTIONAL" AGE
   Vital capacity, breath-holding time, maximal oxygen consumption (VO2 max), kidney function (creatinine clearance), diameter of pupil of eye, visual accommodation, hearing, level of DHEA hormone in blood, tests of mental function.

2. PREDICTIVE VALUE FOR REMAINING LIFE EXPECTANCY
   Vital capacity, heart size, systolic blood pressure, hand grip strength, presence or absence of autoantibodies in blood, immune-function tests, reaction time.

3. DISEASE SUSCEPTIBILITY AND/OR SEGMENTAL AGING
   Glucose-tolerance test; levels of blood cholesterol, LDL, HDL, triglycerides, and homocysteine; systolic blood pressure; blood level of parathyroid hormone.

As you embark upon a life-extension program, stay abreast of the field of human biomarker testing as much as possible. This book will give you the background. A more sophisticated account of both human and animal biomarkers of aging may be found in the book for professional scientists I have written with Dr. Richard Weindruch, *The Retardation of Aging by Dietary Restriction*,[3] as well as other sources.[4]*

Despite certain problems with the reliability of biomarkers, we can hope, at least in the future, to use them for all of five purposes: (1) to determine our "functional" age, (2) to see if the rate of change in the biomarkers over a period of years has been slowed by our anti-aging regimen, (3) to predict on the average how long we might expect still to live, (4) to estimate our resistance to the major killer diseases, and (5) to see if what we are doing to increase our resistance to specific diseases, to cancer, heart disease, diabetes, and other diseases of aging, is having an effect. Are we truly enhancing the state of our health?

It may be instructive to compare your personal biomarker values against the averages for your age. More important, however, is how your values change from the time you started an anti-aging program to wherever you are at later dates.

I'll divide human biomarker of aging tests into two categories: those which you can do yourself, and those which your doctor can do or arrange for you to have done.

TESTS YOU CAN DO ON YOURSELF

These are skin elasticity, the falling-ruler test (for reaction time), static balance, and a simple test for visual accommodation.

Contributing to the development of wrinkles and loose skin (in the neck, for example), loss of skin elasticity begins showing significant changes at about 45 years of age, with large deviations in individual subjects.[5] It reflects deterioration of connective tissue under the surface of the skin. Animal experiments have shown that this type of deterioration can be substantially delayed by a CRON diet.

To perform the elasticity test, pinch the skin on the back of your hand between thumb and forefinger for five seconds, then time how long it takes to flatten out completely. Up until 45 to 50 years of age, only about five seconds is required for the skin to flatten out. But by 60 it will on the average require ten to fifteen seconds; and by 70, 35 to 55 seconds. Because of the large individual variation, the initial test should not be taken too seriously. You are more interested in the rate of change thereafter. Figure 2.2 will give you an idea of how rapidly skin elasticity does change after age 45. This is a good test if you start the CRON dietary regimen in mid or late life. It won't show much change at the younger ages whether you are on the diet or not.

The falling-ruler test measures your reaction time—that is, how long it takes to respond to an outside stimulus, like that red Pontiac that almost clipped you in Chapter 1. Buy a thin 18-inch wooden ruler. Ask a friend to suspend the ruler vertically by holding it at the top. Hold the thumb and middle finger of your own right hand 3 ½ inches apart, equidistant from the 18-inch mark on the ruler. As your friend drops the ruler without warning, you must catch it between your two fingers. Your "score" is whatever inch mark you catch it at. Do this three times and take an average. If you catch it at the 3-inch, 6-inch, and 6-inch marks, your "score" is $(3 + 6 + 6)/3 = 5$. On the average, the score decreases progressively from the 1-inch mark at age 20 to the 6-inch mark at age 60.

The third test is that of static balance. How long can you stand on one leg with your eyes closed before falling over? (As a matter of standardization: left leg if you are right-handed, right leg if left-handed.) This test is clearly the best among the do-it-yourself biomarker measurements. On the average, a fully percent (100 percent) decline occurs from age 20 to age 80. Most young people can hold a one-legged eyes-closed stand for 30 seconds or more, whereas few old persons can hold the pose longer than a few seconds.

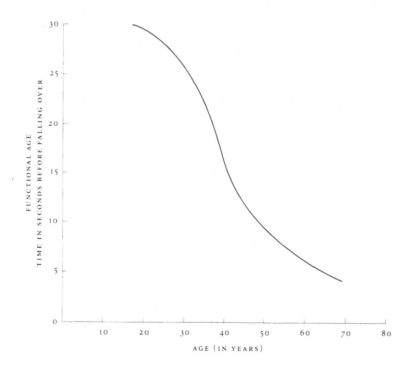

FIGURE 2.1 *Static balance as a biomarker of age. Close eyes, stand on one leg (left if you are right-handed), don't move foot. How long before you fall over? Score = average of three trials.*

Perform the test either barefoot or wearing an ordinary low-heeled shoe. Stand on a hard surface (not on a rug) with both feet together, close your eyes, and lift your foot about six inches off the ground, bending your knee at about a 45-degree angle. Don't move or jiggle your foot; just stand on it with your eyes closed. How many seconds can you stand this way before you have to open your eyes or move your foot to avoid falling over? Have a friend close by to catch you in case you do in fact fall over. Do the test three times and take an average. Values for different ages are illustrated in Figure 2. 1.

The fourth and final test estimates the effect of age on visual accommodation, although it should not replace the more accurate visual tests your eye doctor can do. At 21, an average person can bring a newspaper to within 4 inches of his eyes before the regular-sized print starts blurring; at 30 years, to within 5 ½ inches; at 40, no closer than 9 inches; at 50, 15 inches; and at 60 years, about 39 inches. Do this either without glasses or with glasses corrected for distance—that is, not reading glasses. It's not how well you can actually read the print (you may have astigmatism) that counts, but at what point it suddenly starts to blur.

TESTS YOUR DOCTOR CAN DO OR ARRANGE TO HAVE DONE

Probably the best biomarker now available is the measurement of lung function called "vital capacity." This is the amount of air that can be taken in and breathed out in one very deep breath. It reflects the integrity of the whole respiratory system, the muscles, their central nervous system, control mechanisms, and the elasticity of the lungs. The vital capacity, or VC, of an individual must be adjusted for his or her height in inches. How VC decreases with age is illustrated in Figure 2.2A.

VC has been the most powerful single predictor of subsequent life span in the large, very famous, and still ongoing study involving most of the population of Framingham, Massachusetts. People with low VC for their age did not live as long on the average as those with high VC, and as we have learned, predictability is the most important indicator that a biomarker is measuring true "functional" age. Furthermore, in the Framingham study there was no difference between athletic and sedentary individuals. This means that the VC is not much influenced by physical fitness—an advantage in assessing the basic process of aging, since physical fitness influences average but probably not maximum life span.

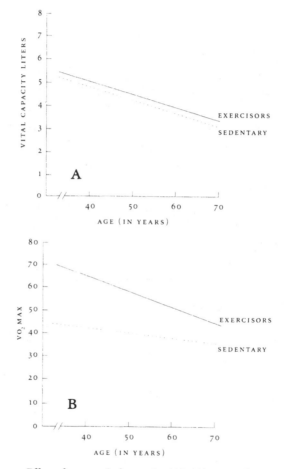

FIGURE 2.2 *Effect of age on vital capacity (A) and on maximum possible oxygen consumption (VO2, max) (B) in men who do frequent aerobic exercise, and in sedentary men (adapted from H. Suominen et al.,* Scandinavian Journal of Social Medicine, *Supplement 14, 1980, p. 225)*

Two measures of heart function often used as biomarkers seem to be indicators more of physical fitness and resistance to several diseases than of the basic aging rate. The first is the "maximum oxygen consumption," also known as VO2, max. It measures the ability of the cardiovascular system to respond to stress. This ability declines with age and/or poor physical fitness, reflecting a lower maximal attainable heart rate combined with a diminished capacity of the tissues to extract oxygen quickly from the blood bathing them.

To measure your VO2 max, your physician will have you exercise at peak rate on a treadmill or stationary bicycle. The amount of oxygen you use per minute is then divided by your body weight. How this ratio varies with age for sedentary men and for those in good physical condition is shown in Figure 2.2B. We see quite clearly by comparing the A and B panels of Figure 2.2 that whereas the vital capacity (VC) is relatively independent of physical fitness, the maximum oxygen consumption, or VO2 max, is greatly influenced by it. For middle-aged sedentary men, the average VO2 max is about 45 millileters of oxygen per minute for every kilogram (2.4 pounds) of body weight; for those men on a good aerobic-exercise program, who jog 15 to 30 miles per week, the value is about 58; for world-class athletes, it's about 75. Because VO2 max is so greatly influenced by physical fitness, it is a good biomarker for age only if the value for the person being tested is compared with control values from people who do the same amount of exercise.

Systolic blood pressure is a second cardiovascular biomarker. Individual variation is great, and the influence of hereditary background, degree of stress, and especially diet (see Chapter 5) makes it less than optimal as a marker for aging. Nevertheless, blood pressure measurements should be part of your personal long-term biomarker program. The way blood pressure tends to increase with age in most populations in the western world is illustrated in Figure. 2.3.

A good measure of kidney function is the Creatinine Clearance Test. The test measures the capacity of the kidneys to clear the waste product creatinine from the blood by filtering it into the urine. From the determination of the concentration of creatinine in the blood and the quantity eliminated in the urine in 24 hours, "clearance" can be calculated. The test can be ordered by your physician in any hospital or clinical laboratory. The steep decline of creatinine clearance after age 30 is illustrated in Figure 2.4. The test is a useful biomarker.

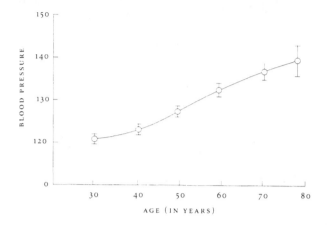

FIGURE 2.3 *Effect of age on blood pressure (adapted from J. D. Tobin, in* Aging: A Challenge to Science and Society, Vol. 1. Biology, *ed. D. Danon et al. [New York: Oxford University Press, 1981])*

A good marker of your blood-sugar metabolism is the Glucose Tolerance Test. When you take glucose (sugar) by mouth, your body absorbs it from your intestines and your level of blood sugar rises sharply. Your pancreas then secretes the hormone insulin, which stimulates the utilization or storage of the sugar. With age these pathways become less effective [6] So-called "insulin sensitivity" is decreased. Instead of being used or stored promptly, the sugar remains longer in the blood.

The Glucose Tolerance Test consists of measuring the level of blood sugar two hours after you have taken a standard amount of sugar on an empty stomach in the morning. This two-hour level is very high in diabetics, and is higher in older "normal" persons than in young normal persons. Examples of the rise and decline of blood sugar (glucose) are given in Figure 2.5 and clearly document the age-related differences. But physical fitness also influences glucose tolerance. A fit person will generally have a lower overall curve and two-hour value than a sedentary person of the same age.

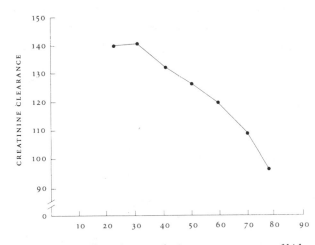

FIGURE 2.4 *The effect of age on the important measure of kidney function known as Creatinine Clearance (adapted from J. W. Rowe et al.,* Journal of Gerontology 31:155 1976)

Some of the biomarkers listed above are not very useful at young ages because the rates of change do not accelerate until late middle age. In the mid-age years, the level in your blood of the hormone DHEA is a good biomarker, since it declines substantially during this period.[7]

Visual accommodation is a good biomarker up to about age 50, after that not so good because the decline levels off. Accommodation—the ability of the lens of the eye to change its shape—is measured in units called *diopters*. It declines in a straight-line fashion from about 13 diopters at age 13 to 1 to 2 diopters at age 50, then remains relatively constant for the rest of your life. I outlined above a simple do-it-yourself accommodation test using a newspaper, but your eye doctor can measure the diopters much more exactly.

Beginning at about age 30, a progressive decline develops in hearing ability. The hearing threshold at a fixed frequency is one of the best ways of estimating this decline, and indeed has a mild predictive value for later life expectancy. The threshold test measures how loud a sound must be at a certain frequency for you to be able to hear it at all (see Figure 2.6). At 4,000 cycles per second, an 18- to 24-year-old person can hear a sound as low in intensity as 14 decibels, whereas a 60- to 70-year-old person generally requires 30 to 50 decibels. At 8,000 cycles per second the young person requires about 18 decibels, whereas the older person needs 50 to 80; this is the best frequency to show the age-related loss.

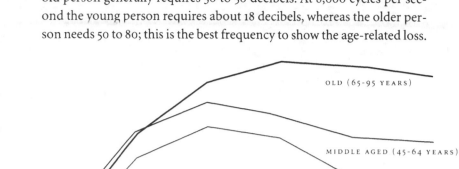

FIGURE 2.5 Glucose Tolerance Test curves for three age groups of normal individuals. Levels of blood glucose are shown at different time intervals after ingestion of a standard amount of glucose in the morning on an empty stomach.

The only immune-function biomarker tests that your physician can readily order are those for anti-self antibodies, called *autoantibodies*. This class of protein molecules react deleteriously with the body's own tissues. Particularly useful are the tests for antibodies to DNA, the well-known "double helix" of hereditary material coiled in each cell, and for the rheumatoid factor. Positive test results increase with age, up to 50 to 70 percent in advanced age. People with autoantibodies in their blood have a shorter life expectancy than those who don't, as was shown by a study involving 10,000 individuals in the town of Busselton, Australia. [8] In animals on the CRON diet, the frequency of autoantibodies is greatly diminished with age, indeed to the point of their being wholly absent. [9]

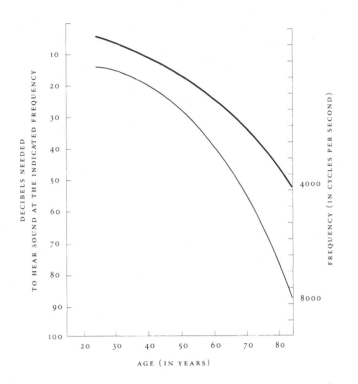

FIGURE 2.6 *Auditory threshold in decibels in relation to age in women, at sound frequencies of 4000 and 8000 cycles per second (adapted from J. F. Corse, in* Lectures on Gerontology, *Vol. 1, part B.,* Biology of Aging, *ed. A. Viidik [New York: Academic Press, 1982], p. 441)*

WHEN AND HOW OFTEN
TO GET THE BIOMARKER TESTS DONE

Have as many of these tests done as possible, either before or a few months after starting the CRON dietary anti-aging, health-enhancement program. Of course, the do-it-yourself tests are easy. The other first-time-around tests include a blood pressure determination, the Glucose Tolerance Test, and the tests for the presence of autoantibodies. You can delay running the other age-biomarker tests until you are a few months into the program, since they don't change all that rapidly. Table 2.2 outlines my suggested overall biomarker battery, along

TABLE 2.2 *Biomarker of aging battery and average values for three age groups*

TEST	AGE GROUP 23–30	40–50	60–70	UNITS/COMMENTS
Skin Elasticity	0–1	2	15	seconds
Reaction Time (falling-ruler test)	12	8	5	inches
Static Balance	28	18	4	seconds
Visual Accomodation (self-test)	4.5	12	39	inches
Vital Capacity	5.5	4.5	3.5	liters
VO₂ Max.:				
EXCERCISER	70	60	48	liters/minute
SEDENTARY	44	40	38	liters/minute
Systolic Blood Pressure:				
MEN	130	138	148	mm. Hg
WOMEN	120	136	155	mm. Hg
Creatinine Clearance	140	126	112	liters/24 hrs.
Glucose Tolerance	118	127	140	mg./100 ml. @ 2 hrs.
Visual Accomodation	13	2	1–2	diopters
Hearing Threshold:				
@ 4000 Hz	4	16	30–50	decibels
@ 8000 Hz	15	24	50–80	decibels
Autoantibodies:				
MEN	10	35	50	% of population
WOMEN	10	45	65	having (+) test
DHEA Hormone Level:				
MEN	3400	1800	900	ng./ml. plasma
WOMEN	2200	1100	800	ng./ml. plasma

with average values for three age groups. Of course "average" is not good enough, and my program is designed to make you much better than average in the course of time, by slowing the age-related decline until you, as it were, "catch up" with younger people, since what is time-related is also relative. Repeat the tests four to six years later. If you are doing the diet properly (see below), the results will show less change than you would expect. Your rate of aging has been retarded. You have added a number of years to your average and maximum life span potentials.[10]*

THE BIOMARKERS OF SUCCESS

The tests outlined above are measures of your *functional or physiologic* age. If you start your CRON diet at the age when you are both chronologically and functionally 40 years old, and stay on it for six years, you will find that you are now *chronologically* 46 years old, but *physiologically* only 43. I make this statement on the basis of evidence in rodents [11] and monkeys.[12] Tests of this nature in humans on CRON diets for very long periods are not yet available. But the combined animal evidence is very convincing indeed.

Of course you will only achieve this slowing down of aging if you are doing the diet correctly, but fortunately you don't have to wait three to six years to find that out. A different battery of biomarkers will change rather quickly if you are following the diet successfully. Six months or even less is ample time to see a substantial change. These tests and changes will be discussed as we go along in this book. However, Table 2.3 gives an initial listing, and also the average percentage change experienced by the eight crew members of Biosphere 2 during the first six to eight months after they were sealed in. (These data have been published in detail in medical journals.[13]) It is worthy of note that whereas restriction of this severity may under the ordinary circumstances of food deprived populations lead to lethargy, forgetfulness, loss of concentration, slow reaction time, peripheral edema (swelling of the ankles),[14] none of these symptoms were observed in the crew members. On the contrary, for the entire two years of being sealed inside, the eight persons (four men, four women) sustained a 70-or-more hour exhaustive weekly schedule during which they ran all aspects of the miniworld of Biosphere 2.[15] We were able to do that because although our caloric intake was reduced, the diet *was optimally nourishing*. Most of the symptoms noted in food deprived populations are due to lack of essential nutrients, not (until after a certain point, of course) to lack of calories.

Again referring to Table 2.3, I should remark that the crew of Biosphere 2 was on a severely reduced-calorie diet, so you should perhaps not expect quite such dramatic changes in your own test values, but moderate changes should occur. If they aren't, give it up, or stick with the diet more closely! [16*]

TABLE 2.3 *Biomarkers of success: average changes in the eight crew members on calorie reduction with optimal nutrition in Biosphere 2. Before starting on CRON, you should get at least the first 6 tests, all 11 if possible. Repeat in 6 months, and every 6 to 12 months thereafter.*

TEST OR DETERMINATION	AVERAGE PERCENT CHANGE (IN SIX MONTHS OR AS INDICATED)
Weight	14% decrease
Systolic blood pressure	18% decrease
Diastolic blood pressure	28% decrease
Blood sugar	21% decrease
Cholesterol	36% decrease
White blood cell count	31% decrease
Insulin	42% decrease
T3 (a thyroid hormone)	19% decrease
Renin	gradual decrease
Glycosylated hemoglobin	gradual decrease
Triglycerides	gradual decrease

CHAPTER 3

SCIENTIFIC BACKGROUND OF THE CRON DIET:

THE ANIMAL EVIDENCE

════

INTRODUCTION TO EVIDENCE

BEFORE WE ESCALATE TO HUMANS, IT'S IMPORTANT that you be convinced beyond any reasonable doubt that in experimental animals the CRON diet works dramatically at slowing the aging process, preventing disease, and enhancing health.

There is now abundant hard evidence—not testimonial evidence, not clinical anecdote, not "make the case" evidence based on plausibility arguments, and not even correlational evidence, although all these exist in plenitude—but hard, well-controlled and steadfastly confirmed experimental evidence that a CRON diet will greatly extend average and maximum life spans, postpone the onset and decrease the frequencies of most or all of the "diseases of aging," maintain biomarkers at levels younger than the chronological age, maintain sexual potency, general vitality, and ability to engage in sports into advanced age, and delay deterioration of the brain.

In 1935 Dr. Clive McCay at Cornell University first demonstrated that if rats from the time of weaning were fed a calorically restricted but healthful diet supplemented with vitamins and minerals, they would live remarkably longer than normally fed rats.[1] By 1,000 days of age, all the normally fed rats had died, but most of the calorie-restricted ones were still alive and active. Their growth rate and body size had been retarded by the severe restrictive regimen, but in other ways they seemed super healthy. If they were allowed a full diet at

1,000 days, they actually began to grow again. The females were sexually active and could reproduce far beyond the normal age. And chronologically old CRON-diet male animals showed higher testosterone levels than normally fed old males. [2]

The maximum life spans of McCay's restricted rats reached out to 1,800 days—equivalent to 150 to 180 human years. Of course McCay's regimen could hardly be applied to humans. The severity of restriction maintained since the time of weaning kept the rats from reaching full body size, and would do the same for humans. But the experiment definitely proved that maximum life span can be greatly extended! The rate of aging is not irretrievably fixed by some unyielding law of nature, as people had tended to think until then. And if maximum life span can be extended at all, perhaps it can be extended more easily, or with a less undesirable side effect on the size of the individual. This has proved to be the case. [3*]

In subsequent years the work of McCay and other early pioneers was confirmed, extended, modified, and carried forward by investigators at the Sloan-Kettering Cancer Research Institute in New York, the University of Texas at San Antonio, the University of Wisconsin, the University of Maryland, the Gerontology Research Center of the National Institute on Aging in Baltimore, the National Center for Toxicological Research in Arkansas, the University of Hull in England, of Sydney in Australia, of Tubingen in Germany, of Akita in Japan, the University of California at Riverside, my own laboratory at the University of California in Los Angeles, and still other places where good science is the rule. A great body of careful documentation, amounting to more than 2,000 articles in leading peer-review scientific journals now exists about the effects of the CRON diet on animals. Why all this work, all these studies? Because to investigate the scientific basis of aging, it helps if you can perturb the system, slow it down. Then you can study it.

Additionally advantageous, as we'll see, is that if you can slow the system down, you know that you are dealing with the basic, fundamental aging process. The CRON diet is the only method that consistently does just that and in a dramatic fashion in higher animals. [4*]

I can only touch on the highlights of the evidence in this chapter, first in rodents, then in monkeys. For detailed information, see the book for professional biologists by Dr. Richard Weindruch and myself, *The Retardation of Aging and Disease by Dietary Restriction,* [5] the volume devoted to aging of the 1995 *Handbook of Physiology,* [6] and Professor Weindruch's excellent 1996 article in *Scientific American.* [7]

There have been five historical phases in the development of CRON-diet research. For several decades following McCay's first demonstration, CRON diets were used to extend life span in various animal species, and (in rodents particularly) to document the diet's remarkable effect in preventing a variety of diseases, particularly different types of cancer. These were the first two historical phases. The third was initiated in my laboratory at UCLA in the late 1960s, when we began to investigate what physiological changes were induced by low-calorie nutrient-dense nutrition (the CRON diet), and (the fourth phase) whether these changes were causally connected to the life span extension and the disease prevention. Our first investigations were directed towards the immune response capacities of mice on CRON regimes. All these phases, but particularly the last two, are now ongoing in many laboratories, and have expanded into biochemistry, endocrinology, molecular genetics, and other branches of modern biology. The quest for the mechanism or mechanisms whereby a selective reduction in calories leads to so many global changes in the body and its life course is considered the major challenge, the Holy Grail if you please, of this field of research. If we knew how calorie restriction works, maybe we could induce the necessary changes more easily, and even to a greater degree, than by restricting our caloric intake. And lastly, the final phase: human application. Will it work in humans? Obviously I believe the answer to this question is a resounding yes, but formally the question has not been answered.

EFFECTS OF THE CRON DIET ON LIFE SPAN

First, a little background. Each species displays a characteristic maximum life span. For humans, it's about 110 years, except for very occasional outliers. That 110 years is more or less a fixed point. A few (not many) ancient Romans lived that long, and hardly anybody today lives

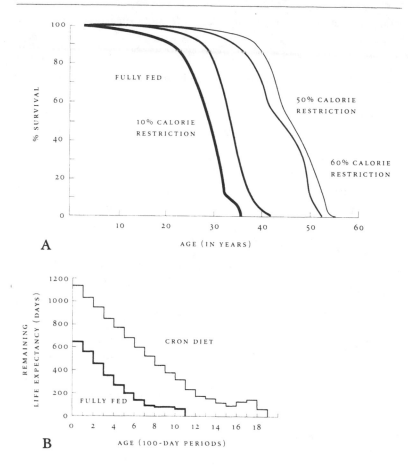

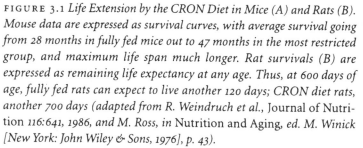

FIGURE 3.1 *Life Extension by the CRON Diet in Mice (A) and Rats (B). Mouse data are expressed as survival curves, with average survival going from 28 months in fully fed mice out to 47 months in the most restricted group, and maximum life span much longer. Rat survivals (B) are expressed as remaining life expectancy at any age. Thus, at 600 days of age, fully fed rats can expect to live another 120 days; CRON diet rats, another 700 days (adapted from R. Weindruch et al.,* Journal of Nutrition 116:641, 1986, *and M. Ross, in* Nutrition and Aging, *ed. M. Winick [New York: John Wiley & Sons, 1976], p. 43).*

any longer. By contrast, *average* life span (the age at which half the population have died off), and *life expectancy* (another phrase for about the same thing) can vary a lot. In ancient Rome it was 22 years, in the modern U.S. it's 73 years for men and 78 for women. The increase is due to better hygiene, better medicine, etc., but it's not due to any retardation of aging. The measure of aging in a population is not the average life span, but rather the *maximum life span*, and that hasn't changed throughout human history —so far!

We'll consider two broad categories of how the CRON diet has been applied in life span studies: caloric reduction begun during childhood, and that begun at various stages in adult life after full growth has been reached.

Look first at the survival information for mice and rats on CRON diets. Figure 3.1A is from a study conducted in my laboratory at the UCLA School of Medicine. The life extension achieved here is especially important because we were dealing with naturally long-lived strains of mice, not strains rendered short-lived by hereditary susceptibility to some particular disease. The fully fed mice displayed a maximum life span of close to 38 months. That by itself is quite long for a mouse. At 10 percent caloric restriction the supplemented diet extended the maximum life span to 43 months, and at 50 percent restriction (corresponding to something close to a 1,200- to 1,500-calorie CRON diet in a human male of average size) to more than 54 months (corresponding to a living human who could remember the Mexican War, the Alamo, and the Gold Rush!).

Figure 3.1B expresses life extension in another but equally fascinating way. Starting at any age, the lines show *remaining life expectancies* for fully fed rats compared with CRON-diet rats. Those animals represented in the first line, zero to 100 days of age, could expect to live another 625 days if fully fed, but 1,125 days if on the CRON diet. At the 1,000 to 1,100 day line, all the fully fed animals had died, but those on the CRON diet could still expect 320 days of life. And a few of the vigorous and venerable diet rats lived an amazing 1,800 days.

These experiments with naturally long-lived strains of animals have been confirmed many times. [8]* It's as though, referring to Figure 1.1, for humans, curve C were being converted into curve D. And with short-lived strains, even more impressive results can be obtained. Here one is not only retarding the rate of aging but inhibiting the development of those diseases that render these strains short-lived. In such strains (and for hereditary reasons you might well belong to the human equivalent of such strains), average life spans have been more than doubled and maximum life spans extended three- to fourfold. [9]

Restriction since time of weaning is not a feasible option for human use because it decreases ultimate body size. But fortunately, the CRON diet prolongs life span and retards aging even if begun in adult life. Studies at the University of Texas have shown that restriction begun at six months of age (young adulthood) in the rat is *just as effective* in extending life span as weaning-initiated restriction. [10] Using the intermittent (every other day) feeding technique in rats, and beginning at either 11 or 18 months of age (equivalent to mid-adulthood and fairly late middle age in humans), scientists at the National Institute on Aging obtained significant average and maximum life span extensions from 20 to 40 percent if begun at 11 months [11]: and in short-lived strains restriction imposed even late in life greatly extended the life span. [12] Roughly speaking, beginning the CRON diet halfway through life will yield half the extension one could obtain by starting in childhood, but without the undesirable side effect of reduced body size. [13]

In terms of human application, it is important to realize that the degree of restriction giving the best results varies with the age at which it is started. [14] Begun in rats at 70 days of age, 6 grams of food per day decreased the death rate to only 35 percent of that of fully fed animals. But when started at 300 days of age, 6 grams actually *increased* the death rate, but 8 grams (just 25 percent more) again decreased it, to 49 percent of that of fully fed animals. And starting at 365 days of age, best results were obtained with 10 grams per day. The optimal restriction level changes with age, and at greater ages should be less severe.

Our experiments at UCLA indicate that in adulthood, caloric restriction works best when slowly imposed. *Body weight should be lost gradually.* Early investigators failed to obtain life extension starting with adult animals because they imposed severe caloric restriction too rapidly. That seems to shorten life span, not prolong it. Crash diets and prolonged fasting in humans probably shorten survival. Your body needs time to adapt, even to a more healthful lifestyle.

A final important observation about CRON diets and life span is that the amount of weight to be gradually lost depends on the set point. The *set point* is the characteristic weight for the particular strain of mouse or rat, or the individual human. It is the weight toward which one naturally drifts if he or she neither under- nor overeats. Set point experiments have been done at several major laboratories.[15] In the strain of mouse fetchingly called "ob/ob," all mice are enormously fat, for hereditary reasons, and their life span is short. When placed on a CRON diet, they lose weight until they stabilize at about what a fully fed mouse of a non-obese strain normally weighs. They are not at all lean in comparison with the usual CRON diet mouse, but they are lean in relation to their own body pattern. And they live 50 to 85 percent longer! So what counts is not the absolute weight or the absolute degree of leanness, but the weight relative to the set point of the strain or individual. This finding will be very important when we come to human application.

EFFECTS OF THE CRON DIET ON DISEASE

All forms of chronic disease and "diseases of aging" are (in most cases dramatically) postponed in time of onset and decreased in overall frequency by a CRON diet. Let's look at a few main categories of disease.

CANCER

In the very first pioneering studies, caloric restriction of rats led to a significant delay in development of all cancers.[16] Soon, a second study by another investigator, using mice this time, confirmed that restriction substantially reduced susceptibility to cancer of the breast, lung, liver, skin, and subcutaneous tissues.[17] Lung tumors occurred in 58 percent of fully fed animals of one mouse strain, but in only 32 percent of CRON diet animals. The incidence of breast cancer was knocked right down to zero in this and also in a much later, modern study.[18] And sharp reduction in breast cancer was confirmed in still another independent investigation.[19] Tumors of the testes, [20] pituitary gland, and lymphatic system[21] are all reduced in frequency by the CRON diet.

Although less dramatically, these effects also hold for animals first placed on the diet in adulthood. In studies in my own laboratory, putting mice on the diet at 12 months of age (equal to 30- to 35-year-old humans) reduced lung cancer incidence from 16 percent in fully fed animals down to 6 percent.[22] And for all types of tumors, the age at which they occurred was from two to five months later in dietary than in fully fed animals (or five to 13 years later in terms of human life span).

Many more studies could be cited, but they all give the same message. The CRON diet is a powerful and effective cancer-prevention and cancer-delaying regimen. If there is a high incidence of cancer in your family, particularly breast cancer, you should certainly consider being on this diet. But to keep some cancer-stricken patient from going off on a foolish self-imposed starvation tangent, I should add that there is no evidence that caloric restriction will help cure cancer once that cancer has occurred, only that it will help prevent the cancer in the first place.

DISEASES OF THE HEART, BLOOD VESSELS, AND KIDNEYS

Here again we can start with McCay. [23] He noted that the calcification occurring with age in the hearts of normal rats was much less severe in animals maintained on low-calorie intakes. Furthermore, their pulse rates, normally a rapid 340 beats per minute, were only 240 beats per minute. Other early studies showed that a 33 percent restriction in calories markedly decreased the occurrence of diseases of the heart, blood vessels, and kidneys.[24] CRON diets lower blood pressure in animals in which it is high,[25] diminish the thickening of blood-vessel walls that occurs with age,[26] and reduce the severity of arteriosclerosis. [27]

Most mammals, including rats and humans, gradually develop kidney disease with age. They lose protein in the urine and sustain a progressive scarring of the multiple small filtration sacs in the kidney, which purify the blood. In humans this lowers the creatinine clearance, which, as we saw in the last chapter, can serve as a biomarker of aging. The CRON diet markedly slows this progressive and deleterious kidney change.[28]

OTHER AGE-RELATED DISEASES

The immune system functions to protect the body. It manufactures antibodies and killer cells against invading bacteria or viruses, and with its armamentarium seeks to recognize and eliminate aberrant cells (like cancer cells) arising from mutation or cellular injury. But it must distinguish "self" from "non-self," and destroy only the latter!

With age the normal immune response declines markedly, down to only 10 to 30 percent of its youthful capacity. The immune machinery becomes perverted, the self/non-self recognition markers fail to work well. And the destructive power of the immune system gradually turns against the body itself, leading to *autoimmunity*, an anti-self destructive process mediated by an immune system gone haywire. [29, 30]*

There is compelling evidence that this decline in normal response and upswing in self-destructive autoimmunity can be greatly reduced by a CRON diet. [31] And the diet even retards formation of anti-brain-reactive antibodies [32]—an intriguing finding if you want to keep your wits about you. [33]*

Important in disease control, the immune system is also one of the "pacemakers" of aging, one of the main systems through which changes programmed at a more fundamental level exert their effect, resulting in what we recognize as aging. It's doubly encouraging, therefore, from the standpoints of both disease susceptibility and basic aging, to know that the integrity of the immune system can be maintained by the CRON diet.

Osteoporosis is yet another age-related and troublesome disease, widespread in humans. Its hallmark is loss of bone calcium, with weakened bone structure and tendency to easy fractures. While the evidence is less compelling, here too the CRON diet may be protective. In animals on calorie-restricted diets beginning in adulthood, the ratio of the strength of the thighbones to body weight is much greater than for fully fed controls. [34] We know that the hormone secreted by the parathyroid glands influences bone and calcium metabolism. And in normal animals the blood levels of this hormone increase with age, and even more so in those animals that sustain the greatest age-related bone loss. However, in animals on the CRON diet, there is no marked increase in the parathyroid hormone with age and little or no senile bone loss. [35]

EFFECTS OF THE CRON DIET ON BIOMARKERS

For purely practical reasons, biomarkers used for studying aging in animals are in many ways different from those applied to humans. It's not easy to estimate vital capacity in a mouse because he won't give you his last breath, and he certainly can't stand on one leg, or tell you at what distance the newsprint is blurring. On the other hand, you cannot sacrifice a human in order to snatch his connective tissue or his spleen, look at the microscopic structure of his kidney, or remove the lens of his eye. So the biomarker batteries are different, although they may overlap. (Both mice and men can be tested for intelligence, blood pressure, glucose tolerance, hormone levels, and other factors.)

Perhaps the most striking example of slowdown in the age-related change of a biomarker comes from work done at the UCLA Medical School using mice from our CRON-diet colony.[36] The study concerned a protein in the lens of the eye called gamma-crystallin. This is a non-turnover protein. Once full growth is attained, no more gamma-crystallin is formed. If any deteriorates and is lost, it is not replaced. In that sense it resembles brain or heart cells, which, once formed, are not broken down and replaced in the normal course of life. What you have now is what you got early on, and that's all!

In the eye lenses of both mice and humans, the amount of gamma-crystallin declines progressively with age. The decline is sometimes associated with cataract formation. We compared the amounts of the protein in the lenses of fully fed and CRON-diet mice at two months, 11 months, and 30 months of age. The results were impressive. The gamma-crystallin was markedly decreased by 11 months in the fully fed mice, and was wholly gone by 30 months, whereas in the diet mice the loss was much less at 11 months, and some was still present even at the advanced age of 30 months. Thus, the aging of this non-turnover protein was remarkably retarded by the CRON diet, and cataract formation was completely inhibited.

Another useful biomarker is "age pigment."[37] Insoluble brown granules accumulate with age in cells of the heart, brain, adrenal gland, and liver. The pigment comes from damaged membrane material within the cells. A low-calorie nutrient-dense diet (the CRON diet) will greatly retard its accumulation. Collagen, which makes up 30 percent of the body's total protein, is the main constituent of connective tissue, the tissue that holds the organs together. Your Achilles tendon, just above your heel, is almost pure collagen. The cartilage in your joints is mainly collagen. A non-turnover protein like gamma-crystallin, collagen forms itself into long parallel fibers. With age these fibers undergo what is called cross-linking. Metabolic products with two hyperactive chemical groups, like a pair of hands, grab onto one collagen molecule with one group and another with the other group, and hold them together. Obviously, having your collagen molecules handcuffed like this is not so good. But aging of collagen is substantially retarded by a CRON diet.[38] This finding is especially important because cross-linking occurs not only in collagen but in other molecules, including DNA, the hereditary material.

Other biomarker tests, and there are many, follow the same positive pattern. The CRON diet prevents the usual rise in blood insulin and blood sugar that occurs with age. It prevents the insulin-resistance of the tissues that develops with age.[39] It delays degenerative changes that take place in skeletal muscles with age.[40] It prevents the age-related rise in serum cholesterol in rats and holds the blood LDL and HDL factors at a younger age level.[41] And it greatly delays the age-related loss in sensitivity of the body's fat cells to several hormones. [42, 43]*

The youthful preservation of these and many other biomarker values by the CRON diet program is unequaled (and not even approached) by any other form of anti-aging or preventive health therapy.

THE CRON DIET AND BRAIN FUNCTION

In normal aging, fully fed animals (and also humans) undergo a considerable decline in what are called *dopamine receptors* on brain cells. Concerned with passage of the nerve impulse, these receptors are necessary for motor behavior, like walking, running, or swimming. The diminished ability with age to perform tasks that require coordination and muscle strength comes in part from gradual loss of these receptors. A CRON diet greatly slows the loss. The concentration of receptors in 24-month-old CRON-diet rats is the same as that of three- to six-month-old fully fed rats.[44] A good test for complex motor function is the "log rolling" test. A slowly rotating rod—like a broom handle—is held some distance off a soft surface, and the test mouse placed upon it. He will "log roll" in order not to fall off. Chronologically old CRON mice do this with the same agility (measured as number of falls) as young-adult, normally fed mice, and far better than age-matched control mice.[45]

Nerve cells in the brain have projections on their surfaces called *dendritic spines*, which are used to communicate with other nerve cells across the spaces between cells. With age these spines flatten out and become nubby. This change seems greatly inhibited by the CRON diet, even if the diet is not begun until 19 months of age in rats (55 years old in a human).[46]

In the "passive avoidance test" for intelligence, a mouse or rat is placed in a lighted chamber connected to a dark chamber. Instinctively, the animal runs immediately into the dark chamber to hide. But in the test, when he enters the dark chamber he receives an electric shock. If you test him again in 24 hours, he will (because he remembers the shock) hesitate longer before instinct propels him into the safe gloom. Younger mice, with better memories, hesitate longer before entering. Mice 38 months old that have been on a CRON diet since youth perform in this test as though they were only 24 months old.[47] Studies at the National Institute on Aging indicate that caloric restriction very favorably influences the ability of rats to navigate a complicated maze.[48] Dieting rats that were 30 months old performed as well as six-month-old fully fed rats, and much better than 22-month-old fully fed rats. CRON-diet mice from our UCLA colony also show enhanced skill at solving maze problems.[49]

THE MONKEY EXPERIMENTS

Monkeys on calorie-reduced, nutrient-dense diets are being studied at two university laboratories (the universities of Wisconsin[50] and Maryland[51]) and at the National Institute on Aging (one of the National Institutes of Health).[52] The studies have been ongoing for about ten years. While the method of restriction is somewhat different for each group, in general it is about 30 percent below what the monkeys would be eating if given free choice. That's less restriction than commonly used in the rodent studies, and less than in the human studies I conducted inside Biosphere 2. Ten years is not long enough for a life-span experiment in such a long-lived species. However, diabetes is already beginning to appear in the fully fed monkeys serving as the controls, but not in those monkeys on the CRON diet, who are the same chronological age as the controls. Now the average age at which the diseases of aging appear is a rather good measure of functional or physiological age, so by this measure the CRON-diet monkeys are physiologically younger than the controls. By this assessment at least, their rate of aging has been reduced.

What about biomarkers? Here the fit is quite good. The hormone DHEA, which declines dramatically with age in normally fed monkeys, declines much less rapidly in calorie-reduced ones: so the latter are functionally younger by this biomarker of aging. Like rodents, calorie-reduced monkeys reveal a decrease in blood lipids (cholesterol and triglycerides), in blood sugar and insulin, in the white blood cell count, in IGF-1 (related to growth hormone); they show an increase in a certain blood enzyme (alkaline phosphatase), just as rodents do. The aberrances are few: in some studies CRON rodents show increased testosterone,[53] but in others, not;[54] monkeys so far do not. In monkeys glycated hemoglobin has not been found to be decreased (but it is in CRON humans, as we shall see). Many items have not yet been tested in monkeys. But as far as tested, they follow a pattern very similar to that of the rodents.

HOW DOES THE CRON DIET WORK?

That's the big question underlying the fourth historical phase of work on CRON nutrition. What is the *mechanism* whereby a *selective* decrease in the amount of calories consumed causes all the beneficial changes I have outlined? In trying to answer we find an embarrassment of plausibilities, because the results of CRON fit very neatly into all the major theories of aging. [55*] It decreases the amount of oxidative damage throughout the body (the free radical theory),[56] decreases blood sugar and insulin and glycated proteins (glycemic theory),[57] augments immune response capacity and inhibits autoimmunity (immunological theory),[58] can be interpreted from an evolutionary perspective in that animals, faced with serious food shortages, may have adapted to withholding energy from growth and reproduction and applying it to maintenance and repair, and so survive the period of food shortage (disposable soma theory),[59] and so on. I won't run through the entire list. CRON fits them all.

Recent studies from a rather unexpected source, studies on the tiny vinegar worm, *C. elegans*, apply to our inquiry. When properly manipulated, a particular gene set called daf-2 and daf-10 (never mind the origin of the quaint terminology) increase the worm's life span by 300 percent.[60] These genes plays a key role in the insulin-glucose metabolic pathway. There are similar genes also in mammals. Such across-species findings lend support to the glycemic theory's interpretation of the mechanism of CRON's effect. However, one can make almost as good a case for interpretation via the free radical theory.[61] Perhaps they are all involved, interweave, and aging itself and its retardation by CRON may reflect a situation of emergence, complexity, and chaos dynamics that requires a mathematical interpretation, as suggested by Hibbs and myself. [62]

A recent notable advance in our understanding of aging and its retardation by caloric restriction comes from the laboratories of Richard Weindruch and Tomas Prolla at the University of Wisconsin. [63] Using the advanced technology of microarray systems, they were able to measure simultaneously the activities of 6,347 genes (5 to 10 percent of the total mouse genome) from muscle of young and old normally fed, and same-age calorie restricted mice. With normal aging, 58 genes showed increased expression and 55 showed decreased expression. Of the four major gene classes that displayed age-associated alterations, fully 84 percent of these alterations were either completely or partially counteracted by calorie restriction. These findings prove beyond any doubt that calorie restriction retards aging at the most basic biologic level. The nature of the gene findings also suggest that protein modification and protein damage play a significant role in aging, and that calorie restriction acts in part by increased protein turnover, and by altered expression of genes that mediate insulin sensitivity.

Basically, however, CRON is not a *theory*. It's an *experiment* , which, if properly carried out, always works. The theories are still in the making.

SUMMARY

Beyond any reasonable doubt, a CRON diet extends maximum life span in rodents, retards their rate of aging, and inhibits and delays the onset of the major diseases of aging. It holds the biomarkers younger than the chronologic age of the animals, and it keeps their brains functioning at a younger age level. Not only do the animals live a lot longer, they live younger! And these are not the fuzzy concoctions of fringe philosophers and faddists, but evidence from the world's top scientific laboratories engaged in aging research.

Studies of monkeys on CRON diets have not been ongoing for nearly as long as the rodent experiments, not long enough to evaluate life span, since monkeys live 20 to 35 years or so, depending on the species. However, the monkeys clearly show biomarker changes closely similar to those of the rodents, and a major disease of age in monkeys, diabetes, appears inhibited in the CRON monkeys compared to the controls on normal diets. It's all going in the right direction.

We are now ready to consider human application.

CHAPTER 4

THE CRON DIET FOR HUMANS:

FIRST PRINCIPLES

PARAMETERS OF THE CRON DIET FOR HUMANS

AS WE HAVE SEEN, MUCH HIGHLY SPECIFIC AND SOPHISTI-cated information has accumulated about the effects of a CRON diet in animals. Based on inference from that data, I was convinced in 1986 (when the first edition of this book was published) that with a high order of probability such a diet would produce the same beneficial results in humans. Subsequent work in animals, now including monkeys, and my own human studies in Biosphere 2 have further strengthened that belief. Most contemporary scientists conversant with the field now largely share my views, although there is much disagreement over whether a calorie-reduced diet of this nature is "practical," which reflects the viewpoint that most people cannot follow it. Of course, since the rate of *long-term* failure on weight loss programs is over 95 percent,[1] most people can't stick with any diet; they yo-yo back-and-forth and end up where they started. Americans, in the process, collectively spend about $40 billion per year on weight-loss treatments.[2] There is at least much greater incentive to stick with the CRON diet than merely the desire to look better, although that's included. If followed for a long period of time, the CRON diet will retard the rate of aging from whenever in life it is begun—and even rejuvenate the functions of some (not all) of your bodily systems. It will greatly extend maximum as well as average life span, help maintain mental function, enhance health, increase vitality, improve looks, and cut disease susceptibility by at least half. I will show you—not stories and anecdotes and testimonials—hard evidence, published in leading scientific journals, to back up all these claims.

My application of the CRON diet principles to humans is based in part upon extrapolation from years of extensive work with nutritional modulation of the aging process in animal populations, knowledge of what others have done, data from a few published human studies, and the specific investigations I performed during the two-year experiment inside Biosphere 2. These records must all be taken into account in structuring how to implement the diet. Simply launching oneself on a hit-or-miss, long-term, low-calorie diet would not work well. It might even shorten your life span.

The program calls for gradual weight reduction over a period of six to nine months or longers, in short slowly, avoiding the danger of malnutrition inherent in most weight-loss regimes that continue this long. You should proceed until you reach, stabilize, and remain at a weight 10 to 25 percent below your personal set point, where set point is measured in pounds. Or, if set point is measured in Body Mass Index,[3]* proceed until you are three to four index points lower than your personal norm; and you must do this on a nutrient-dense diet that provides, with limited but targeted supplementation, all essential nutrients, known and—to the extent made possible by the broadness of the diet —not yet known. It's a strenuous regime, but it's clear-cut, quite doable, and the rewards are extraordinary.

The eventual degree of leanness required depends on where you begin. When fully fed, the genetically "ob/ob" obese mice I described in Chapter 3 weigh on the average 60 to 65 grams. A fully fed genetically normal mouse weighs only 35 to 45 grams. If we put normal mice on a severe calorie-restriction program and cut their weights down to 25 grams, their life spans will be greatly extended. On the low-calorie regime an "ob/ob" mouse will not become obese but will level off at about 40 grams. It will have a very extended life span, because it is weighing in at less than its set point, even though it weighs as much as or more than a normal fully fed mouse. Below their set point, normal mice look razor thin; "ob/ob" mice, below *their* set point, just look normal, or even slightly obese, but their life spans are greatly extended.

Set point is a critical concept in weight control. Heredity and early feeding experience fix a set point for each individual, which is then defended by adaptive processes within the body. Multiple feedback loops maintain the body at its set point by shunting messages through the blood and the nervous system, between the brain, digestive tract, muscle, and fat.[4] Fat itself secretes hormonal signals. Unless he or she grossly overeats or undereats, each person tends to maintain a particular characteristic weight, which may be considerably above or below the actual "average weight" for that person's height. The body defends its individual set point by shifting the efficiency of its metabolic machine. Take in fewer calories and your body increases its metabolic efficiency; up your intake and your efficiency decreases. This tends to stabilize your weight, although your set point can gradually change (increasing with age, for example). The average American adult gains about 20 pounds between the ages of 25 and 55. Formerly regarded as "normal," this weight gain is now seen as an unhealthy trend, according to insurance company statistics.

The underlying control mechanisms for metabolic efficiency are not entirely known. However, there are so-called "uncoupling proteins" (UCPs) that dissociate the reactions that break down food from those that produce the body's chemical energy.[5] By so doing, they raise the body's metabolic rate. Originally thought to be present only in the specialized brown fat that hibernators use to maintain core body temperature in frigid weather, UCPs are now known to be present in humans. Measurements of the amount of oxygen that humans consume when they metabolize food show that anywhere from 25 to 35 percent is being used to compensate for the "uncoupling" that is going on at all times. It is caused by the UCPs. Decreasing food intake decreases the UCPs, "coupling" is tighter, and metabolic efficiency is increased. *Increasing* the UCPs increases the metabolic rate. That may tend to reduce obesity, but it probably generates more free radicals. That's not the way to go.

Evidence exists that a high fat diet may turn up the production of UCPs, and protect mice against obesity by increasing the metabolic rate.[6] If that's in part how the high fat diets now being touted function to cause weight loss, they are not what you want. "Burning it off" as a substitute for a low calorie intake may be okay for cosmetics, but not for life span.

Efficiency, then, refers to the percentage of your caloric intake that goes into making usable energy. The rest is simply burned off as heat. *Usable* means providing energy for manufacturing proteins and other bodily constituents, for doing muscular work, or performing fundamental processes like transporting calcium or sodium atoms across cell membranes. Normally, metabolic efficiency is about 33 percent. The top efficiency that we can possibly reach is 50 percent. We can approach this upper limit by holding our weight 10 to 25 percent below our "natural weight" or set point. Like an "ob/ob" mouse on the CRON diet, one can be well below one's personal set point and still not be razor thin.

A study of 54 farmers in Java revealed that metabolic efficiency, expressed as work done in relation to energy intake, was actually 80 percent higher for the ten farmers with the lowest intake (1,535 calories) than for those with the highest intake (2,382 calories).[7] Heights and weights did not differ, and the two groups performed the same amount of labor. The one group had "adapted" to the lower intake and were metabolically more efficient.

A major secret of health and longevity is to be always below your set point, maintaining yourself on a high enough quality diet that you are not deficient in any essentials, and to operate at maximum metabolic efficiency. This is, in fact, the central idea of my longevity program.

REACHING FOR MAXIMUM METABOLIC EFFICIENCY

From the most primitive cell to the most advanced organism, living matter needs energy to do its work and to make and maintain the structures giving form to life. It also needs energy to move itself about, to procreate, and to compete with other life forms. Life depends upon energy.

In the early days of our planet, before oxygen was freely available in the atmosphere, life forms derived energy from what is called glycolysis, the conversion of sugar into lactic acid in the tissues. We still derive part of our energy this way. When you become sore and ache from vigorous exercise, it's because lactic acid has built up in your muscles.

Chemically, glycolysis is not a very effective way to generate energy, so when oxygen started percolating into the earth's early atmosphere, mutant organisms that could derive energy from oxygen by means of respiratory metabolism had an evolutionary advantage. The term *respiratory metabolism* does not refer to breathing, but to a collection of processes, mostly taking place within the energy factories (mitochondria) of our cells, and resulting in the formation of a high energy compound known as ATP (short for adenosine triphosphate). This basic source of energy for the process of life has come down more or less unchanged since remote geologic time.

Thus our human bodies do not obtain energy directly from food, but mostly from ATP formed by respiratory metabolism. (A little still comes from residual glycolysis.). And we must manufacture ATP from carbohydrates, fats, and proteins before our cells can use the ingested food for energy. A specific amount of energy remains locked up in the chemical bonds of carbohydrates and fats. Only some 50 percent of this "potential" energy can be converted into ATP. The rest is dissipated as heat or stored as fat. When you overeat, *less* of the energy from your food is channeled through the body-building ATP, and *more* when you undereat. For an average adult American or European male, the 50 percent maximum of "potential" energy that can be converted, or the *energy efficiency*, is probably reached at about 1,800 calories daily. At 2,500 calories, the so-called "caloric RDA" for average adult males, the efficiency drops to 37 percent; at 3,300 calories, to 30 percent.

This existence of so-called "futile cycles" is also important in energy regulation. A futile cycle is one in which the ATP stored in the body can be degraded without actually providing any body-building energy. It produces heat without work (that is, without usable energy). Metabolic efficiency is lowered. Of course, futile cycles can be useful! If it's cold and we need to generate body heat, increasing the futile cycles will act like an internal furnace. Futile cycles may also be turned on when we overeat on junk food, serving as additional safety valves to drain off excess food energy.

By appropriate studies one can determine how much energy a person is using at rest (the Basal Metabolic Rate), how much goes for the thermal effect of feeding, what the overall energy cost of physical activity is, and the efficiency at which the person converts chemical energy into physical work.[8] All these make up the total energy expenditure. When people drop their weight by 10 percent, their energy expenditure declines by 15 percent. The majority of the change occurs in the energy cost of physical activity itself. In terms of energy output, it costs less to run a mile if you are below your set point.

To summarize all the above: maximum metabolic efficiency means achieving the highest possible initial conversion of carbohydrates and fats into ATP, minimizing both fat storage and the breakdown of ATP by futile cycles, and doing your physical activities at a reduced energy cost. The CRON diet is designed to achieve all of these goals.

THE CONCEPT OF NUTRIENT DENSITY

An important feature of the CRON diet is that every calorie must be nutrition packed. Otherwise, gradual weight loss on a long-term basis may cause deficiencies in essential nutrients, and of course that will not prolong life span but shorten it. And do not suppose you can reach your goal by eating a low-calorie mediocre or even nutritionally poor diet supplemented with vitamins and minerals. That would be dangerous and foolhardy. Too much remains unknown about essential nutriments—what forms they should be in, how they interact, how many are still undiscovered . . . but you can bet you are not going to find acceptable combinations simply in refined white flour, hot dogs, and cola drinks plus a handful of pills. Calcium in the form of a calcium carbonate pill, for example, has value as a supplement, but it exerts a partially suppressive effect on bone remodeling; the same amount of calcium in milk has no suppressive effect.[9] Certain forms of fiber in the diet will help lower blood cholesterol, but only if it is a component of the actual food or else carefully mixed with the food. Just taking the fiber as an extra supplement may have no effect. According to a *Consumer Reports* study of vitamin fortified cereals,[10] the added vitamins' availability to the body is questionable. Supplementation has a place in the CRON diet program, but good nutrient-dense food selection is essential.

The average American diet is anything but nutrient dense. The calorie level is inflated, 2,400 to 3,200 for men (depending on age) and 1,650 to 2,150 for women—but it is often deficient in essentials. Large surveys have been run of what Americans eat: the National Food Consumption Survey of 7,500 families conducted by the U. S. Department of Agriculture, and the National Health and Nutrition Examination by the Department of Health and Human Services. They found that meat, fish, or poultry was consumed daily by 90 percent of the families, dark green vegetables by only 9 percent, yellow vegetables by 8 percent, fruit by 33 percent, and whole grain cereals by 16 percent. Fully half of the 7,500 families were below what the National Academy of Sciences has set as the Recommended Daily Allowances (the RDAs) of one or more nutrients, especially calcium, vitamin A, vitamin C, iron, thiamine, and riboflavin. The RDA for magnesium was reached by only 25 percent of individuals; of vitamin B6, 20 percent; of iron, 43 percent; of vitamin A, 50 percent.[11] Magnesium levels in the average diet have dropped from 475 milligrams per person per day in 1900 to 245 milligrams today. One survey revealed deficiencies in iron, copper, zinc, and chromium.[12] According to another, the vitamin B6 content of meals served in 50 American colleges averaged 1.43 milligrams per person per day; thus, over 80 percent of the meals served in these colleges were below the vitamin B6 RDA of 2.0 milligrams per day.[13] It is shocking to realize that even on the high-calorie diet of the richest nation in the world, our own United States, borderline nutritional deficiency is widespread. The average American diet is not nutrient dense, but the opposite.

Simply eating less of the same old things would restrict calories, but it would also bring on malnutrition as a potentially devastating side effect. This is the danger of many weight-loss diets, including most of the popular ones.[14]*

Even well-educated, financially comfortable people may show nutritional deficiencies. Protein, vitamin C, and various B vitamins (folic acid, niacin, pyridoxine, riboflavin, thiamine, and vitamin B12) emerged as the nutrients most often deficient in 5 to 10 percent of a population of 256 affluent individuals surveyed by scientists at the University of New Mexico.[15] And those persons deficient in water-soluble vitamins tested lower than nondeficient partners on tests for abstract thinking and memory! Either borderline malnutrition affects brain function, or else dumber people select worse diets.

Vitamin and mineral deficiency is even more common among the elderly. In one study, fully 50 percent of elderly patients consumed less than two-thirds of the RDA for zinc.[16] Iron and possibly chromium have also been found deficient in the diets of the elderly. Intake of vitamins C and A and niacin has been reported to be less than two-thirds of the RDAs in over 25 percent of subjects in more than 50 percent of published reports on nutrition in the elderly. Even as conservative an authority as the late pioneer-physiologist Dr. Nathan Shock of the National Institute on Aging recommended for the elderly, supplementation with RDA amounts for vitamins and trace elements.

THE PARABLE OF ROSS'S RATS

Many people suppose that animals would instinctively select what is good for them nutritionally if given the chance, and that humans would too, if they were not heavily influenced by advertising and cultural and ethnic conditioning. This is a delightful idea. Rousseau would have loved it. But Dr. Morris Ross's introduction of dietary self-selection into the study of aging and disease showed it to be quite naive.[17, 18] Among four populations of rats, one received a diet of 10 percent protein throughout life; a second, 22 percent protein throughout life; a third, 51 percent. The rats of the fourth population were allowed to select what they wanted from among the three available diets. Dr. Ross measured growth rates, body sizes, life spans, and frequencies of different diseases in all four populations. The rats that self-selected—that is, the fourth population—grew more rapidly and attained a greater body size than all the rest. They instinctively self-selected food combinations that would optimize growth and development; but—and here is what made the experiment unique and fascinating—that very self-selection resulted in a far higher incidence of tumors and other diseases. As shown in Table 4.1, the actual data are striking. Note that the prevalence of disease was considerably greater than 100 percent if you add up most of the columns. By the time of death many animals had multiple afflictions. Indeed, 66 percent of those on the self-select diet had at least three of the four diseases listed. (Notice, incidentally, the difference in tumor incidence between the 10 percent protein and both higher protein diets [We shall return to this in a later chapter], which suggests what fate might await those sticking long-term to the currently popular Atkin's diet.)

TABLE 4.1 *The frequencies, by percentage, of diseases in male rats kept on either fixed or free choice (self-selected) diets (adapted from M. H. Ross and G. J. Bras, Nature 250:263, 1974)*

| | FED THROUGHOUT LIFE ON ONE DIET CONTAINING EITHER 10%, 22%, OR 51% PROTEIN | | | FREE CHOICE DAILY FROM 10%, 22%, OR 51% |
DISEASE	10%	22%	51%	PROTEIN DIETS
Cancer	26	29	28	62
Kidney disease	38	56	73	90
Heart disease	11	42	48	67
Prostate disease	5	10	12	62
TOTALS	80	137	161	281

Now here's my parable. Given free choice, an animal will instinctively choose a diet that leads to quick growth and development and to reaching sexual maturity as soon as possible. This tendency promotes survival of the species in the wild, but is at the same time highly counterproductive for individual long life. In terms of innate self-selection hungers, the welfare of the species and of the individual are in murderous conflict. Animals are instinctively programmed to choose what will make them grow fast and have lots of offspring, even if that choice brings them frequent disease later on. This direct conflict between species and individual survival may be unprecedented in biology.

The behavior of Ross's rats suggests that some of the crazy and self-destructive things we do are the result of species-survival instincts acting through us without our knowing what is really going on. These instincts were of course formed in prehistoric times, during the process of evolution, and they may not be appropriate at all in today's world, even for species survival itself, much less our long-term personal survival. Whatever the value of these speculations, it seems most unlikely that we can trust our instincts to select what is good for us as individuals.

NUTRIENT-DENSE FOOD COMBINATIONS

It's difficult to devise low-calorie menus that are not deficient in essential nutrients. If you think it's easy (and many dietitians and physicians do seem to think so, judging from such bland offhand advice as "Select items from the five food groups."), just try it. Using the tables in Appendix B, try to make up a 1,500-calorie, one-day menu that approximates or exceeds the RDAs for most or all nutrients. Without the right guidelines, it's not easy.

Initially, about 14 years ago, I fed nutrient information on hundreds of foods into a main-frame computer and asked for combinations containing less than 1,500 calories but approximating or exceeding the RDA levels recommended by the National Academy of Sciences for each major nutrient, with calories derived from fat between 8 and 20 percent of the total, and total protein 60 to 90 grams per day. My original diet was based on these computer-optimized food combinations. The computer programming was carried forward to become the software package known as *The Interactive Diet Planner* we used to chart our meal planning inside Biosphere 2.

Because it permits such a ready and graphic comparison of the nutrient values of foods (without eyeballing of endless pages of tables), the computer approach can be instructive and surprising. For example, we hear a great deal these days about the nutritive value of pasta, cereals, and grains, from the Pritikin program, the macrobiotic enthusiasts, and conventionally qualified academic nutritionists. These constitute the base of the famous "food pyramid," and are what you are advised to eat the most of. But calorie for calorie, and especially if you wish to restrict fat intake, vegetables are far and away the most nutritious foods. Table 4.2 tells the tale. On both a weight (4.2A) and a calorie (4.2B) basis, it compares nutritive values of some of the most nutritious vegetables with top candidates from the legumes, cereals, grains, red meat, fish, and even yeast.

As an additional help in your own dietary planning, Table 4.3 lists foods from all five food groups that have high nutrient density, or because the foods have an exceptionally large amount of some essential nutrient that is not present in large amounts in other foods.

TABLE 4.2A *Comparative nutritive components of selected high-quality foods on a weight basis*

Weight basis percentage of RDA per 100 grams	TURNIP GREENS	KALE	BROCCOLI	SOY BEANS	LIMA BEANS	BROWN RICE	MILLET	BUCK WHEAT	LIVER	BEEF	SALMON	HALIBUT	YEAST
AMINO ACIDS													
Tryptophan	26	27	25	291	102	46	122	81	166	144	125	111	388
Isoleucine	14	20	19	279	163	41	77	55	138	159	156	149	333
Lysine	21	18	22	326	190	41	47	62	201	266	272	244	458
Valine	16	23	22	238	153	47	71	92	142	145	142	127	321
Methionine	5	6	9	87	55	30	40	30	75	90	108	98	133
Threonine	22	26	27	262	171	53	71	75	160	173	173	158	410
Leucine	21	29	18	302	177	67	160	71	182	187	176	156	333
Phenylalanine	23	17	18	348	180	70	46	76	171	171	159	134	395
VITAMINS													
A	152	178	50	1	0	0	0	0	450	0	6	8	0
D	0	0	0	0	0	0	0	0	3	0	38	11	0
K	928	0	285	271	0	0	0	0	128	0	0	0	0
C	231	208	183	0	0	0	0	0	60	0	15	0	0
E	22	53	4	153	4	13	0	36	13	1	13	8	0
B1	14	0	7	78	34	24	52	42	14	6	12	5	1142
B2	23	15	13	17	9	2	22	8	158	11	4	4	235
B6	13	15	10	40	30	27	37	15	35	20	35	21	125
B12	0	0	0	0	0	0	0	0	2000	61	133	33	0
Niacin	4	11	5	12	10	27	12	24	61	28	38	46	222
Folic acid	23	15	17	42	27	4	0	0	55	1	6	3	975
Pantothenic acid	9	25	30	42	25	27	0	37	200	12	32	7	300
Biotin	0	0	0	60	9	12	0	0	100	0	5	8	110
MINERALS													
Calcium	20	15	8	19	6	2	1	9	0	1	6	1	17
Magnesium	15	9	6	66	45	22	40	63	0	5	7	5	57
Copper	4	4	0	5	9	18	42	21	250	2	10	11	265
Zinc	0	0	1	24	18	12	12	5	26	27	6	4	73
Chromium	0	0	60	0	120	0	0	0	120	60	0	0	320
Potassium	4	20	20	90	81	11	22	24	14	18	22	23	101
Iron	10	12	6	44	43	10	37	17	50	17	5	3	94
Manganese	56	22	2	112	21	68	76	83	6	0	0	0	16
Selenium	0	4	0	120	0	78	0	36	86	0	0	0	142
Calories per 100 gm.	28	38	32	403	345	356	327	335	140	143	217	100	283
% calories from fat	10	19	8	40	4	5	8	6	32	38	54	11	3

TABLE 4.2B *Comparative nutritive components of selected high-quality foods on a calorie basis*

Calorie basis percentage of RDA per 100 Calories	TURNIP GREENS	KALE	BROCCOLI	SOY BEANS	LIMA BEANS	BROWN RICE	MILLET	BUCK WHEAT	LIVER	BEEF	SALMON	HALIBUT	YEAST
AMINO ACIDS													
Tryptophan	93	73	78	72	29	13	37	24	118	101	57	111	136
Isoleucine	52	54	59	69	47	11	23	16	98	111	71	149	116
Lysine	77	47	69	81	55	11	14	18	142	186	125	244	160
Valine	57	62	68	59	44	13	21	27	101	101	65	127	112
Methionine	19	17	28	21	15	8	12	8	53	63	49	98	46
Threonine	80	70	86	65	49	15	21	22	114	121	79	158	143
Leucine	78	76	57	75	51	19	49	21	129	131	80	156	116
Phenylalanine	84	46	57	87	52	19	14	22	122	120	73	134	138
VITAMINS													
A	542	468	156	0	0	0	0	0	319	0	2	8	0
D	0	0	0	0	0	0	0	0	2	0	17	11	0
K	3315	0	894	67	0	0	0	0	91	0	0	0	0
C	827	547	573	0	0	0	0	0	42	0	6	0	0
E	78	140	14	38	1	3	0	10	9	0	6	8	0
B1	51	0	22	19	9	6	15	12	10	4	5	5	400
B2	83	40	42	4	2	0	6	2	112	7	2	4	82
B6	46	39	31	10	8	7	11	4	24	14	16	21	43
B12	0	0	0	0	0	0	0	0	1420	43	61	33	0
Niacin	15	30	15	3	3	7	3	7	43	20	17	46	77
Folic acid	84	39	54	10	7	1	0	0	39	1	2	3	341
Pantothenic acid	33	65	93	10	7	7	0	11	142	8	14	7	104
Biotin	1	1	1	15	2	3	0	0	71	0	2	8	38
MINERALS													
Calcium	74	39	26	4	1	0	0	2	0	0	3	1	6
Magnesium	53	24	18	16	13	6	12	18	2	3	3	5	20
Copper	16	11	1	1	2	5	13	6	177	1	4	11.	92
Zinc	0	0	5	6	5	3	3	1	18	19	2	4	25
Chromium	0	0	187	0	34	0	0	0	85	42	0	0	111
Potassium	14	53	63	22	23	3	7	7	10	13	10	23	35
Iron	35	32	19	11	12	2	11	5	35	12	2	3	33
Manganese	202	57	7	28	6	19	23	24	4	0	0	0	5
Selenium	0	12	0	30	0	21	0	10	61	0	0	0	49
Calories per 100 gm.	357	263	313	25	29	28	31	30	71	70	46	100	35
% calories from fat	10	19	8	40	4	5	8	6	32	38	54	11	3

TABLE 4.3 *Top quality foods according to nutrient density per portion (+ Best, ○ Next)*

Food	WT. (GMS)	CALS	VIT. A	VIT. C	VIT. D	VIT. E	VIT. K	THIAMINE	RIBOFLAVIN	NIACIN	B6	PANTOTHENIC ACID	B12	FOLACIN
RANGE OF RDA PER PORTION (+)		+	91–100	79–199	100	66–100	85–100	67–100	100	61–100	34–43	60–100	100	42–97
RANGE OF RDA PER PORTION (○)		○	30–50	55–71	31–55	25–60	30–62	26–52	15–37	33–46	20–31	25–42	58–73	15–32
Beef (lean)	100	143									○	○		
Chicken (dark)	100	130							○			○	○	
Chicken (light)	100	117							+	+				
Liver	100	140	+	○			+		+	+	+	+	+	+
Pork (lean)	100	165						+			○			
Veal	100	156		○						○				
Cod	100	78												
Mackerel	100	191			+				○	○	○	+		
Oysters	50	33			○							+		
Salmon	100	217			○					○	+	○	+	
Sardines fresh	50	78			+							+		
Sardines can	100	200												
Squid	100	84												
Tuna	100	127			+					+	○	+		
Skim milk, cup	244	85							○					
Buttermilk	244	100							○					
Yogurt	244	156							○			+		
Ricotta skim	124	174					○							
Sunflower seeds	15	84				+								
Broccoli	200	45	+	+			+		○		○	+		○
Chard	112	28	+	○										
Kale	100	38	+	+		+			○			○		○

TABLE 4.3 *(Continued) Top quality foods according to nutrient density per portion (+ Best, ○ Next)*

Food	WT. (GMS)	CALS	BIOTIN	CA	MG	POTASSIUM	IRON	CU	MN	ZN	SE	CR	LYSINE	METHIONINE
RANGE OF RDA PER PORTION (+)			60–100	18–36	32–66	69–100	34–50	83–100	44–100	97–100	60–100		72–100	75–100
RANGE OF RDA PER PORTION (○)			10–31	12–16	15–28	25–53	15–26	17–42	21–24	16–31	36–48			30–50
Beef (lean)	100	143				○			○				+	+
Chicken (dark)	100	130											+	+
Chicken (light)	100	117											+	+
Liver	100	140	+		+	+	+			○	+		+	+
Pork (lean)	100	165								○			+	+
Veal	100	156				○			○				+	+
Cod	100	78							+	+			+	+
Mackerel	100	191								+			+	+
Oysters	50	33				○			+	+				
Salmon	100	217											+	+
Sardines fresh	50	78	○								+		+	
Sardines can	100	200		+										
Squid	100	84						+					+	+
Tuna	100	127				○					+		+	+
Skim milk, cup	244	85	+										+	
Buttermilk	244	100	+										+	
Yogurt	244	156	+	○									+	
Ricotta skim	124	174	+										+	
Sunflower seeds	15	84					○							
Broccoli	200	45	○											
Chard	112	28		○	○	○		+						
Kale	100	38	○											
Mushrooms	70	20	○	+	○	○			○				+	
Parsley	100	44		○		○	+	○						
Spinach	100	26		○	○	○				○		○		

TABLE 4.3 *(Continued) Top quality foods according to nutrient density per portion (+ Best, ○ Next)*

Food	WT. (GMS)	CALS	BIOTIN	CA	MG	POTASSIUM	IRON	CU	MN	ZN	SE	CR	LYSINE	METHIONINE
RANGE OF RDA PER PORTION (+)			60–100	18–36	32–66	69–100	34–50	83–100	44–100	97–100	60–100		72–100	75–100
(○)			10–31	12–16	15–28	25–53	15–26	17–42	21–24	16–31	36–48			30–50
Sweet potato	180	205						⊦						
Turnip greens	115	32		+	○	○			+	○	+		+	+
Garbanzos	100	360	○	○	+	○	+	○	+	○			+	○
Lentils	100	340		○	○	+	○		○					○
Lima beans	100	345							○	○				○
Soybeans	100	403	+		+	+	+		+	○	+		+	+
Banana	150	127				○								
Cantaloupe	200	60				○								
Papaya	100	39												
Millet	100	327			+		+	○	+					
Rice brown	100	356	○		○				+		+			
Rice wild	100	353			⊦	○					○		+	
Wheat germ	10	40												
W/wheat pasta	80	266			○						+			
Kombu	8	19	○	○										
Nori	8	20	○	○		○	○							
Wakami	8	20	○	○		○								
Yeast	10	28	○					○					○	
Yeast	20	56	○					○					+	

WHEN TO GO ON THE DIET

I definitely do not recommend that anyone begin a CRON diet until they are fully grown. After that, the sooner the better. Beginning the program halfway through life should yield about half the degree of life extension as starting in young adulthood, and proportionately for

TABLE 4.3 (Continued) Top quality foods according to nutrient density
per portion (+ Best, ○ Next)

Food	WT. (GMS)	CALS	VIT. A	VIT. C	VIT. D	VIT. E	VIT. K	THIAMINE	RIBOFLAVIN	NIACIN	B6	PANTOTHENIC ACID	B12	FOLACIN
RANGE OF RDA PER PORTION (+)			91–100	79–199	100	66–100	85–100	67–100	100	61–100	34–43	60–100	100	42–97
(○)			30–50	55–71	31–55	25–60	30–62	26–52	15–37	33–46	20–31	25–42	58–73	15–32
Mushrooms	70	20							○			+		
Parsley	100	44	+	+					○					○
Spinach	100	26	+	+			+							+
Sweet potato	180	205	+	○	+							○		○
Turnip greens	115	32	+	+		○	+	○						○
Garbanzos	100	360									○	○		+
Lentils	100	340						○			+	○		
Lima beans	100	345				+		○				○	○	○
Soybeans	100	403				+	+	+	○			+	○	+
Banana	150	127									+			
Cantaloupe	200	60	+	+										
Papaya	100	39	○	+										
Millet	100	327						○	○		+			
Rice brown	100	356									○	○		
Rice wild	100	353						○	○	○		○		
Wheat germ	10	40				+	○							
W/wheat pasta	80	266						○						
Kombu	8	19			○							○	○	
Nori	8	20	○		○							○	○	
Wakami	8	20			○						○			○
Yeast	10	28						+	○					
Yeast	20	56						+	○	○		○		

other time periods.

Caloric restriction beginning in childhood would yield the greatest extension of maximum life span, but remains an unacceptable option for humans. Substantial restriction in very young animals may cause an increased infant or early age mortality, even though the survivors do go on to enjoy remarkably long lives. We could not sacrifice a small percentage of young humans to ensure long lives for the survivors. Also, restriction during the growing years in animals is often associated with a smaller final body size. In humans, this could mean being six to ten inches shorter than you otherwise would have been.

Do not take these caveats to mean that a somewhat lower-calorie, higher-quality diet would not potentially increase life span for today's children. Indeed, translating this animal data into human terms, Dr. Morris Ross[18] estimated that a difference in daily intake of merely 100 to 125 calories during the period of human growth would influence the duration of life by 2.5 years. Empty calories for children—so-called "energy snacks" and the like—are bad news for their health later on in life.

HOW TO LOSE WEIGHT

The CRON diet works very well for rapid weight loss. In fact, because of its nutrient density, it is probably the best of all diets for that purpose. At an equivalent caloric intake, it will leave you better nourished than other diets. But a word of caution is needed here. In Western societies, enormous subliminal and not so subliminal pressure is exerted on everyone to be as slim as starlets and models. We are made to feel we should be not merely "not fat" but positively slender. Responding to this pressure, people plunge desperately into quick weight reduction regimens. A popular diet book promising rapid, painless slenderizing comes out almost every other month. No check-out-counter tabloid is without one. From the standpoint of health and longevity, quick weight loss is harmful.

It had been known since 1935 that if you kept animals on a low-calorie diet from time of weaning, you could dramatically extend life span and decrease susceptibility to disease. But nobody could make the method work if it was started in adulthood. Indeed, in the early experiments this actually *shortened* the life span. Studying these early experiments, Dr. Richard Weindruch and I noted that the investigators had put the animals suddenly, or over a very short period, on the lower-calorie diet. This sudden switch, we reasoned, may have injured them metabolically. Then, in our own investigations we found that if a CRON diet was begun very gradually in adult animals, leading to a very slow weight loss (equivalent to weight loss in humans over a four– to six-year period), life span could be greatly extended and disease incidence reduced.[19] If this applies to humans, then the quick weight loss promised by most modern diet books may be dandy for your immediate cosmetic appeal, but across-the-board bad for your ultimate health, and even for the long-term cosmetic appeal of looking younger than you are. Anyway, almost everyone knows that all these diets don't work very well. You lose weight and then you gain it back. Then you buy another highly promoted diet book, and do it again. The whole cycle is discouraging, irrational, and unhealthful.

Based on further work in animals and on the Biosphere 2 experience, I now believe the time period for weight loss in humans can be reduced from four to six years to six to nine months or, better still, up to one or two years. You may ask, "What's wrong with going faster?" There are two reasons not to! The first is that the Biosphere 2 crew members sustained the major part of their substantial weight loss during the first six to nine months, yet remained healthy; so one to two years seems conservatively safe for humans in terms of what we learned from the animal experiments. Thus, one to two years is ample to allow for metabolic adaptation. Less might also be all right, but I am not entirely sure.

The second reason for losing weight slowly concerns the release into the blood of toxic materials, such as pesticide residues, out of your own stores of bodily fat. Certain pesticide residues like DDE (from DDT), as well as dioxin and the PCBs, plus others, are not broken down very rapidly by the detoxifying enzymes of the body. However, because they are fat soluble, they are prevented from doing harm by being absorbed into the body's fat. It's a bit like storing nuclear

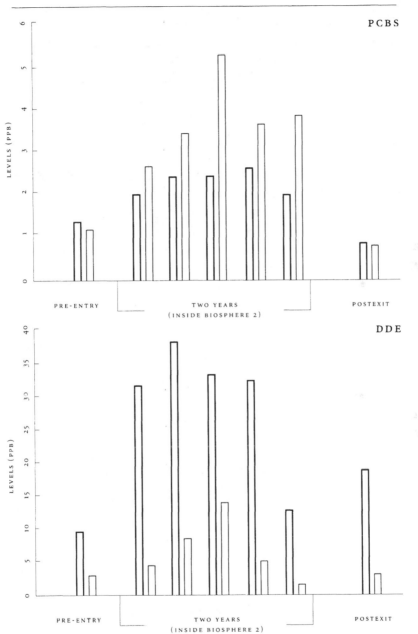

FIGURE 4.1. *Levels of DDE (a breakdown product of DDT) and of PCBs in the blood of two crew members before entry, during residence in, and after exit from Biosphere 2 (adapted from Walford et al.,* Toxicological Sciences, *1999 [in press])*

wastes in underground salt domes, only in this case it's in fat. Because Biosphere 2 was a totally closed system and there was no chance of DDT or PCBs blowing in with the dust or other sources and influencing the pesticide levels in the crew's blood, we were able to follow those levels under constant environmental conditions. We discovered that with the rapid loss of weight (and therefore fat mass) the levels *increased.*[20] Furthermore, because the body's detoxification system does not handle fat-soluble residues very rapidly, they *remained elevated* for a year or longer. (see Figure 4.1.) Therefore, you should lose weight slowly enough for the released toxins to be cleared without getting too high. And yo-yo dieting is particularly bad, as it may wash toxic material in and out and in and out of the blood stream.

What level of toxic residues is too much? The answer is, any level is too high, but a certain amount cannot be avoided because of the environment in which we live. The government has established so-called "allowable limits." These seem generally okay. On the other hand, in 1996, 11-year-olds in Michigan exposed in the womb to only slightly higher levels of PCBs than the U.S. average were found to have measurably lower IQs.[21]

What calorie range suffices to enable you to lose weight slowly over a one- to two-year period, placing you below your set point? It will vary from person to person. For example, the caloric RDA for a 120-pound woman is given as 1,700 to 2,500. That means that *some* 120-pound women will stay at that weight on a 1,700 calorie intake, but others will require 2,500. The amount is very individually specific. Nevertheless we can form a general idea from a study performed not long after World War 2 by scientists at the University of Minnesota.[22]* They placed 32 young male conscientious objectors on a strict 1,600-calorie per day diet for six months. The subjects lost weight fairly rapidly, and the loss leveled off to a maintenance value of 75 percent of the original weight. Once lost, the weight was not regained unless more than 2,000 calories per day were given.

Start your own program with about a 2,000-calorie CRON diet if you are an average-size man, 1,800 calories if a woman, and see if this induces gradual weight loss and at the same time enhances your sense of physical well-being. If so, continue. If you are losing weight too fast or too slowly or not at all, adjust your intake accordingly. The food and menu combinations given in Appendix A are pitched to approximate or exceed the RDAs for all important nutrients at a level of 1,500 or fewer calories. Unless you have a medical reason for wanting quick weight loss, add about 300 to 500 calories of intake to any of these daily regimens. Choose whatever you like for these extra calories, but keep in mind what I shall outline in the next chapter about susceptibility to the major killer diseases.

What should be the quantities and ratios of the macronutrients (protein, carbohydrate, and fat) in your diet? This question has evoked great and continuing controversy, particularly about the proper percentage of fat in the diet. The low-fat enthusiasts are supported by the following: obesity is rare in experimental animals kept on a low-fat diet, and common in animals maintained on high fat diets.[23] In numerous studies in humans, total energy intake—and therefore obesity—was higher when the subjects consumed high fat diets. The amount of body fat is also higher when the excess energy comes from fats rather than from proteins or carbohydrates. However, it is difficult to separate the fat effect from an energy density effect. People tend to eat a constant weight of food, and the energy density of fat is over two-times that of the other macronutrients. The picture has been complicated by the fact that an increasing number of processed "low-fat" foods have—because of low fiber and water content and addition of sugar—an energy density per weight as high as fat.

On the other side of the question: not all experts agree that dietary fat promotes development of obesity. On a population basis, obesity prevalence has greatly increased in the last decade whereas the percentage of energy intake from dietary fat has decreased.[24] Studies of diabetes and diabeteslike syndromes suggest that when high-carbohydrate diets are compared to high mono-fat diets, subjects show better physiologic responses with the latter.[25]

However, it is noteworthy that most of the above information, especially that from humans, comes from relatively short-term studies, and it is well established that long-term calorie reduction may yield results different than short term.[26*] For our purposes the best cohorts to study—unfortunately, they are few in number—are those reduced obese individuals who have stayed reduced for five years, i.e., the small percentage of really successful dieters. They report that their success in weight-loss maintenance stems from consumption of a low-fat, low total energy intake, accompanied by high levels of regular physical activity.[27]

FASTING

One should be aware that while total fasting *increases* UCP (uncoupling protein) activity in the rat, merely restricting food intake by 50 percent actually *decreases* UCP expression.[28] When totally deprived of food, the body acts to maintain temperature by turning up the UCPs, thereby decreasing its metabolic efficiency and burning its fat. On the other hand, responding to *partial* food deprivation, it may just turn down the thermostat. Indeed CRON humans, as well as monkeys, tend to display a body temperature one or more degrees lower than normal.[29] That's what you want.

It's acceptable to cut caloric intake by frequent fasts, if that's the easiest way for you to go, as long as the fasts are short, no more than one or two days. Some of the animal studies have entailed "intermittent fasting", giving the animals as much as they want of a high-quality diet, but only every other day, and on alternate days they receive nothing. The overall weekly caloric intake turns out to be less, slow weight loss ensues, and life span is extended.

In human societies fasting has an extensive history, dating back to antiquity. Many cultures and religions have incorporated it into their writings and practices. North American Indians and Eskimos fast prior to being ordained for their priesthood. Muslims fast for many reasons (before prayer, when ill, or when they wish to conjure). Eastern yogis fast to achieve spiritual enlightenment. Jesus fasted forty days and nights.

Technically, you are "fasting" only if you consume nothing but water. Such fasting is short-term starvation. Fasting under proper supervision (especially if long-term, which for the reasons given I do not recommend) differs from actual starvation in that the diet is supplemented with vitamins and minerals. Without this, symptoms of frank vitamin deficiency develop in totally fasting individuals in considerably less than two months. On the other hand, very obese people have gone without food (properly supplemented and in a hospital, where they could be observed) for as long as 249 days without apparent harm. [30, 31]*

Short-term fasts of one or two days per week, with more generous amounts of high-quality foods on the eating days, are just as effective in inducing gradual weight loss as simply eating less each day. It depends on what is comfortable for you. An occasional short-term fast is also good because it will change your perceptions of hunger and energy. Hunger is partly habit. And skipping or cutting down on meals does not rob you of energy: in fact, the reverse. In one study, five men were subjected to five two-and-a-half day fasts at five- to six-week intervals. [32] Their ability to undertake hard physical labor during the fast periods was measured. Between the first and final periods, reaction times and pattern recognition (a test of intellectual function) actually improved. Glucose-tolerance tests showed an increased ability to regulate blood sugar. Short-term fasts may aid metabolic adaptation; however, they are not a necessary part of the CRON diet program.

APPETITE AND ITS CONTROL

Following weight loss resulting from low calorie intake, the concentrations of the hormones insulin and leptin (a recently discovered hormone released from fat tissue itself) decrease, and glucocorticoid concentrations increase. This combination of changes activates pathways that stimulate appetite and promote weight gain, while inhibiting pathways having the opposite effect. [33] This so-called "lipostatic model" is currently favored to explain appetite and the set point. It links food intake to the amount of stored energy (fat mass) in the body. Animals modify their eating pattern so that sufficient calories are consumed to maintain a constant amount of fat stores. Other gut-derived "satiety factors" can alter the size of individual meals, but they have limited influence on overall adiposity. Resting levels of insulin are proportional to total fat mass. By contrast, posteating insulin levels are proportional to the rise in glucose following a meal. Glucocorticoids secreted by the adrenal cortex antagonize the actions of the fat-derived hormone leptin and of insulin in the control of energy balance. Glucocorticoid increase (as occurs to a mild degree in people on a CRON diet) decreases the ability of insulin and leptin to promote appetite suppression and weight loss. The interaction of these various factors makes losing weight difficult, which is why most diets don't work.

In any long-term dietary program leading to gradual, substantial, and sustained weight loss, appetite control is a problem. You will ask, "Am I going to be famished all the time?"

You won't feel as full as a gorged lion, but on a CRON diet you won't be as hungry as you might imagine. The type and quality of food itself also influences appetite. Rats on a low-protein, high-carbohydrate diet voluntarily restrict their intake and live longer.[34] Rats fed a high-fat, "junk food" diet gain a great deal more weight than normally fed rats. A study at the University of Alabama[35] revealed that volunteer humans allowed to eat as much as they liked achieved full satisfaction from as little as 1,500 calories a day from whole foods, but it took 3,000 calories of refined and processed foods to satisfy them. The "whole" foods included fruit, hot cereals, skim milk, soups, salads, non-meat sandwiches, pasta, fish, chicken, rice, vegetables, and whole-wheat toast and rolls. The "refined" foods included bacon, eggs, juice, buttered toast, fast and fried foods, roast or steak, buttered vegetables, whole milk, cake, and ice cream.

One hypothesis of appetite regulation maintains that unrefined foods with a low energy density will induce a feeling of fullness at a low energy intake.[36] *Low-energy density* means a lot of bulk per calorie. There is no contradiction between high *nutrient* density and low *energy* density: turnip greens, for example, are bulky, packed with nutrients but low in calories (See Table 4.2.)

Fiber material such as guar gum added to a meal significantly prolongs the time after eating before hunger returns. An addition of 10 grams of guar gum to meals twice daily decreased appetite by delaying gastric emptying time, with a significant weight loss over ten weeks in obese persons, accompanied by a decrease in LDL fats in the blood and an improved glucose-tolerance curve.[37]

Refined sugar in the diet stimulates appetite. Persons eating highly refined and processed foods have been shown to consume 25 percent more calories than persons on a more natural diet.

The CRON diet is a high-nutrient density/low-energy density formulation. As such, it will give you greater satiety per calorie than any other diet.

Drugs that decrease appetite are not a good answer for long-term gradual weight loss. A number of complex events occur in the body that result in its asking, "What's to eat?" These involve metabolic rates, the energy enzymes of the body, insulin, blood sugar, and a portion of the brain called the hypothalamus. Trying to handle all these events with a pill doesn't make sense. Like suppressing a toothache with codeine, it'll work for a while . . . but your tooth will rot.

You can make a rat eat by pinching its tail.[38] The pain causes the release of chemicals (opioids) in part of the brain (the hypothalamus) that block the sensation of pain, but also stimulate hunger. Like opium or morphine, these opioids (also known as endorphins) are addicting. Pinch a rat's tail frequently for ten days and it will release opioids and overeat. That's one way (not a very nice one) to get a fat rat. Suddenly stop pinching its tail, opioids are not released, and the addicted rat will go into a fit—the same reaction as a heroin addict. Mental pain or stress may also augment endorphin or opioid release and so stimulate hunger. Avoidance of stress will aid in appetite control. In this sense, weight gain and obesity may be thought of as a kind of auto-addiction.

The best answer to hunger turns out to be high-quality nutrition and rational self-restraint. And don't let anybody pinch your tail!

WILL IT WORK?

TRANSLATABILITY

Granted that the CRON diet works well in animals, how do we know it will work in humans? Of course the final, absolute proof will not come until people on a CRON diet are seen to live extraordinarily longer than the norm, and the outlook of traditional, conservative medicine would be to wait for this ultimate demonstration. But, of course, if we do wait before going on the diet, we probably won't be around to see what happens. We'll have died before the final answer comes in.

However, in medicine it is not uncommon to recommend measures not yet "proved" but for which substantial evidence exists. As mentioned earlier, many doctors have for years been recommending the lowering of blood cholesterol because this would probably help prevent coronary heart disease, but this was not "proved" until 1984, and then for only a selected category of patient. And only in early 1985 did a panel of 13 experts convened as part of a National Institutes of Health "consensus conference" conclude "beyond a reasonable doubt" that lowering elevated blood cholesterol levels would reduce the risk of heart attacks. "Beyond a reasonable doubt" in fact means "with a high order of probability." Surely this is not *formal* proof. It's a consensus decision. Many more examples could be cited. The key question for much good medical advice is not whether proof is at hand, but what is the order of probability that the advice is correct.

Existing evidence indicates not absolutely but with a very high order of probability that the same CRON diet that extends life span in all the varieties of nonhuman species so far tested will do the same for man. One reason for thinking so is that we are dealing with a very general process. Experiments involving the overall operation of the immune system, the nature of DNA repair, and the various types and causes of cancer indicate that these *general* phenomena are quite similar across the species barrier. Nutritional modulation of the aging process seems to be such a general phenomenon, involving common processes across wide species barriers. In my view this animal work is entirely translatable to humans.

It is occasionally asserted, as evidence against translatability of calorie-restriction experiments, that in underdeveloped countries or situations where people are underfed, there is no increase in longevity.[39] I find it astonishing that those who express this view never pause to consider that these underfed populations are also malnourished. Their caloric restriction is often accompanied by inadequate vitamin, mineral, protein, and other intake. Nobody claims that undernutrition with malnutrition increases life span.

DIRECT EVIDENCE

Aside from the question of translatability, there is in fact a modest amount of *direct* evidence beyond what I have already set forth, that the CRON diet will exert the same effects in humans as in animals.

Long-term (three to nine months) low-calorie supplemented diets have been investigated in the treatment of obesity and diabetes.[40] These diets yield metabolic effects in humans that closely resemble some of those seen in animals on similar diets: a decrease in cholesterol, an improved insulin response, and a better regulation of blood sugar.

Anorexia nervosa is a dreadful, sometimes fatal psychological disease in which (usually) young women, often overachievers, develop a compulsive urge to control their weight. They literally starve themselves slowly, sometimes even unto death, as did the popular singer Karen Carpenter in late 1982.

Despite the disastrous nature of the disease, certain things about it are interesting for our purpose. Anorexics typically restrict their intake of fat and carbohydrates but allow themselves relatively more protein in vegetables and low-fat cheeses. They undergo drastic weight loss but with considerably less comparative malnutrition than is seen in typical semistarved individuals from famine or poverty areas. So it's a bit like a high-quality low-calorie diet except it's carried to excess. And for a while, anorexics do remain surprisingly well despite their growing emaciation. They do not usually get into serious problems until up to 30 to 40 percent of their body weight has been lost.[41] Despite an extremely low calcium intake, they do not experience an automatic increase in parathyroid hormone levels and reabsorb calcium from bone.[42] They do not show any increased susceptibility to infections. And quite unlike the results of malnutrition caused by famine or poverty, the immune system in anorexics is generally preserved until weight loss is far advanced. Indeed, in early stages the immune responses may be better than control values.[43] The same phenomenon of heightened immune response is of course found in rodents subjected to caloric restriction commencing in adulthood.[44]

In *Maximum Life Span* I discussed two populations world famous for fabulous longevity, the people of the former Soviet Georgia and the villagers of Vilcabamba, Peru. Alas, they are not really long-lived! They possess no secrets of longevity at all, and their maximum life span is no longer than anybody else's. Yogurt advertisements notwithstanding, in the absence of reliable birth records, no knowledgeable gerontologist believes the Georgian myth. The same is true for the villagers in Vilcabamba, who for about a dozen years received a great deal of press coverage because they supposedly had many super-centenarians in their society. But it's just not true. According to the most recent evidence, the oldest person in Vilcabamba is only 96.

But there is one population today who just might be breaking the maximum life span barrier, and it is not in a mysterious place, but on the Japanese island of Okinawa.

THE OKINAWAN EXPERIENCE

In Japan, large-scale and quite accurate nutritional surveys have been conducted yearly since 1946 by the Ministry of Health and Welfare.[45] Accurate information is available about weight, body size, health, and disease incidences of the different areas of Japan. The numbers of centenarians are also known throughout Japan, since accurate legal birth records have been kept there since 1872.

On the island of Okinawa and in a few other areas of Japan, there are 15 to 37 centenarians per 100,000 persons over 65 years of age (the highest incidence is in Okinawa!), whereas in most of Japan the number ranges from one to nine. One way to estimate maximum life span of a population, besides finding the age of the oldest tiny cohort of survivors, is to calculate the average age of the last surviving 10 percent of the population. This is called the *tenth decile* of survivorship. With so many more actual centenarians in the population (and therefore also a lot more people over 90) than elsewhere,[46] it seems likely that the tenth decile is significantly higher in Okinawa than elsewhere in Japan. It's not just average age that's longer there, but maximum survival too.

Now, the daily caloric intake of Okinawan schoolchildren, though adequate in vitamins and animal protein, is only 62 percent of the "recommended intake" for Japan. Average sugar and salt intake for

Okinawans is lower than the national average, while consumption of green/yellow vegetables and meats is higher. Although it is not nearly so rigorous as the one spelled out in this book, the Okinawans, compared with the rest of the Japanese, seem to be on a CRON diet.

The frequencies of cancer, heart disease, high blood pressure, diabetes, and senile brain disease are lower by 30 to 40 percent in Okinawa than elsewhere in Japan. And the average heights and weights of the population are lower.

The increased number of centenarians among Okinawans, the quality and caloric content of their diet, the lowered incidence of the major diseases of aging, and their smaller body size are exactly what one finds in laboratory animals on a CRON diet since early life. Professor Yasuo Kagawa of Jichi Medical School, who has studied the Okinawans, attributes their longevity and health to caloric restriction.[47]

DR. VALLEJO'S EXPERIMENT

The high-low diet idea was tackled in an experiment performed in Madrid.[48] An over-65 population of 180 men and women in an old-age home were divided into two equal groups. One group was placed on a diet of 2,300 calories one day and 885 calories the next. The control group received 2,300 calories every day. Over the three years of the experiment, the subjects receiving the fewer calories spent only 123 days in the infirmary, compared with 219 days for the fully fed subjects. And their death rate was only half that of the control group. While Dr. Vallejo's experiment was not large enough, long enough, or careful enough to be regarded as definitive proof, it is still of considerable interest.

TWO VENERABLE GENTLEMEN

The Renaissance Italian gentleman Luigi Cornaro, a member of the minor Italian nobility, led a gluttonous life that resulted in dangerous ill health by age 37. Then, on his doctor's advice, he adopted a very temperate dietarily restricted regimen, which seems to have been equivalent to about 1,500 calories per day. The diet was also of good quality, considering the primitive state of nutritional science at that time. We know all about Signor Cornaro because he wrote a famous autobiography called *The Art of Long Living*. He died in 1567 at the age of 103. A few hundred years later Dr. A. Guenoit, president of the Paris Medical Academy, elected to follow a similar regimen. He died in 1935 at the age of 102.

SUMMARY

You will recognize, I hope, that the histories of Cornaro and Guenoit constitute merely anecdotal evidence. Does it really mean much that among historical figures who followed a (for their times) carefully selected high-quality, low-calorie diet, two out of two lived to become centenarians? No, not a great deal by itself. But note carefully where we now stand, even leaving aside the pleasant histories of our venerable gentlemen.

Overwhelming evidence proves the CRON diet will increase maximum life span in animals, and the biology involved is of such a general nature it ought to apply to humans. In humans and their close neighbors, the monkeys, low-calorie nutritious regimens yield biomarker changes similar to what a CRON diet produces in rodents. And while the experiments have not gone long enough to assess long-term survival, in the monkey populations a decrease in the diseases of aging is already being observed. One existing well-documented human population on a low-level approximation of the CRON diet appears to show an excess number of centenarians and less disease. In an experimental human population, and even beginning in old age, three years on intermittent calorie deprivation seemed to decrease the rates of illness and death.

For these reasons I am convinced that a CRON diet by itself (and the one you'll find in this book is finer tuned than any of the above) will greatly retard human aging and extend maximum survival.

CHAPTER 5

PREVENT WHAT IS GOING TO KILL YOU

AGING WITHOUT SICKNESS

YOU NOT ONLY WANT TO LIVE LONGER, YOU WANT TO remain as healthy as possible and free of disease throughout that extended time. Although the CRON diet will take you most of the way toward achieving this two-pronged goal, we can further target our program toward additional preventive measures for many of the diseases that might otherwise afflict us during the course of our 120-plus years of life. I don't want to die at 100 if I'm still functionally young, still chasing the apples of desire. Neither do you. We all want to die of "old age" rather than cancer, which means we'll be healthy until our 120th-plus year, and then succumb rather quickly to some minor irregularity, pneumonia from exposure to skiing weather, say, or complications arising from a motorcycle spill on the way to a game. In the poem "The Deacon's Masterpiece" by Oliver Wendell Holmes, all parts of the wonderful one horse shay were built to endure exactly 100 years, ever smooth and shining, and then turn to dust all together. Poof! And blow away! It won't happen with us quite that way, of course, but that's a goal to strive for as we manipulate the human survival curve. Extend it and bend it, this is the idea. (See Figure 1.1.)

I am talking now about increasing the average life span, the part of the survival curve influenced mainly by disease. The CRON diet will increase *maximum* life span, and to a considerable extent carry average life span along with it, but other measures may further help to square or rectangularize the survival curve. These measures deal with fat, fiber, and fitness, with having larger amounts of certain vitamins and minerals in our diet than the official Recommended Daily Allowances (RDA), adding other chemical agents to the diet (a very controversial but potentially important matter), and avoiding stress and noxious environmental agents. In this and the next several chapters, I will discuss all but the last two of these, which are out of my area of expertise.

As we grow older, partly because of the increasing vulnerability that comes with normal aging, and partly because poor health habits gradually catch up with us, we tend to develop a number of diseases: arteriosclerosis, cancer, high blood pressure, diabetes, osteoporosis, and others. You won't develop lung cancer from smoking for one year, but after 30 years your chances of contracting lung cancer will be 15 to 20 times that of nonsmokers. There may be a history of hypertension in your family, but you may not have a high-pressure blowout until you've eaten too much salt or an excess of calories for 20 to 30 years.

A genetic predisposition to develop a disease may not show itself until played upon by environmental factors over a long period. In other words, genetic component + environmental component = disease. Medical science now believes that lifestyle and environment are significantly involved in up to 75 percent of the major killer diseases in the Western world. In addition to smoking, the main influence is what we eat, or fail to eat.

Besides some discussion of certain micronutrients (vitamins and minerals), we shall be focusing much of our attention in this chapter on the macronutrients, namely, fat, carbohydrate, and protein, and to what extent these may influence disease and aging. The general recommendations of many health professionals for low-fat, high-carbohydrate diets have in the past five or so years swung miraculously in the opposite direction, towards high-fat, low-carbohydrate diets. And recommendations to eat complex carbohydrates rather than simple sugars have now changed towards advocating carbohydrates with low glycemic indexes (*glycemic index* will be defined presently) regardless of their complexity. Recommendations about fats have shifted from focus on polyunsaturated fatty acids to monounsaturated fatty acids, or PUFA to MUFA, to use the common abbreviations. (In part this is because excess PUFAs, while decreasing the incidence of coronary heart disease in comparison with controls, may stimulate cancer, particularly of the gastrointestinal tract, breast, and lungs.[1])

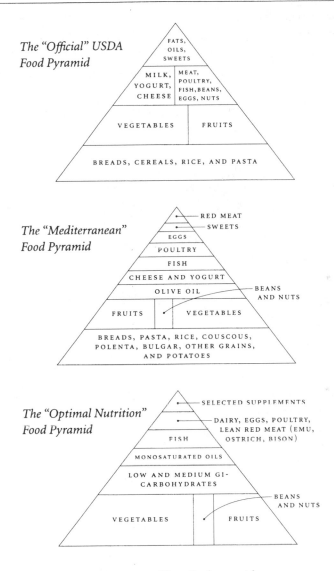

The "Official" USDA Food Pyramid

FATS, OILS, SWEETS

MILK, YOGURT, CHEESE | MEAT, POULTRY, FISH, BEANS, EGGS, NUTS

VEGETABLES | FRUITS

BREADS, CEREALS, RICE, AND PASTA

The "Mediterranean" Food Pyramid

RED MEAT
SWEETS
EGGS
POULTRY
FISH
CHEESE AND YOGURT
OLIVE OIL — BEANS AND NUTS
FRUITS | VEGETABLES
BREADS, PASTA, RICE, COUSCOUS, POLENTA, BULGAR, OTHER GRAINS, AND POTATOES

The "Optimal Nutrition" Food Pyramid

SELECTED SUPPLEMENTS
DAIRY, EGGS, POULTRY, LEAN RED MEAT (EMU, OSTRICH, BISON)
FISH
MONOSATURATED OILS
LOW AND MEDIUM GI-CARBOHYDRATES
BEANS AND NUTS
VEGETABLES | FRUITS

FIGURE 5.1 *Three food pyramids*

One reason for the above confusion is that the academic nutritional and medical communities (particularly in the United States) are obsessed with the notion that they must keep it simple, that they cannot stray too far and too rapidly in their recommendations from what people habitually eat, otherwise patients will be confused and non-compliant. But recent U. S. Department of Agriculture figures show that simply asking Americans to focus only on reducing total fat intake, as the health professionals have done during most of the past 10 to 15 years, has backfired. People limit fat intake but feel thereby free to eat low-fat foods in unlimited quantities, resulting in an average increase in daily calorie consumption of 200 calories per day, and an upsurge in obesity.

In my view, it is better to lay out what is optimally healthy and life-span-promoting, rather than arrogantly deciding what people can bear to hear. A good example is the—by now rather famous—so-called Western "food pyramid." At the bottom of the pyramid, i.e., what you are supposed to eat the most of, are rice, pasta, potatoes, etc., rather than vegetables and fruits, which should be there on the bottom, but are in fact one tier up. And behold, at the top of the pyramid are the sweets: cakes, pies, ice cream. In short, it appears "recommended" that you consume small quantities of these unhealthy materials. I myself occasionally eat ice cream or other sweets; but I certainly would not give them an official "recommendation." They do not belong on top of a food pyramid. They belong on top of a tombstone. Figure 5.1 shows three pyramids: the "official" USDA pyramid, a pyramid representing the so-called "Mediterranean Diet," and what I consider an "optimal nutrition" pyramid.

THE AVERAGE AMERICAN DIET:
QUANTITY WITHOUT QUALITY

By 1925 we had cornflakes, hot dogs, processed cheese, and bright white bread; by 1950, baby foods and cake mix; by 1975, fast foods, frozen dinners, and kids who drank more pop than milk. Today's American diet is long on quantity and sadly short on quality—much more so than health authorities admit. Until not long ago the major role of diet in disease susceptibility had not been appreciated. Its role in cancer for both men and women is strikingly illustrated in Figure 5.2. Add to this the fact that diet, impinging upon the aging process itself, is by all odds the main cause of arteriosclerosis and heart disease, and significantly contributes to diabetes and other late-life diseases. What a shame it is that with such an abundance of food in the stores, supermarkets, and restaurants, people are not eating what is good for them, but the contrary, and accepting their heart attacks, their strokes, their diabetes, and cancers as pretty much "normal" events in the course of life.

From 1910 to 1980, fat consumption in the United States increased from 125 to 156 grams per day, and in 1990 was about 175 grams per day.[2] It declined somewhat in the next eight years, but is on the rise again. In the 1980s the average American diet derived 42 percent of its whopping 2,400 (for women) to 3,200 (for men) calories from fat, with a polyunsaturated to saturated fat ratio of 0.5:1. At that time most authorities believed the ratio should be close to 1:1. The current favored distribution is 10 percent saturated, 10 percent polyunsaturated, and 80 percent monounsaturated. The past 50 years have seen an increase in the consumption of processed vegetable fats: margarines, oils, and vegetable shortenings that contain significant quantities of chemically altered unsaturated fatty acids. (Some commercial vegetable oils contain up to 17 percent, some margarines 47 percent, some vegetable shortenings 58 percent of trans- instead of the natural cis- double bonds.) Protein intake has remained at about 103 grams per day since 1910, but with growing emphasis on animal rather than vegetable sources. Carbohydrate consumption fell from 490 grams daily in 1910 to 390 grams by 1980, but has substantially increased since then, with a shift from complex carbohydrates to sugars. Consumption of corn syrup, for example, is up 500 percent, and consumption of refined cane and beet sugar 25 percent. About a fourth of the calories consumed by the average person come from sugar, mostly hidden in processed foods and beverages. Our total sugar intake has increased 25-fold during the past few hundred years. Since these, nutritionally, are empty calories, the value of our diet has obviously decreased.

The consumption of processed foods has shown a fantastic increase in the past 70 years. And 18 percent of our meals and 25 percent of the money we spend on them goes for eating away from home. The annual $8 billion or more in sales of McDonald's, the world's largest

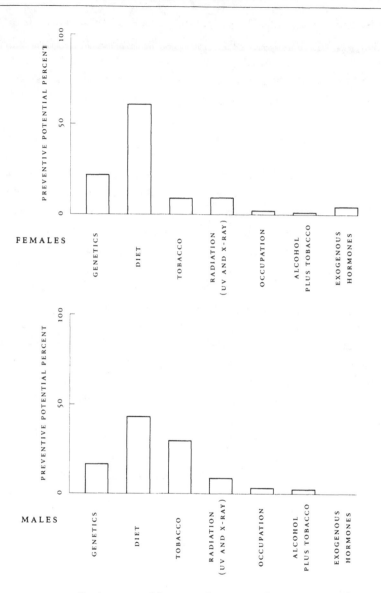

FIGURE 5.2 *Environmental factors and cancer. Only 10 to 20 percent of cancers are genetically determined, as shown by the first vertical bar. The rest are due to environmental influences, of which diet is by all odds the most important factor (adapted from G. B. Gori,* Cancer *43:2151, 1979).*

fast-food purveyor, far outstrips the number two contender, the United States Department of Agriculture itself, which in 1980 dispensed merely $3 billion worth of food to schoolchildren and the elderly.

The big trends in our diet have been, throughout most of the twentieth century, to maintain the level of calories (but with an increase in the last ten years) even though as a nation we are much more sedentary than we were in the early part of the century and don't need as many, and to increase fats and refined sugars, to increase animal and decrease vegetable proteins, to sharply decrease fiber intake, to shift from natural to processed foods, and to create nutritionally ghastly diet and food-preference habits. What is more revolting healthwise than the thought of eating a killer Twinkie? Or more criminal than feeding one to a child!

THE SCALE OF OBESITY

According to a 1995 report by the National Academy of Science's Institute of Medicine, 59 percent of the adult population of the U.S. meet the current definition of being overweight. [3] And even the best-intentioned attempts to eat less and exercise more have, in well-controlled trials, all failed to reduce the weight of more than a small fraction of the obese participants by at least 10 percent for five years.

"Let me have men about me that are fat," pleaded Julius Caesar in Shakespeare's play. Caesar thought fat men were less dangerous. Right or wrong, if he lived in the United States today, Caesar would have his wish. We are definitely fatter than we once were. Since the American Civil War our average weight has increased fully 16 percent. It's more important as an individual to concentrate on your personal set point than to struggle with how your weight compares with your neighbor's or your ancestor's. But to grasp the relations between fatness and disease we must understand the prevalence and measurement of obesity as it relates to the "average" body weight for sex, height, and body frame. And certain controversies about body weight and life expectancy must be cleared up. Generally, *obesity* means a weight 20 percent or more above average, or a body fat content exceeding 30 percent for women and 20 to 25 percent for men.

The actual proportion of the body consisting of fat can be estimated by various methods. I'll mention four. The first is easy but not very accurate, and involves measuring skin fold thickness. In most places the skin of the body is but 1 millimeter thick, so the distance between folds in different locations is due to fat. By measuring this distance at selected sites, we can estimate body fatness from tables or equations. The proportion of body fat in young adults at what insurance companies generally regard as "desirable weight" is about 12 percent for men, 19 percent for women. Several easy-to-use instruments are available for estimating skin-fold thickness. (See Readings and Resources.) Central obesity can be estimated by measurement of the skin-fold thickness between your shoulder blades, and peripheral obesity by the skin-fold thickness on the back of your upper arm (triceps).

A second method involves using a scale with electrical impedance capabilities. (See Readings and Resources.) You enter your sex and height into the scale, stand on it, and it reads off your weight and percent body fat.

A third and much used but indirect method involves calculation of the so-called Body Mass Index, or BMI. The BMI is defined as the ratio of body weight to height-squared. You can find out yours by looking at Table 5.1. Or you can calculate it as follows: (1) Multiply your weight in pounds by 0.45, (2) multiply your height in inches by 0.025, then (3) square that number, (4) and divide the result of number one by that of number three, to get your BMI. For the average person, the BMI gives a good indirect measurement of obesity, but in some instances it can be way off, too high for example in bodybuilders, who tend to have low body fat but increased muscle mass. Arnold Schwarzenegger as seen in his first movie, *Pumping Iron*, or in *Conan the Barbarian*, would have a very high BMI but a percentage of body fat of perhaps merely 5 to 7 percent. Nevertheless, in large population studies the BMI is a useful and easy-to-get measurement.

Currently, while 59 percent of U.S. citizens are *overweight* (BMI over 25), 23 percent are actually *clinically obese* (BMI over 30), compared to only 13 percent in 1962 and 15 percent in 1980.[4] Obviously a big fat leap occurred in the '80s and '90s. This ongoing "obesity epidemic" affects even children.

TABLE 5.1 *Body Mass Index (BMI)*

	100	105	110	115	120	125	130	135	140	145	150	155	160	165	170	175	180	185	190	195	200	205
5'0"	20	21	21	22	23	24	25	26	27	28	29	30	31	32	33	34	35	36	37	38	39	40
5'1"	19	20	21	22	23	24	25	26	26	27	28	29	30	31	32	33	34	35	36	37	38	39
5'2"	18	19	20	21	22	23	24	25	26	27	27	28	29	30	31	32	33	34	35	36	37	37
5'3"	18	19	20	20	21	22	23	24	25	26	27	27	28	29	30	31	32	33	34	35	35	36
5'4"	17	18	20	20	21	21	22	23	24	25	26	27	27	26	29	30	31	32	33	33	34	35
5'5"	17	17	19	19	20	21	22	22	23	24	25	26	27	27	28	29	30	31	32	32	33	34
5'6"	16	17	19	19	19	20	21	22	23	23	24	25	26	27	27	28	29	30	31	31	32	33
5'7"	16	16	18	18	19	20	20	21	22	23	23	24	25	26	27	27	28	29	30	31	31	32
5'8"	15	16	17	17	18	19	20	21	21	22	23	24	24	25	26	27	27	28	29	30	30	31
5'9"	15	16	16	17	18	18	19	20	21	21	22	23	24	24	25	26	27	27	28	29	30	30
5'10"	14	15	16	17	17	18	19	19	20	21	22	22	23	24	24	25	26	27	27	28	29	29
5'11"	14	15	15	16	17	17	18	19	20	20	21	22	22	23	24	24	25	26	26	27	28	29
6'0"	14	14	15	16	16	17	18	18	19	20	20	21	22	22	23	24	24	25	26	26	27	28
6'1"	13	14	15	15	16	16	17	18	18	19	20	20	21	22	22	23	24	24	25	26	26	27
6'2"	13	13	14	15	15	16	17	17	18	19	19	20	21	21	22	22	23	24	24	25	26	26
6'3"	12	13	14	14	15	16	16	17	17	18	19	19	20	21	21	22	22	23	24	24	25	26
6'4"	12	13	13	14	15	15	16	16	17	18	18	19	19	20	21	21	22	23	23	24	24	25

The most accurate way to estimate body fat (your doctor would have to arrange this) is by the density method. It was originally discovered by the ancient Greek mathematician Archimedes while sitting in his bath. Archimedes had the task of finding whether the king's crown was pure gold or whether the crown maker had adulterated it with baser metal. Seeing how his own body caused the water level in the tub to rise, Archimedes perceived that the amount of water he displaced equaled his own volume. By the same criterion, he could measure the crown's irregular volume, and thus see if the proper weight of gold displaced exactly as much. "Eureka!" he shouted, "I have found it!"—and in his excitement leaped from his bath and ran naked through the town.

To estimate your percentage of body fat, you are submerged in a tank of water and weighed after you have completely exhaled. Just as though you were a crown of gold, dividing your weight by the amount of water you displace (that is, by your volume) will determine your density. As the density of fat is 0.9 and of the nonfat parts of the body about 1.1, the percentage of you that is fat can be read from tables. If it is substantially less than 12 percent (for males, more for females), you will not look bad running naked through the town, although you may encounter stricter laws than Archimedes did.

BODY WEIGHT AND OVERALL MORTALITY

How does obesity, relative body weight, or degree of leanness affect the overall death rates of a population? Does being fat or slim influence your survival chances? The question became highly controversial for a time, with the 1983 publication of insurance company statistics indicating that the lowest death rates coincided with being mildly overweight in terms of average values. Other studies about the same time also seemed to indicate that mortality was lowest for those at 10 to 25 percent above average body weight for ages 40 to 49 years and 30 percent above average weight for ages 50 to 59, and that only after age 65 is mortality least for mildly underweight persons.[5] These findings contrasted sharply with earlier (1959) insurance company data showing that lowest mortality coincided with being about 10 percent *under*weight.

What is one to make of these surprising data of the early 1980s? They seemed to show that if you want to live longer, it's best to be mildly overweight.

The answer was that all sets of data were correct, and that appropriate biological interpretation could reconcile them. The data were only superficially contradictory. To begin with, insurance company data on the weight/mortality relationship have changed from time to time over the years. They reflect what is going on at any particular period. In the first half of the nineteenth century, insurance companies insisted that thin people pay a higher premium. At that time tuberculosis, the number one killer, caused 20 percent of all deaths. Because tuberculosis is an emaciating disease, its high frequency influenced the weight aspect of the mortality picture. It was not "thinness" itself that caused higher death rates, but that many thin people had undiagnosed tuberculosis. Today there is far less tuberculosis in Western societies, so this association no longer holds true.

In the first half of the twentieth century, the insurance company tables found mortality to be highest in the *heavier* segment of the population, who were therefore charged extra premiums for their insurance. The pattern keeps changing.

According to obesity expert Dr. Albert Stunkard of the University of Pennsylvania School of Medicine[6] most of the 1980s data were not adequately controlled for smoking, which is second only to poor diet in damaging health. In the famous study in Framingham, Massachusetts, the proportion of smokers in the population was 55 percent in the most overweight group and over 80 percent among the most underweight.[7] So it was not that fat people were healthier and so lived longer, but that thin people smoked more and so lived less long. It was also considered that a higher death rate among thin middle-aged men might reflect hidden disease (especially cancer) rather than leanness in itself. Even at that time, however, in one ten-year study lean middle-aged men who maintained the same weight they had had as young men enjoyed the lowest mortality of all.[8]

Other better controlled studies confirmed that any level of obesity is disadvantageous. A major conference sponsored by the National Institutes of Health's Nutrition Committee and the Centers for Disease Control concluded that *the weights associated with the greatest longevity are below average weights of the population,* as long as such weights are not associated with illness.[9] In the justly famous Nurses' Health Study of 110,000 women,[10] the lowest mortality rate was found in those with BMIs of less than 19. That's very skinny. Fashion models, for example, have BMIs around 18. In the Nurses' Health Study, the risk of death from all causes increased by 20 percent as the BMI increased from 19 to 25, by 60 percent as it rose to 28, and by more than 100 percent for BMIs of 29 and higher.

The distribution of fat on the body also affects mortality and disease susceptibility.[11] Abdominal fat, characterized by the bulging belly of middle age, increases the risk of cardiovascular disease and diabetes, compared to fat distributed on the thighs and lower body (the pear-shaped body).

You might still hear smug claims from the pro-obesity lobby, but don't believe them. It's in to be thin, and stout is still definitely *out* in terms of health.[12]

DIET AND THE KILLER DISEASES

Poor nutrition is the chief factor in most of the major diseases in First World societies. Let us single out these diseases and see how susceptibility to them might be diminished by adjustment of our eating habits in ways additive to simply lowering the amount of calories.

First, however, because we are entering controversial areas, we require a few definitions. The *glycemic index* (GI) of foods has important implications for the major causes of sickness and death in western countries, including obesity, heart disease, and diabetes.[13]* The GI classifies foods according to how much they raise blood glucose following ingestion of an amount of the food that contains 50 grams of carbohydrate. High GI foods include, for example, white bread, potatoes, regular rice; low GI foods include pasta, soybeans, and many fruits and vegetables. It's hard to predict where a food will fall. You simply have to measure its effect. Bananas, watermelon, and carrots have high GIs; apples and peaches, low. (See Table 9.3.)

High-GI diets generate a demand for insulin, and hyperinsulinemia is linked with all facets of the *metabolic syndrome* (insulin resistance, hyperlipidemia, hypertension, and visceral obesity). It seems also to be the case that high-protein, high-fat foods stimulate a greater insulin response than predicted by the level of glycemia,[14] and an Insulin Index of foods may eventually prove as or more helpful than the Glycemic Index. In the *glycemic theory of aging* it might after all be the insulin that is at fault.[15]

While the GI concept has been taken up by nutritionists in most other Western countries, this has been much less true in the U.S. Therefore, much of the gathering present-day disillusionment[16] on the part of health professionals with the low-fat, high-carbohydrate diets they have been pushing for the last 15 to 20 years may well be because in the U.S. high-carbohydrate habits are customarily directed towards high-GI carbohydrates, with adverse effects on blood lipid (triglyceride and HDL) levels. But these effects are *not* seen with consumption of low-GI carbohydrates. After all, the much vaunted Mediterranean diet[17]* (rich in fruits, vegetables, whole grains, legumes, and fish, and omega-3 fatty acids, which are those fatty acids that have the first double bond between the third and fourth carbon atom of the carbon chain) is high carbohydrate, but the carbohydrates have low GIs, in contrast to the carbohydrates in the usual American diet. (In the U.S., consumption of white and whole wheat flour, both high-GI, has increased about 40 percent since 1970.[18]) Furthermore, the fixation for some years on low-fat nutrition led food companies to respond to the fat phobia by marketing a plethora of fat-free and fat-reduced products. The result was an overdose of high-GI carbohydrates, like the wrong kinds of bread, fat-free pretzels, crackers, cookies, etc. If they were "fat-free," you could eat them with impunity, and people did just that, and got fat and unhealthy. These fat-free foods contained a lot of high-GI carbohydrate calories.

In any case, the proper use of the glycemic index is to compare foods within categories of similar nutrient profile, not so much across profiles. Apples to oranges is okay, but apples to steak is not. High-fat foods may be seen as falsely favorable if only the GI is considered, in that large amounts of fats in food reduce glycemia by slowing emptying time, but glucose tolerance to the subsequent meal is impaired. And while insulin responses follow the rank order of the glycemic responses, high-protein and high-fat foods stimulate greater insulin responses than predicted by the level of glycemia; and like too much glucose in the blood, too much insulin is bad.

Now some comments on fat. Many studies have shown that the prevalence of obesity is higher in people with high-fat diets as a percentage of energy intake;[19] the same holds for animal studies. Body fat storage occurs at a greater rate when excess energy comes from fat than when it comes from carbohydrate or protein. And reducing fat intake appears to have been the most successful strategy in promoting *long-term* weight loss in that small percentage of humans who are able to persevere in weight reduction, those who lose weight and keep it off.

Despite the above, admittedly older but at the same time abundant and careful data, fat intake has shifted from being totally bad to being totally innocuous, so long as it is monounsaturated fats (MUFA), and to being positive so long as it comprises the omega-3s.

The argument in favor of MUFA is that both high-MUFA and high-carbohydrate diets lower LDL to the same degree, but high-carbohydrate diets increase blood glucose and insulin and result in increased triglycerides and lower HDL (i.e. are atherogenic and diabetogenic). However, reducing the GI of the carbohydrates has about the same effects as emphasizing the MUFA content. The Pritikin diet is low fat (10 percent of calories), low protein, high carbohydrate, and is able to ameliorate the elevated blood sugar levels of diabetics—but will not do so without the low-fat, low-protein components.[20]

The evidence keeps shifting, and official recommendations may well be different a decade from now. At the present time, for the macronutrients I prefer the middle ground of a moderately low-fat diet, but with emphasis on MUFAs and omega-3s, moderate protein intake, and the rest mostly low-GI carbohydrates. (The diet of Paleolithic man derived 20 percent of its calories from fat.)

ARTERIOSCLEROSIS AND HEART DISEASE

Arteriosclerotic heart disease is the greatest epidemic mankind has ever faced, carrying off a larger percentage of the population than the Black Death in the Middle Ages. (See Figure 5.3.) Every 33 seconds someone in the United States dies of heart disease—about a million people each year. Yet it's by no means an inevitable factor of life. We almost entirely bring it on ourselves by our lifestyles. And we start young. Many of the supposedly healthy American soldiers killed in Vietnam were found, on autopsy, to have arteriosclerosis.

Experimental evidence shows that high-GI foods promote higher day-long insulin levels, which promote carbohydrate oxidation at the expense of fatty acid oxidation, thereby enhancing synthesis of the very low lipoprotein cholesterol (VLDL), which you don't want.[21] This happens to a much lesser extent with low-GI carbohydrates. As stated earlier, the GI index was found to be an important risk indicator for heart disease in the Nurses' Health study. In healthy people as well as diabetics, high carbohydrate diets worsen the blood lipid pro-

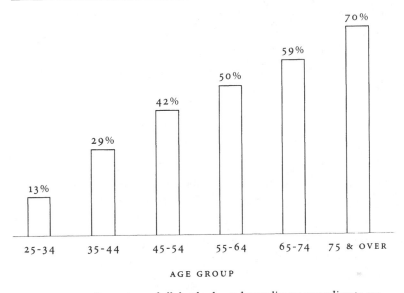

FIGURE 5.3 *Percentage of all deaths due to heart disease according to age groups*

file, including triglycerides, VLDL, and HDL, but these effects are almost certainly linked to the rate of absorption of the carbohydrates, as strategies that slow digestion and absorption (high soluble fiber, low-GI), improve these parameters. Also, slower digested carbohydrates are associated with higher satiety.

In the Nurses' Health Study,[22] total fat consumption did not affect coronary risk, but the kinds of fats did. Each 5 percent increase in calories from saturated fat (meat and dairy) increased coronary risk by 17 percent. And each 2 percent increase in *trans*-fat calories raised their risk by 93 percent. Also, those with the highest intake of the omega-3 fatty acid alpha-linolenic acid (see Chapter 9) enjoyed a 50 percent lower risk of fatal heart attacks compared to women consuming the least amount.

Epidemiological (population) studies are both clear-cut and cloudy. They show that arteriosclerotic heart disease is lowest in populations eating diets high in complex carbohydrates and low in fat and cholesterol. The Japanese are a modern, industrial, high-stress, heavy smoking society but enjoy a relatively low incidence of heart disease—

unless they emigrate to the United States and adopt American dietary habits. The typical diet in Japan is low in fat, albeit high in omega 3s (raw fish), especially in saturated animal fat. Red meat, with its high saturated-fat content, is not a traditional Japanese dish. But a major component, rice, is a high-GI grain.

The vegetarian Hunzas of India, whose diet consists of whole grains, vegetables, and fruits and is high in fiber, have very little heart disease or diabetes. The Seventh-day Adventists, also mostly vegetarians, enjoy a much lower incidence of heart disease than the average American population. The "diseases of affluence"—heart disease, large-bowel cancer, diabetes, and others—are rare in Polynesian communities until these people emigrate to New Zealand and fall victim to a Western way of life.[23] By contrast to the above, Finland suffers from the world's highest death rate from heart disease, and has the highest saturated-fat and cholesterol intakes.

Diet and disease patterns of a few special populations do seem to conflict with the above picture. The Masai tribes of Africa, cattle-raising nomads, have a high animal fat, high-cholesterol diet, living as they do on milk and cattle blood, but very little arteriosclerosis. This may in part reflect a unique genetic endowment that shuts down their own cholesterol synthesis when there is a lot of cholesterol in the food. (Ordinarily, your liver manufactures its own cholesterol, so your blood level reflects an interplay between internal synthesis and diet.) The Masai also seem to have yearly periods of low-calorie but rather high-quality food intake, a sort of stretched-out version of a CRON diet.[24] Finally, Masai cattle are grass-fed and lean, whereas U.S. cattle are fattened with grains and high-protein feed for four to five months before slaughter. Free-roaming cattle have much less total body fat than domestic cattle, and probably a different blood-fat pattern. And in free roaming cattle, up to 40 percent of the fat they do have is polyunsaturated, whereas in our U.S. domestic cattle it's only 4 percent.[25] So the fat intake pattern in the Masai may resemble that or close to what we in advanced countries are genetically programmed to consume but don't.

Eskimos, who subsist almost exclusively on fish, seal, whale, and caribou, with an average daily intake of 3,400 calories, including 377 grams of protein and a whopping 162 grams of fat, show little or no arteriosclerosis. But the fat in their diet is unlike that in the typical American diet. It is rich in polyunsaturated fatty acids derived from fish oil, especially in omega-3 acid, which protects against arteriosclerosis.[26] It was largely this odd pattern of diet in relation to disease among the Eskimos that called researchers' attention to the omega-3s. When Eskimos adopt a Western-style diet, they too become arteriosclerotic.

The correctional evidence has been good enough that many doctors for many years recommended cholesterol-lowering diets to their patients. Not every doctor agreed with this, saying that it had not been formally shown in a large, well-controlled clinical study that lowering blood cholesterol would also lower the frequency of actual heart attacks. Finally, direct experimental evidence became available. A $150 million tracking study supported by the National Heart, Lung and Blood Institute established that lowering cholesterol in blood reduces coronary risks. A total of 3,800 men between the ages of 35 and 59, with no history of hypertension or heart disease but with abnormally high blood cholesterol levels, were divided into two groups. Both were placed on a low-cholesterol diet. In addition, one group received the cholesterol-lowering drug cholestyramine for a period of seven to ten years. This drug binds to the bile acids in the intestines and enhances their excretion from the body. There is a double effect here. Bile acids are needed to emulsify ingested fat so it can be absorbed in the intestines. If they are bound by the gritty cholestyramine resin, less fat is absorbed. Also, bile acids are manufactured in the liver out of cholesterol. Normally they are reabsorbed, used over again, recycled. Bound to cholestyramine, they are eliminated.

In this study, the group receiving cholestyramine averaged an 8 percent greater reduction in cholesterol and a 12 percent greater reduction in LDL than the other group—and 24 percent fewer cardiac deaths. In those individuals who faithfully took the drug (five to six packets per day) for the entire period—with decreases of 25 percent or more in total blood cholesterol and 35 percent in LDL—the incidence of heart attacks was less by 50 percent.

Food clearly affects the levels of blood fats, particularly cholesterol,

LDL (low-density lipoproteins), and HDL (high-density lipoproteins). In the body, cholesterol is packaged in envelopes of protein for
moving through the blood and tissues. The packages are the LDL and
HDL molecules. LDL is like an oil truck. It carries 70 to 80 percent of
the cholesterol in the blood plasma, and delivers fat and cholesterol to
the cells. The cells manufacture "receptors" on their surfaces that serve
as docks for the LDL trucks to make their deliveries. When cells contain an excess of cholesterol, reflecting too much animal and dairy fat
in the diet, they manufacture fewer receptor docks, and the undeliv-
ered loads of LDL cholesterol pile up in the blood.[27] If breaks occur in
the inside lining of the vessel wall (smoking and high blood pressure
are the commonest causes of such injury), the crowded LDL oil trucks
drive through them and dump their cargo into the tissues, as industrial polluters do on the back roads of our fair land. That's the beginning of arteriosclerotic plaques. HDL trucks, on the other hand, go in
the opposite direction. They help remove cholesterol from the blood
and tissues, reducing the risk of arteriosclerosis. A ratio of total blood
cholesterol/HDL of 5 carries an average risk of heart disease; a ratio of
3.5 only half the average risk.

Some years ago the National Institutes of Health strongly recommended that you reduce your dietary fat and cholesterol, although it is
now recognized that dietary cholesterol is not a significant factor in
the level of blood cholesterol.[28, 29] Total plasma and LDL-cholesterol
levels are directly associated with consumption of saturated fat and
inversely with total calories.[30] Total cholesterol levels are also directly
associated with total fat, the specific fat oleic acid, and animal fat in
the diet, and inversely with carbohydrate intake.

Blood cholesterol levels in the U. S. population by age groups are
shown in Table 5.2. In the famous Framingham study in Massachusetts,
the risk of coronary disease was fairly low if the cholesterol was under
200 (and the lower the better). Keep yours below 180 and you very likely
will never have a heart attack. Below 150, you almost certainly will not.
Unless you have a strong genetic predisposition toward a high blood
cholesterol level, the CRON diet will bring you into that range.

Most recently, the level of blood homocysteine has been found to
be an independent risk factor for the further, rapider progression of

arteriosclerosis and heart disease.[31]* If the lining of a blood vessel wall is damaged, its cells fail to turn the homocysteine into a useful (vasodilatory) product, and auto-oxidation of the homocysteine may occur, leading to free radical damage to the lining cells.

TABLE 5.2 *Blood cholesterol levels in American men and women. Average values for the total population at each age group are shown, also the average values for the 5% of the population with the lowest and the 5% with the highest cholesterol levels (adapted from* Hospital Practice, *May 1983).*

AGE (YEARS)	MEN			WOMEN		
	AVERAGE ALL	AVERAGE LOWEST	VALUES HIGHEST	AVERAGE ALL	AVERAGE LOWEST	VALUES HIGHEST
0–4	155	114	203	156	112	200
5–9	160	121	203	164	126	205
10–14	158	119	202	160	124	201
15–19	150	113	197	157	120	200
20–24	167	124	218	164	122	216
25–29	182	133	244	171	128	222
30–34	192	138	254	175	130	231
35–39	201	146	270	184	140	242
40–44	207	151	268	194	147	252
45–49	212	158	276	203	152	265
50–54	213	158	277	218	162	285
55–59	214	156	276	231	173	300
60–64	213	159	276	231	172	297
65–69	213	158	274	233	171	303
70+	207	151	270	228	169	289

Change your blood-fat factors for the better: Lowering total dietary fat will lower blood cholesterol.[32, 33] The type of fat is also important. Most saturated fats promote arteriosclerosis and polyunsaturated fats inhibit it. Remember that even though Eskimos do eat an enormous amount of fat, their diet is high in polyunsaturated fish-oil fats; they have low LDL, high HDL, and very little heart disease. Vegetable oils such as corn oil, and seed oils such as sunflower-seed oil, are more or less polyunsaturated. About 2 grams of polyunsaturated oils is required to neutralize the cholesterol elevation caused by 1 gram of saturated fats.[34] In one study, adding polyunsaturated fats to the diet in the amount of 20 percent of total energy (a polyunsaturated to saturated fat ratio of about 1 to 1), led to a 20 to 23 percent drop in cholesterol, with the main effect being on LDL. [35]

As emphasized in the 1986 edition of this book, the fatty acids called linolenic and eicosapentaenoic acid (again the Eskimos) are especially important as they influence the metabolism of some remarkable body chemicals called prostaglandins, which in turn influence blood vessel contraction and blood clotting. The prostaglandins PGE1 (made by your body from linolenic acid) and PGE3 (from eicosapentaenoic acid) are the ones you want to have more of; and PGE2 (made from arachidonic acid), less of. Cod-liver oil and mackerel contain large amounts of eicosapentaenoic acid. In clinical trials, adding fish oil rich in eicosapentaenoic acid to the diet decreased blood viscosity, decreased blood clotting, increased bleeding time, increased HDL, and somewhat decreased LDL.[36] All these changes are to the good. One of the available products, if you decide to take eicosapentaenoic acid as a supplement, is called MaxEPA. Ten grams of MaxEPA contains about 3 grams of eicosapentaenoic acid. One to two grams of MaxEPA per day would be a conservative dose. Salmon oil is also acceptable. Neither of these contains the excessive amounts of vitamins A and D present in fish-liver oils,[37] which should be avoided (see Osteoporosis section later in this chapter). Evidence strongly supports the idea that diets high in fish may help prevent coronary heart disease.[38] The consumption of as little as one or two fish dishes per week may be of preventive value.

Other dietary components besides actual fats and oils will influence your levels of blood fats and susceptibility to arteriosclerosis. These include the kinds of protein you eat, as well as carbohydrates, sugars, minerals, trace elements, and fibers. And a small amount of aspirin, such as one baby aspirin every second day, may favorably affect the prostaglandin pattern.

Replacement of animal with vegetable protein in the diet will lower plasma cholesterol and LDL and favorably influence both the onset and the course of arteriosclerosis. This effect is not merely due to the greater fat intake associated with animal protein, since it can be seen

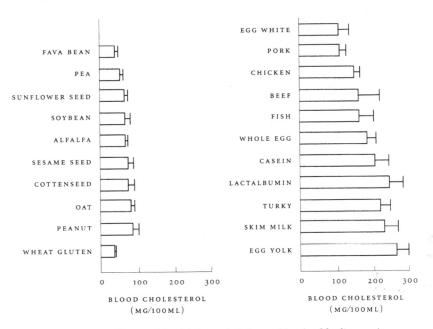

FIGURE 5.4 *Effects on blood (plasma) cholesterol levels of feeding various protein preparations to rabbits maintained on cholesterol free diets (adapted from K. K. Carroll,* Federation Proceedings 41:2792, 1982)

(in animals) with low-fat, cholesterol-free, semipurified diets in which milk and soybean proteins are compared.[39] Figure 5.4 dramatically illustrates the effects on blood cholesterol of feeding various types of protein for 28 days to rabbits maintained on cholesterol-free diets. We see that *all* plant proteins are better than *any* animal proteins, and that within the two classes, some influence the bunnies' cholesterol more than others. But don't let these data necessarily scare you totally off animal proteins. They are just one more item in the balance.

With regard to carbohydrates: refined sugars, especially sucrose (the sugar in your sugar bowl), may increase blood cholesterol. A significant part of your blood cholesterol is synthesized by your liver. Refined sugar increases this internal synthesis. It also lowers HDL in animals and humans, and animals that receive sugar as part of their carbohydrate source don't live as long as partners fed cornstarch (a complex and lower-GI carbohydrate) at the same calorie level.

Dietary changes in zinc, copper, chromium, and magnesium may influence susceptibility to arteriosclerosis. Copper deficiency increases blood cholesterol, and the average copper intake in the United States is only about 1 milligram per day, well below the RDA of 2 milligrams per day. An excess of zinc in the diet (unlikely unless the diet is oversupplemented) will further increase the cholesterol-raising effect of copper deficiency.

Chromium deficiency may play a role in both arteriosclerosis and diabetes. In rats, when the diet is low in chromium, the levels of both blood cholesterol and glucose are abnormally high. The tissues of American adults show on the average only about 2.4 micrograms of chromium per 100 grams of tissue, whereas in other North American mammals—cattle, sheep, rats, squirrels, foxes, and so on—the level averages 21 micrograms. In a study of ten adult American males and 22 females, 90 percent habitually ate less than the minimum suggested "safe and adequate" amount of chromium.[40]

Why are Americans deficient in chromium? *Raw* sugar contains 36 micrograms of chromium per 150 grams of sugar, *refined* sugar only 3 to 4 micrograms. On the average we consume 200 grams of refined sugar a day, including the large amount in many processed foods. Whole wheat contains 175 micrograms of chromium per 100 grams, refined white flour only about 22. The high intake of refined sugar and white flour in today's average American diet simply does not supply enough chromium. This causes the body to use its own stores in order to help insulin handle the rise in blood sugar that follows a sugar rich meal. Part of this mobilized chromium is then excreted through the kidneys, and the deficiency increases. A good way to stimulate chromium deficiency is to drink tea and coffee all day long with plenty of refined sugar and eat toast with jam on it, processed breakfast food with sugar, white bread, and sugary desserts. And taking chromium in pill form may not help: less than 1 percent is absorbed unless you take it as Glucose Tolerance Factor pills. Shellfish and chicken as well as some forms of brewer's yeast are good sources of usable chromium.

Long term inadequacy of magnesium in the diet will contribute substantially to heart disease.[41] Those parts of the United States where the drinking water is low in dissolved minerals experience a higher death rate from heart disease than where the ground water is hard. The responsible element seems to be magnesium. Magnesium balances the effects of calcium on the heart. Calcium keeps the heart in a highly electrically stimulated state, and increases the heart rate; magnesium relaxes and slows the heart. Patients with coronary heart disease tend to have lower blood magnesium levels than well persons.

Magnesium intakes in the United States have been declining since 1900 in the face of sharp rises in nutrients that increase the need for it, such as vitamin D (in fortified milk) and phosphorus (high in soft drinks). Alcohol decreases magnesium absorption and increases magnesium excretion. A factor in the long average life spans of the Hunzas may be their drinking of "glacial milk," essentially an aqueous extract of rocks. The moving glacier grinds up rocks in its bed and percolates its melting waters through the mineral-rich mush.

Studies of fiber intake in relation to fat metabolism have given interesting but variable results. In part this is due to there being many different kinds of "fiber."[42] Just as vitamins were treated as a single entity when first discovered, so with fiber. Strictly speaking, dietary fiber refers only to the cell-wall material of plants, including nondigestible cellulose and such noncellulose sugars as the galactomanins. Pectin, gum tragacanth, gum arabic, guar gum (a galactomanin extracted from the Japanese konjac root, a member of the yam family), locust bean gum, and carrageenin are chemically similar to components of the plant cell wall, and pectin is an actual component of the cell wall (although it is water-soluble and gelatinous); but some of these materials are produced by secretory cells. In truth the gums are not fibrous at all. A statistical meta-analysis of 67 trials of fiber indicated that 2 to 10 grams of soluble fiber daily lowered total cholesterol and LDLs by small but significant amounts.[43]

Most brans and other particulate fibers in cereal grains (the fibers in All-Bran, for example—which, however, contains 19 percent sugar[44]) are high in nondigestible cellulose. They increase fecal bulk and fluidity, but they have no effect at all on blood cholesterol.

The other kinds of fibers, the gel-forming pectins and gums, lower LDL and blood cholesterol[45] by interfering with fat absorption from the intestines, slowing the rate of sugar absorption, and binding with and increasing the secretion of bile acids. Table 5.3 compares how wheat bran, guar gum, and the cholestyramine used in the National Heart, Blood, and Lung Institute study bind bile acids, cholesterol, and fat. In general, vegetable but not cereal fibers exert an antiblood fat effect. Guar gum and other vegetable gums are often used in low-fat salad dressings. They impart an oily feel but are not oils.

TABLE 5.3 *Percentage of binding of bile acids, cholesterol, and fat by dietary "fibers" and by the drug cholestyramine (adapted from K. K. Carroll,* Federation Proceedings *41:2792, 1982)*

DIETARY SUBSTANCE (40 MG.)	BILE ACIDS	% BINDING OF CHOLESTEROL	FAT
Wheat bran	4	0	11
Alfalfa meal	7	1	19
Guar gum	36	23	23
Cholestyramine	82	95	92

The average-sized person should be (but usually isn't) consuming at least 40 grams of total fiber per day, including cereal, pectin, and gums. Few people do, and 60 grams is even better. High fiber combined with low-fat diets very favorably affect the blood lipid picture, with an average 32 percent lowering of blood cholesterol in long-term usage. Table 5.4 gives fiber contents of different foods in normal size portions. These values are only approximations as different sources vary widely, depending on just what has been included under the designation fiber.

Avoid arteriosclerosis: Obesity in and of itself is a major risk factor for arteriosclerosis. In a long-term follow up of Framingham participants, the degree of obesity on initial examination predicted the 26-year frequency of heart attacks in men regardless of age, cholesterol, blood pressure, or other risk factors.[46] Weight gain after the young-adult years brought a considerably increased risk of heart disease, with change from a slim youth to an obese adult being especially bad. By contrast, change from an obese youth to a thin adult greatly lowered susceptibility.

The amount and type of fat in your diet is the single most important risk factor. Much over 20 percent of calories from fat or oil, but depending on the degree of saturation, probably promotes arteriosclerosis. Much under 8 percent may interfere with the absorption of fat-soluble vitamins, including anticancer vitamins like vitamins A and E, the carotenes, and other beneficial phytochemicals derived from plants.

TABLE 5.4 *Fiber content of some common foods*
expressed as grams of fiber per 100 grams (3 ½ oz.) of food, and
as amount of fiber in one average, uncooked portion

FOOD	GM. FIBER PER 100 GM.	UNCOOKED PORTION	GM. FIBER PER PORTION
FRUITS			
Apple	3	1 medium	4
Apricot	2	3 medium	2
Banana	2	1 medium	4
Blackberries	7	½ cup	5
Cherries	2	10	1
Orange	2	1 medium	3
Peach	2	1 medium	3
Pear	2	1 medium	4
Pineapple	1	½ cup	1
Plums	2	3 medium	2
Prunes, dry	14	3–4	5
Raisins	7	¼ cup	3
Strawberries	2	½ cup	2
VEGETABLES			
Asparagus	3	4 spears	2
Beets	3	½ cup	2
Broccoli	3	½ cup	4
Brussels sprouts	3	4	2
Cabbage	2	½ cup	4
Carrots	4	1 medium	2
Cauliflower	2	½ cup	1
Celery	2	1 stalk	1
Corn	5	½ cup	3
Cucumber	1	½ cup	1
Onions	1	¼ cup	½
Potatoes, white	2	1 medium	3
Potatoes, sweet	4	1 medium	4

TABLE 5.4 *(Continued) Fiber content of some common foods expressed as grams of fiber per 100 grams (3 ½ oz.) of food, and as amount of fiber in one average, uncooked portion*

FOOD	GM. FIBER PER 100 GM.	UNCOOKED PORTION	GM. FIBER PER PORTION
Spinach	4	½ cup	2
Tomato	1	1 medium	2
Zucchini	3	½ cup	2
LEGUMES			
Black beans	6	½ cup	6
Kidney beans	5	½ cup	5
Lentils	4	½ cup	4
Lima beans	5	½ cup	4
Pinto beans	5	½ cup	5
Peas, fresh	3	½ cup	3
Peas, split	4	½ cup	4
White beans	5	½ cup	6
Soybeans	6	½ cup	5
CEREALS & GRAINS			
Bread, white	3	1 slice	1
Bread, whole wheat	12	1 slice	3
Barley	2	½ cup	2
Bran, wheat	53	1 tbsp.	2
Bran, oat	26	1 tbsp.	1
Oats	11	¼ cup	3
Rice, brown	6	¼ cup	3
NUTS & SEEDS			
Almonds	14	¼ cup	5
Peanuts	6	¼ cup	3
Sunflower seeds	14	¼ cup	5
Walnuts	5	¼ cup	2

Around 80 percent of the fats or oils in your diet should be monounsaturated (olive oil, canola oil, avocado), 10 percent or more polyunsaturated (the omega-3s fall in this group), and the rest can be saturated. If you are an average American, you should increase the ratio of fish to red meat in your diet, increase vegetable protein in relation to animal protein, increase the ratio of low-GI to high-GI carbohydrates, cut back sharply on refined sugars (especially sucrose), make sure your copper and chromium intake are not greatly below the RDA levels, raise your magnesium intake over the current average amounts, and let the ratio of your calcium/magnesium intake be 1 to 1 (instead of the 2 to 1 found in many mineral supplements currently on the market). Increase your intake of gel-forming fibers. All of these measures are included in the CRON diet formulation. Additional measures, including vitamin and mineral supplementation and the right quality and quantity of exercise, will be described in later sections of this book. If you follow these combined protocols, you will be far less likely than the average person to be among that 50 percent of the population who end their lives with the stabbing pain of a cardiac death.

"THE BIG C"

Operated on for lung cancer and initially doing well, John Wayne thought he was cured. "I licked the Big C," he boasted. But he hadn't—not even the Duke. Neither did Babe Ruth, Humphrey Bogart, Yul Brynner, Julian Beck, and a long string of tough and not so tough other guys. After arteriosclerosis of the heart and brain, cancer is public enemy number one. And as we've seen, 80 to 90 percent of cancers are due to environmental factors, of which diet is the most important.

Overwhelming evidence shows that diet plays a role in cancer. Studies comparing worldwide cancer frequencies between cultures with different dietary patterns, of changes in frequency of different types of cancer as people migrate from one culture to another and adopt new eating habits, of cancer frequencies in particular populations within one culture that have different eating habits from the rest of the population, and of experimental animals—all these point to diet as a leading cancer culprit. Figure 5.5 shows the distribution of the different types of cancer and (in parentheses) the breakdown of deaths from cancer. Because some cancers can now be cured, there is a difference in distribution between percentage of occurrence and percentage of deaths. Lung cancer constitutes 22 percent of all cancers that occur, but since it is rarely curable, it makes up 35 percent of all fatal cancers. The greatest single killer-cancer, it causes upwards of

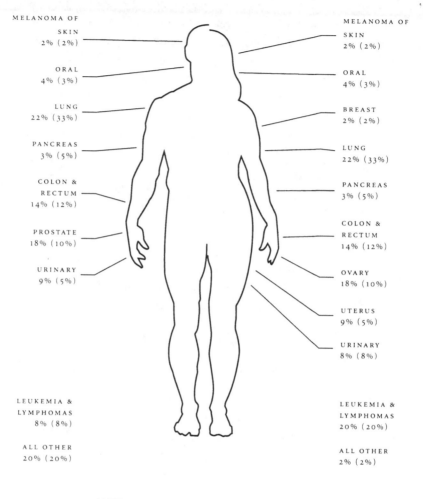

MELANOMA OF
SKIN
2% (2%)

ORAL
4% (3%)

LUNG
22% (33%)

PANCREAS
3% (5%)

COLON &
RECTUM
14% (12%)

PROSTATE
18% (10%)

URINARY
9% (5%)

LEUKEMIA &
LYMPHOMAS
8% (8%)

ALL OTHER
20% (20%)

MELANOMA OF
SKIN
2% (2%)

ORAL
4% (3%)

BREAST
2% (2%)

LUNG
22% (33%)

PANCREAS
3% (5%)

COLON &
RECTUM
14% (12%)

OVARY
18% (10%)

UTERUS
9% (5%)

URINARY
8% (8%)

LEUKEMIA &
LYMPHOMAS
20% (20%)

ALL OTHER
2% (2%)

MEN   WOMEN

FIGURE 5.5 *Distribution of all cancers occurring, cured or not, and (in parentheses) distribution of cancers among persons who die of cancer. The number in parentheses is greater for those cancers that cannot now be very effectively treated. All percentages, both inside and outside the parentheses, can be substantially reduced by the CRON diet.*

120,000 deaths per year in the United States. By contrast, cancer of the prostate constitutes 18 percent of cancers that occur, but only 10 percent of fatal cancers. It can often be cured.

The cancers in which diet plays a significant role are those of the colon, breast, and stomach for sure, probably those of the uterus and prostate, and maybe oral cancer. Frequencies of breast and prostate cancer in relation to total fat intake for different world populations are shown in Figure 5.6. Total fat is a better predictor of cancer than specific types of fat, animal or vegetable, saturated or polyunsaturated. It should be stated, however, that recent and very good studies have failed to confirm any relation between intake of fat, whether it be total fat or types of fat, and risk of breast cancer in women.[47] And if you look at the values for Italy (fats largely MUFA), compared to Finland (high saturated fat intake), you will perceive that high MUFA, while okay in relation to heart disease and diabetes, seems no better than saturated fat for cancer. Greece does better (high omega-3s), but no better than Mexico. In fact no clear-cut pattern emerges beyond the relationship to total fat intake.

When people migrate from one country to another, they or their descendants acquire the cancer pattern of their new country. Japan has one of the highest rates of stomach cancer in the world, five times the U.S. rate. This may be due to nitrates in the Japanese diet or drinking water, low consumption of fruits and vegetables, and excessive consumption of salt-cured fish. Emigrants from Japan to Hawaii continue to be at high risk for stomach cancer, but their children, those who adopt Western dietary habits, are not. In contrast to stomach cancer, cancers of the colon, breast, and pancreas are low in frequency in native Japanese, but high in their descendants in the United States. The genetic background is the same, but the cancer pattern changes as the diet changes.

Many types of cancer require an "initiating event" that involves alteration of DNA, the genetic material inside each cell. Initiation is irreversible, but by itself does not lead to cancer. It must be followed by "promotion," which is reversible and seems to act either by stimulating inappropriate cell division or by stimulating cells to manufacture large amounts of the injurious chemicals known as free radicals.[48] High-fat diets exert a strong promotional effect.

BREAST CANCER

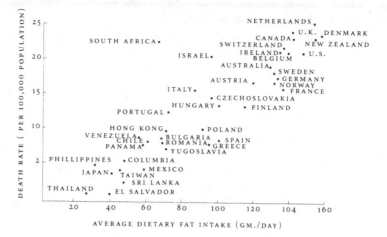

PROSTATIC CANCER

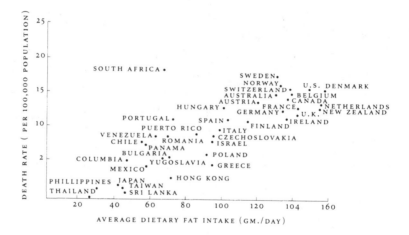

FIGURE 5.6 *Relationship of death rates for female breast cancer and for male prostatic cancer to consumption of fat by different populations (adapted from B. S. Reddy,* Advances in Cancer Research *32:237, 1980)*

Not long ago a high fiber intake was thought to inhibit the development of colon cancer. Since bile salts are, under the right circumstances, tumor "promoters," a protective effect of fiber against colon cancer was theorized to depend on its capacity to bind bile acids in the intestinal tract. The daily fiber intake in Third World countries, where colon cancer is much less frequent than in the West, is over 60 grams per day, largely derived from the insoluble cell-wall fibers of starchy foods, compared with only about 20 grams per day in the West, largely from fruits and vegetables (pectins and gums). A special importance for fiber intake in preventing colon cancer, derived from these findings in Africa, was reinforced by the observation that in Finland, where the food intake is high in both fat and fiber, the frequency of colon cancer is in fact low. The benefit from fiber, at least for colon cancer, seemed to cancel out the ill effects of fat.

Despite the above, fiber is no longer thought to be protective against colon cancer,[49] according to a study analyzing about 90,000 women for 16 years. Those who ate 25 or more grams of fiber per day were just as likely to develop colon cancer as those eating less than 10 grams. (This is no reason to swear off fiber, because evidence that it fends off heart disease remains strong, and it may have other benefits like preventing diverticulitis, constipation, etc.)

Vitamin C intake may influence cancer susceptibility. The National Research Council now specifically recommends eating plenty of vitamin C containing materials—in fact amounting to more, although no precise amount is stipulated, than the RDA of 60 milligrams per day. Extra quantities of the element selenium and of some of the carotenes may also offer protective action against cancer, and will be discussed later. A 19-year study suggested that colon cancer is increased in persons with a diet too low in calcium and vitamin D. [50]

The association of a diet high in intake of vegetables and fruits with decreased cancer incidence was first reported in 1985.[51] Large amounts in the diet of Brussels sprouts, cabbage, turnips, broccoli, and cauliflower, all vegetables of the Brassicaceae family, may decrease the incidence of colon and rectal cancer. All these vegetables, when they are fresh, contain chemicals called *indols* that may raise intestinal levels of enzymes (the mono-oxygenase enzymes) that inactivate some of the cancer-causing agents.[52]* Women who eat two to three servings of fruits and vegetables per day have been reported to have less than half the risk of mouth and throat cancer of those consuming less than one and one-half servings. There is a twofold decrease in the risk of developing lung cancer associated with a high fruit and vegetable diet (although not very impressive compared to the twentyfold drop in risk associated with quitting smoking). The role of dietary phyto-chemicals in combating cancer will be discussed in Chapter 9.

Avoid cancer: The low calorie intake of the CRON diet yields far more protection than anything else. Beyond that, the lowered fat intake, particularly saturated fats, recommended for arteriosclerosis holds also for cancer prevention. Increased amounts of vitamin C, selenium, certain carotenes, and vegetables like cabbage and broccoli plus other vegetables and fruits are indicated, and at least RDA amounts of calcium and vitamin D.

HYPERTENSION AND STROKE

On April 12, 1945, as World War II was drawing to a close, 63-year-old President Franklin D. Roosevelt was sitting quietly for his portrait during a much-needed rest at Warm Springs, Georgia. Suddenly he said, "I have a terrible headache," and fell forward, unconscious. He had had high blood pressure for a long time, and now had sustained a massive brain hemorrhage, a stroke. He died a few hours later.

Blood pressure is usually given in two numbers, such as 140/90. The upper number, called the systolic pressure, is the pressure the blood exerts on the walls of the arteries during the heart beat. The lower one, the diastolic pressure, is the pressure remaining in the arteries between heart beats. In adults a blood pressure exceeding 140/90 is abnormal, the lowest rung of hypertension. At any level of increased blood pressure, the younger the person, the greater the decrease in his life expectancy. By 65 to 74 years of age three-fourths of U.S. adults have either definite or borderline hypertension.

Intelligence itself may be influenced by hypertension. At the Duke University Center for the Study of Aging, individuals in their sixties were divided into three groups: normal, borderline, and frank hyper-tensives—and their intelligence levels were tested regularly for ten years. Those with normal blood pressure suffered no decline, but con-siderable decline occurred in those with frank hypertension.

Most authorities believe that excessive salt (sodium chloride) plays a major role in causing hypertension. While not perfect, the evidence is good enough that the American Medical Association, the American Heart Association, the National Academy of Sciences, the Food and Drug Administration, and the U.S. Department of Agriculture have all recommended a decrease in salt intake for the U.S. population.

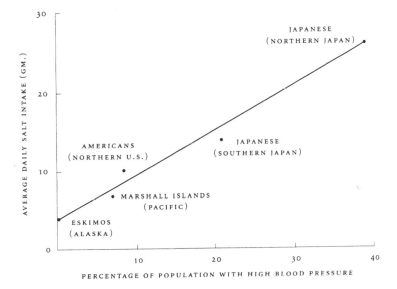

FIGURE 5.7 *Salt intake and the frequency of high blood pressure in different populations*

Salt has an ancient history in its interactions with human culture. The connotations of the word in English include worthiness ("to be worth one's salt") and excellence ("salt of the earth"). The word *salary* comes from a salt allowance *salarius*, given to Roman soldiers. Jews seal covenants by exchanging salt. Desert Arabs will not attack a man whose salt they have eaten. Bread and salt are gifts in Slavic countries. Kings in countries such as Babylon, Egypt, China, Mexico, and Peru ruled by salt monopoly. One of Mahatma Gandhi's most dramatic maneuvers was against the British salt tax. He walked 200 miles to the seashore, evaporated a pan of water, ate the residue of salt, and paid no tax to the British.

Despite its romantic history, an excess of salt is unhealthy, and the average American consumes 12 or more grams a day when less than 1 gram is all he or she needs. Surveys of many cultures, from Greenland Eskimos to nomads of southern Iran to South Sea Islanders, indicate that hypertension is virtually absent in populations that use only small amounts of salt. Figure 5.7 shows the relation between average daily salt intake and the percentage of hypertensives in five different populations.

Why do we crave so much salt? Primitive man didn't get enough in his diet and experienced a chronic salt hunger. He would fill up on it when it was available. Perhaps we have the same hunger even though salt is now abundant.[53] That's one possible reason. But a large part of our salt hunger today is no doubt culturally induced. The exposure of infants to saltiness, which is of quite recent origin, induces a taste for salt later in life. Breast milk contains much less salt than cow's milk, and before 1900 nearly all infants were breast-fed. Also, babies are now started earlier on solid foods, and are more likely to be fed high-salt commercial foods than low-salt dishes cooked at home.

Probably the sodium rather than the chloride in salt is related to hypertension, although opinions differ. As a result of widespread use of processed and prepared foods, often high in sodium chloride, Americans commonly consume 5 to 20 times as much sodium as they need. One hundred grams of fresh peas contains only 2 milligrams of sodium; canned peas, about 590 milligrams. A bowl of Campbell's Chicken Noodle Soup contains 1,140 milligrams of sodium; 3 ounces of Chicken of the Sea tuna packed in water, 400 milligrams sodium; a Big Mac, 1,510 milligrams; one serving of Minute Rice's Long Grain & Wild Rice, 570 milligrams (1 milligrams is naturally there, 569 milligrams are added); 1 ounce of Kellogg's Corn Flakes, 260 milligrams sodium . . . and so on and on and on.

Some processed-food companies are now putting out two versions of their products, one with the old amount of salt and a low-salt equivalent. Campbell's Chunky Vegetable Beef Soup in the "regular" variety has 935 milligrams of sodium; in the "low-salt" variety, 90 milligrams. Its low-salt Chicken Noodle Soup has only 130 milligrams of sodium, in contrast to the 1,140 milligrams given in the above list. Unfortunately, in the low-salt products the companies have substantially increased the fat content. A can of Campbell's regular French Onion Soup contains 2.6 grams of fat; its low-sodium equivalent contains 5 grams.[54]

Evidence of a relationship between salt and hypertension is less convincing if one compares data *within* populations rather than *between* them. In the United States, for example, some people eat a great deal of salt and others not so much, but the amount does not seem to correlate very well with who actually develops hypertension. The probable explanation has been termed the *saturation effect*, which postulates that about 20 to 50 percent of us have a tendency to develop high blood pressure in response to increased salt intake. The other percent will not develop it regardless of intake. Under these conditions, if nearly everyone in the population consumes excess salt, no relation will be found between salt intake and hypertension because nearly everyone is far above the threshold.

Nevertheless, a reduced salt intake can lower blood pressure in more than 50 percent of humans who are already hypertensive. In fact, a low-sodium diet can lower blood pressure even among people with normal blood pressure,[55] and increasing the salt intake in middle-aged men has been shown to raise blood pressure regardless of hereditary background.[56] In the 1940s and early 1950s doctors tried using drastic reduction of sodium intake to treat hypertension, and this frequently worked, but few patients would tolerate the monotonous diets. The patient had to be talked into it—and scared enough to stick to it—not an easy prospect. However, I recall that when I was an intern in Gorgas Hospital, in the Canal Zone, I cured a young woman who experienced a sudden onset of severe hypertension, with hemorrhages into the eyes, by placing her on what was then called the *rice diet*, which consisted basically of nothing but rice. She recovered completely in two weeks.

But salt is not the only factor, and the nationwide preoccupation with excessive salt has clouded the role of other factors in hypertension. Switching to a vegetarian diet may lower blood pressure. Weight reduction often brings significant decreases in blood pressure. Weight change from thin youth to obese adult gives a high incidence of hypertension, and from obese youth to thin adult a low incidence. Reduction of fat intake can lower high blood pressure,[57] and may even lower blood pressure in normal persons.[58] Finnish scientists[59] divided 114 subjects with normal or high blood pressure into three groups. Group one ate a low-fat diet for six weeks; group two, a low-salt diet. Group three served as controls. Only group one experienced a decline in blood pressure.

TABLE 5.5 *Sodium and potassium contents in representative fresh, frozen, and canned foods*

FOOD	PROCESS	PORTION	SODIUM (MG.)	POTASSIUM (MG.)
Corn	fresh	1 ear	1	364
	frozen	3.5 oz.	4	188
	canned	½ cup	239	144
Peas	fresh	½ cup	1	157
	frozen	3.5 oz.	88	126
	canned	½ cup	246	79
Potato	fresh	1 medium	5	587
	canned	½ cup	376	304
	instant	½ cup	280	287

Potassium, magnesium, and calcium deficiencies may play roles. Potassium is particularly important because the balance between potassium and sodium in the diet is intertwined and delicate.[60] Thanks to more abundant supplies of fruits and vegetables, people of Southern Europe have twice the potassium intake of those in the North—and less hypertension. Diets of modern-day primitive societies with low incidence of hypertension are not only low in sodium, they are high in potassium. Their intake averages 4 to 7 grams as potassium chloride, so the ratio of potassium to sodium is two to one or greater, whereas in a typical American diet with its high proportion of commercially prepared and processed foods the ratio is one to two, the exact reverse.

Commercial freezing and canning processes often increase the sodium to potassium ratio, as illustrated in Table 5.5. Frozen peas are not necessarily right out of the pod. Sometimes they are presorted by the use of sodium chloride solutions at different concentrations. Some vegetables are skinned in sodium hydroxide solutions before being frozen.

Calcium deficiency may also be important in hypertension. Low calcium intake has been associated with hypertension in epidemiological studies, and may be linked with the salt-sensitive form(s) of hypertension.[61] Calcium supplementation of 1 gram per day for 22 weeks has been shown to lead to a decline in blood pressure, even in healthy young persons without hypertension.[62]

Avoid hypertension: Reduce your sodium intake (from all sources, not just salt, and not just salt from the salt shaker but also from processed foods) to less than 2 grams per day (0.3 to 0.5 grams is all you really need). Lemon juice can replace the taste of salt in some foods: add a tablespoon to salt-free tomato juice and try it. Salt reduction will automatically also change your potassium to sodium ratio to a more appropriate level. If you are of normal size, consume 1 gram of magnesium and 1 gram of calcium per day, using supplements if necessary. Most important, lose weight. Adopt the CRON diet. It has a remarkable effect on blood pressure. (See Table 2.3.)

ARETAEUS OF CAPPADOCIA NAMED IT *DIABETES*

Diabetes is Greek for *siphon*, coming from a word that means *to pass through*, and indeed Aretaeus of Cappadocia described it as "a strange disease that consists in the flesh and bones running together into the urine." Severe untreated diabetes fits this imaginative description well: a copious flow of urine along with great thirst and resulting in the wasting away of both muscle and fat to produce severe emaciation, ending in coma and death. The untreated patient literally starves to death because his body is unable to derive energy from glucose, either because his ability to make insulin is faulty (type 1, or "juvenile," diabetes, accounting for about 10 percent of cases) or because the insulin receptors on the organs of his body are greatly diminished (type 2, or late-onset, or insulin resistant, diabetes, which occurs in older persons). In late-onset diabetes, the intake of carbohydrates causes the blood glucose to rise, and insulin is released by the pancreas to help the tissues utilize the glucose; however, the deficit in tissue receptors for insulin prevents a normal rate of utilization. Blood glucose and insulin both remain abnormally high. Glucose piles up in the blood and spills into the urine. (A clever medieval diagnostic trick was to see if the patient's urine was attractive to ants. Ants like the sweetness of diabetic urine.)

The type 2, late-onset diabetes afflicts 5 percent of the U.S. population, including 5 million diagnosed and an estimated 2 ½ million undiagnosed cases. The likelihood of developing diabetes doubles with each decade of life, going from 0.1 percent for people under 20 years old to about 15 percent for those over 60. The likelihood also doubles with every 20 percent gain in body weight above average. Even among the nonobese, it is much commoner in those who are now of average weight but were previously very lean. One person in 14 in the U.S. either has diabetes or will develop it.

Diabetes is the third leading cause of sickness and death in the United States if one includes its many complications: arteriosclerosis, cataracts, and nerve and kidney damage. Diabetics have five times the normal risk for a major heart attack. Diabetes is the leading cause of blindness in the developed nations of the world. Of the people with advanced kidney disease, 40 percent have diabetes.

Broadly speaking, diabetes is attributable to a failure of the body to appropriately metabolize glucose.[63] The clinical picture, the *phenotype*, is a sort of end-phenomenon. The underlying cause can be any of many genetic mutations. Disruption can occur anywhere in the long pathway from the synthesis and release of insulin to the complete oxidation of glucose by the target cells. There are many steps, involving many enzymes, and alterations in the code for any of these will cause diabetes. Altogether, the various disorders that yield the phenotype of diabetes constitute the largest group of genetic disorders found in humans. Both nuclear and mitochondrial mutations may yield the phenotype. Indeed the number of mutations that may lead to the phenotype exceeds 200. For their part, environmental factors— for example obesity—have a strong influence on the development of the phenotype, which is diabetes.

Diabetes is of special interest to us because it shows many, albeit not all, of the features of accelerated aging. In this sense it is unlike the diseases we've previously talked about, which occur more often in older people but are not necessarily associated with biomarker changes denoting accelerated aging. Diabetics are functionally older than their chronologic age. A decline in immune function is seen in them earlier. Changes in their connective-tissue proteins (collagen) are characteristic of older persons. They lose gamma crystallin from their eye-lens proteins at an accelerated rate. And the number of times their connective-tissue cells will divide is considerably curtailed, just as in aging.[64]

Diabetics usually display high blood cholesterol, a decrease in the beneficial arteriosclerosis-preventing HDL factors, and greater susceptibility to arteriosclerosis. Cataracts occur earlier than normal, as do heart disease, kidney damage, and nerve disorders. Many of these adverse effects are due to the fact that the diabetic's elevated blood sugar is itself damaging to cells. High concentrations are especially detrimental to those proteins that are slow to be replaced (low-turnover proteins): those in the lens of the eye, the lining of blood vessels, and the insulating material around nerve cells. Exposed to glucose over a long period, proteins develop so-called "cross links," or *Advanced Glycation End Products*, and an insoluble brown pigment is formed.[65] However, this is not the whole story about the toxicity of glucose. Hyperglycemia also increases the levels of enzyme systems that cause damage to small– and large-caliber blood vessels and peripheral nerves.[66]*

The CRON diet will retard these age-related defects in normally aging persons. In one experiment in humans, when mildly overweight men and women lost an average of 24 pounds, the researchers observed an improvement in glucose metabolism and an impressive decrease in the insulin levels following a glucose meal. And CRON-diet treated, 12-month-old rats give glucose and insulin responses similar to those of untreated two-month-old rats.[67]

Long-term animal studies show that high-GI foods increase fasting insulin levels and promote insulin resistance, more rapid weight gain, higher body fat levels, and increased triglycerides.[68] Low-GI meals improve glucose and insulin metabolism and lead to lower glycosylated proteins, one form of Advanced Glycation End Product. (High MUFA in diabetes does not affect these glycosylated proteins.)

Supplementing the diet with gel-forming fibers such as guar gum or pectin may favorably affect glucose metabolism and insulin requirements.[69] But the fiber must be either a part of or intimately mixed with the food. Guar gum taken two minutes before the meal has no effect; it must be incorporated into the meal, as in bread or cookies. The way a rich supply of fiber, if actually a part of the meal, affects the glucose curve is illustrated in Figure 5.8.

Responsible for the biological activity of the so-called glucose tolerance factor, or GTF, the trace element chromium may play a role in late-onset diabetes. Glucose metabolism can be improved in the elderly not only by fiber but by addition of a small quantity of organic chromium, or brewer's yeast, which contains GTF, to the diet, or even inorganic chromium.[70] In one study, adding supplemental chromium to the diet of diabetics caused a drop in blood glucose levels and a significant rise in the anti-arteriosclerosis HDL factors in the blood.

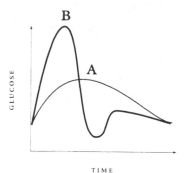

FIGURE 5.8 *A rich supply of fiber in the meal will allow a smooth glucose curve as in A. With a low-fiber, high-starch meal, a large peak and over-correction occurs as in B.*

Avoid diabetes: Don't let yourself be or become above average weight. If you were lean when younger, stay lean when older; don't let your weight increase to average as you grow older because for you—if you were previously lean—that would be relative obesity. While late-life diabetes is partially hereditary, remember that weight gain will complete the equation and bring on the disease. Keep physically fit (see Chapter 8) and include enough of the proper kinds of fibers in your diet as well as at least RDA amounts of usable chromium. If you are genetically susceptible to developing this debilitating, troublesome, ultimately killer disease, you should certainly adopt the CRON diet. It prevents the development of diabetes in genetically highly at-risk mice, and may well do the same for you. Studies of long-term regimes of moderate calorie reduction in humans suggest that a CRON diet should improve the insulin response and control of blood sugar not only in diabetics but in the normal elderly.[71]

OSTEOPOROSIS

No one knows just why George Bernard Shaw climbed a few feet up a tree when he was 93 years old; but he did, and falling from the tree, he broke his hip and subsequently died. It was known as far back as Pliny the Younger, in ancient Rome, that older people tend to break their bones rather easily. In writing about his old adviser, Verginius Rufus, Pliny tells us in his letters, "He was rehearsing the delivery of his address of thanks to the Emperor for his election to his third consulship, when he had occasion to take up a heavy book, the weight of which made it fall out of his hands, as he was an old man. He bent down to pick it up, and lost his footing on the slippery polished floor, so that he fell and fractured his thigh."

People think of bones as inert structures, like wooden beams, but bone is a living tissue constantly being remodeled. After age 35, on the average a little more bone is lost each year than is gained during this remodeling. Between 40 and 50, men characteristically lose 0.5 to 0.75 percent of bone mass yearly, while women lose it at more than twice that rate. Bones that once were sturdy may become lighter, more fragile, their interiors resembling lacy honeycombs. The rate of natural loss increases substantially after age 50. If it's severe enough, the thinned-out bones become porous, and you develop *osteoporosis* — which literally means *bone porosity*.

Twenty-five to 30 percent of white women and 15 to 20 percent of men over 50 have osteoporosis severely enough to involve some compression of the vertebrae of the spinal column. Women's bone loss accelerates at menopause. Fractured vertebrae from osteoporosis produce the stoop unkindly called *dowager's hump*.

Osteoporosis is one of the major problems of old age. It afflicts 20 million Americans; leads to 190,000 hip fractures yearly; 100,000 broken wrists; 180,000 "crush fractures" in which vertebrae collapse. It kills 300,000 citizens annually, and costs the nation $3.8 billion a year in medical bills. Osteoporosis is more widespread than arthritis and about three times as common as diabetes. If you have osteoporosis, small incidents like slipping on a rug, lifting a bag of groceries, even a friendly hug can break a bone.

The causes of osteoporosis are complex. Absorption of calcium from the gut is regulated by a biologically active form of vitamin D. With age, a deficiency develops in the body's ability to convert regular vitamin D to this active form. Decreased absorption of calcium results, leading to lowered blood calcium. This small drop in blood calcium triggers an increased release of a hormone from the parathyroid glands located on each side of the neck. This parathyroid hormone, or PTH, raises the blood calcium by drawing calcium from the bones, because the blood calcium has to be kept normal for the rest of the body's machinery to function. Excess PTH is then removed by the kidneys. One reason for osteoporosis in late life is that the blood level of PTH may increase secondary to the decline in kidney function that occurs with age. Also, with menopause in women, the amount of estrogen in the blood decreases, and estrogen makes bone less sensitive to dissolution by PTH. Still another hormone, called *calcitonin*, secreted by the thyroid gland, serves to inhibit bone resorption; its level is normally greater in men than in women, but decreases in both with age. All these factors contribute to a developing porosity of bones.

A diet too low in calcium also contributes. Calcium requirements increase with age, whereas calcium absorption in the intestines decreases. In most premenopausal women and in men, at least 800 milligrams of calcium per day is required to maintain body calcium, and 30 to 40 percent of men require up to 1,200 milligrams.[72] Except for those on estrogen therapy, postmenopausal women need 1,200 to 1,500 milligrams daily—about the amount contained in 1 ⅓ quarts of milk. More than 50 percent of American women typically consume less than 500 milligrams of calcium daily, and 25 percent ingest less than 300 milligrams

Protein intake affects the daily calcium requirement. An increased intake speeds calcium excretion. The intake of sulfur-containing amino acids may be the determining factor here. These are much higher in meat than in vegetable proteins. Thus the high-meat diet in

Western societies may be a factor in accelerating bone loss.

According to some authorities, the ratio of calcium to phosphorus in the diet should be greater than one to one to help prevent bone loss. It is often much lower, because most soft drinks contain large amounts of phosphates.

Ideally, you should have a bone-mass assessment when you are in your thirties. Heavy-boned persons are much less liable to develop osteoporosis. They still lose calcium with age, but they start with more. Weight-bearing exercise stimulates the development of heavier bones. Tennis players aged 55 to 65 have much more bone mass than the average person. And more bone in the racquet arm than in the other! At age 55, long-distance runners display a much greater bone density than semisedentary people of the same age, and osteoporosis is almost unknown in societies in which continued high levels of physical activity are customary.[73] The denser your bones are before you reach 35 the less susceptible you'll be later on. In fact, increasing your bone mass before age 35 is one of the most important preventive measure against osteoporosis.

Avoid osteoporosis: The causes of this terrible malady are even more complex than I have outlined here. They involve interactions between calcium, phosphorus, fluoride, vitamin D, estrogens, calcitonin, parathyroid hormone, and the proteins of the bone matrix itself. Until the many complexities are better understood, these are my recommendations: Ensure an adequate calcium intake, in the diet itself if possible (milk, yogurt) or at least by supplemental calcium. Calcium supplements may exert a partial suppressive effect on bone remodeling, whereas the calcium in milk does not, so milk is preferred.[74] Engage in a reasonable amount of weight-bearing exercise (swimming, while an excellent aerobic sport, does not qualify on this score); pay attention to your vitamin D intake; and avoid excessive phosphates in your diet. Recent studies indicate that gamma-linolenic acid (GLA) and eicosapentaenoic acid (EPA) enhance calcium absorption, reduce excretion, and increase calcium deposition into bone.[75] I will survey the general effects of these fatty acids in Chapter 9.

What is the effect, if any, of the CRON diet in relation to osteoporosis? We know that ordinary semistarvation leads to accentuated bone loss, but CRON as you recall implies *optimal nutrition*. The reduced calories are selective, every essential nutrient, macro- or micro-, is adequately represented. In well-controlled rodent studies a CRON diet was shown to substantially slow down and even prevent the age-related loss of bone.[76] In still-growing monkeys food restriction slowed overall growth, including skeletal growth, but the skeleton was otherwise normal.[77]

ALZHEIMER'S AND PARKINSON'S DISEASE

Aging greatly increases susceptibility of the neurons in certain regions of the brain (the hippocampus) to the degeneration induced by the neurotoxic agent TMT. CRON reduces the susceptibility to TMT.[78] Adult rats placed on a CRON diet for two to four months showed increased resistance of their (hippocampal) neurons and their (striatal) neurons to degeneration induced by two toxins that strike at the mitochondria (the energy factories of the cell). These same CRON rats also showed increased resistance to drug-induced deficits in performance in learning and memory tasks. All of these experiments suggest that CRON increases resistance of the brain to insults involving metabolic compromise, oxidative stress, and what is called *excitotoxicity*, all of which may play major roles in neurodegenerative diseases such as Alzheimer's and Parkinson's.[79] In a study of over 2,000 elderly persons, those with lower calorie intake showed a reduced tendency to develop Alzheimer's.[80]

A LESSON FROM BIOSPHERE 2

The current developing dogma in the medicine/nutrition community is that low-fat, high-carbohydrate (especially high-GI) diets cause triglycerides to go up, HDLs to go down, insulin resistance to worsen. And while total LDLs remain unchanged, there is a shift from large buoyant LDLs to small, dense LDLs—the baddest of the bad guys.[81]

TABLE 5.6 *Types and quantities of foods eaten by each crew member per day during eight consecutive 3-month periods for two years inside Biosphere 2 (Each column represents an average of 8 to 9 random days during the 3-month period.) (Adapted from Walford et al, J. Gerontology [in press])*

	1ST	2ND	3RD	4TH	5TH	6TH	7TH	8TH
FRUIT								
Banana	233	218	346	197	256	366	438	340
Fig	3	45	13	32	4			
Guava	3				9	6	3	
Lemon	2	2	15	2	30	5	21	10
Kumquat		2	1			1		
Papaya	104	91	160	231	233	100	107	143
NUTS								
Peanuts	18	21	14	15	9	17	18	26
GRAINS								
Rice	59	56	37	73	57	48		30
Sorghum	5		17	31	26			20
Wheat	100	111	145	107	114	85	92	133
Millet							12	6
LEGUMES								
Green beans			2	29	18			21
Hyacinth beans	7	34	42	26	11	4	15	19
Pinto beans	7	3			6	89	36	25
Red beans				2	7		50	
Soybeans	11				4	20	53	20
Split peas	17	5						
MEAT, DAIRY, EGGS								
Chicken		13						
Pork		8	13	16			11	15
Goat	8			8	10			12
Fish (tilapia)	7	3						
Goat milk	103	79	75	146	136	99	95	166
Eggs	6	4	2	3	3		6	
VEGETABLES								
Beets	131	269	34			10	209	140
Beet greens	56	17				29	50	27
Bok Choy				11	13			
Cabbage	28	94					56	34
Carrots	7	42	19	27		25	48	78

TABLE 5.6 *(Continued) types and quantities of foods eaten by each crew member per day during eight consecutive 3-month periods for two years inside Biosphere 2 (Each column represents an average of 8 to 9 random days during the 3-month period.) (Adapted from Walford et al, J. Gerontology [in press])*

	1ST	2ND	3RD	4TH	5TH	6TH	7TH	8TH
Chard	52	25	55	24	53	30	110	24
Corn		5			7			
Cucumber			5			5	35	34
Eggplant	74	25	8	33	46	27	9	48
Herb greens	4	4	6	4	4	5	4	5
Jicama		2	7	10				
Kale	4	8	16					
Lettuce	39	62	19	21	46	30	46	27
Onions	10	88	105	33	20	12	7	13
Parsley	2	2	2	2	2	2	2	2
Pepper, green	11	20	27	31	71	40	34	20
Pepper, red	2	1					24	45
Potato, sweet	313	110	240	512	472	318	188	538
Potato greens, sweet			11	81	98	19		
Potato, white	49	224	143				18	
Raddish	4		2	2		22	7	
Squash, summer	93	177	161	203	248	29	38	140
Squash, winter			18	36	34			
Tato	26	33	70			15	26	13
Tomato	54	182	131	116	33	7	35	27
Calories, kcal	1735	1834	1926	2109	2017	1914	2107	2402
Protein, gm	54	62	59	67	63	64	84	81
% cals. from protein	12%	13%	12%	12%	12%	13%	15%	13%
Total fat, gm	23	24	20	25	21	25	33	36
% cals. from fat	12%	11%	9%	10%	9%	11%	13%	13%
Carbohydrate, gm	351	369	408	429	424	386	404	471
% cals from carb.	76%	76%	80%	77%	79%	76%	72%	75%
Fiber, gm	33	50	40	42	38	51	62	56

Let us look at the results from Biosphere 2 in the light of the above remarks, and of what I have said elsewhere in this chapter. The types and quantities of foods eaten inside Biosphere 2 are given in Table 5.6, along with data on the macronutrient composition of the diet. While the total calorie count may not appear very reduced, balanced against the intense work load, it was sufficiently low that the four male crew members lost 18 percent of body weight within six to eight months, and the women 10 percent. The diet was high in micronutrient (vitamins, minerals, etc.) quality, but low in fat, relatively low in protein, and very high in carbohydrate, including both high-GI (bananas, wheat) and low-GI foods.

What I observed in my study of the crew members[82, 83, 84] were large-scale declines in blood pressure, blood cholesterol (pre-entry average of 195 becoming 123 within six to eight months), blood glucose (21 percent decline), insulin (42 percent), glycosylated hemoglobin (15 percent). Initially tryglicerides actually increased mildly, but then went gradually down (40 percent decline within 20 months).

Clearly it's calories that count. The rest may add a little thereto but is not something to obsess about. Keep the calories down and the diet nutrient dense, and you will gradually slip into the adaptive response that produces the CRON effects. In terms of the subject of this chapter, you will have greatly reduced your risk of getting the major killer diseases that land 75 percent of U.S. citizens in the morgue.

Among those persons who stick to the program, I believe that many will break the present 110 year maximum life span barrier. Depending on how young they are when they start, a few should reach 140 to 150 years of age, by which time, if not sooner, other, probably molecular genetic, manipulations will have extended the life span still further, and the CRON practitioners will have bridged the gap between ours and the era of "the long-living society."

CHAPTER 6

THE COMPLEX
PHILOSOPHY OF
SUPPLEMENTATION

INTRODUCTION

ONE OF THE MOST CONFUSED AREAS WE MUST TRY TO make sense of is that of dietary supplementation. Vitamins, antioxidants, chemicals, hormones, minerals, mini-doses, mega-doses, the Recommended Daily Allowances—dietary supplementation is a battleground, in large part because it involves big business, the supplement companies with their products in the health food stores, the pharmaceutical companies who perceive the supplement companies as threats, the Food and Drug Administration, with their rules and regulations, and of course the diet book industry, to name a few of the often conflicting interests. In this field of strife one finds amazing legions of lay and semilay faddists promoting their pseudoscientific advice with little understanding of or regard for valid evidence. Equally occupying the field roam cadres of otherwise quite good scientists and physicians who, because establishment medicine has been dead set against any additives in excess of the holy RDAs— they are gradually seeing the light, however, but rather slowly— accept mediocre evidence uncritically if it seems to support their consensus views. The serious layman will find himself between shifting hostile lines, the troubled air filled with out-of-sight promises and dire warnings.

My current position with regard to this controversy, and in relation to the CRON diet, can be stated briefly: (1) On the diet you should take small amounts of the essential vitamins and minerals, to avoid borderline deficiencies. This precaution is supported by the animal studies and has been recommended for low-calorie diets by many authorities. (2) Taking substantially more than the Recommended Daily Allowances (but not really mega-dose amounts) of *selected* nutrients will, with a *moderate* order of probability (according to the evidence), enhance your average survival prospects. It will do so by increasing your resistance to a variety of diseases, including some types of cancer, very probably heart disease, and other maladies. The CRON diet will yield these same benefits to a far greater degree, and against a wider variety of diseases. Whether the effects are additive or in some cases subtractive is virtually unknown. According to existing evidence based upon survival curves (the only unassailable evidence, to my way of thinking), it remains quite unproven that any supplement or combination of supplements, or hormone replacement, will extend our species' maximum life span.

The chief danger of getting involved in "the supplement culture" is that you will be caught in the endless babble of controversy, which might cause you to focus too much on what is marginal and problematic and possibly to neglect basic nutrition and good health habits. For these reasons I am reluctant to become further involved in the whole supplementation area, but I think I must. If you are going to undertake a life-extension program, I want to forewarn you against overzealous promotion on the one hand and obstinate prejudice of the establishment on the other. We must take a fresh look.

CRITERIA FOR LOOKING

How shall we assess the evidence when there are so many claims and controversies, when only in the past few years books by credentialed persons have appeared like *The Omega Plan*, *Enter the Zone*, *The Antioxidant Miracle*, *The Glucose Revolution*, and they all go confidently in somewhat different directions—to say nothing of less credible books such as *Eat 4 Your Type* or *Dr. Atkins' Diet Revolution?*

First, there should be a background of publications in the regular, peer-reviewed scientific literature about the proposed supplements or procedures—not merely privately printed pamphlets put out by a business, nor printed material, including books, based on someone's personal experience (like a celebrity's), or upon "60,000 satisfied patients," as Atkins claims. None of that, for God's sake! Ideally the pertinent scientific literature should present both animal and human data. The animal work should feature controlled experiments, the human data are often less controlled but may be satisfactory if pointing in the same direction as the animal work. Conjugated linoleic acid (CLA) is a good example of what I mean. Numerous studies in rodents have shown that CLA inhibits breast and skin cancers, reduces cholesterol, reduces fat stores, and increases muscle mass by altering the way the body uses and stores energy. However, only two studies in humans have been conducted, one involving 10 and the other 28 persons. They gave opposing results in terms of short-term weight loss.[1] No studies are on record as to the effects of CLA on cancer, heart disease, or cholesterol in humans. In what humans eat, CLA is chiefly present in meat and dairy products, which are hardly known for anti-carcinogenic effects. Yet CLA is touted as the new "good fat" for human consumption. It might well be, in view of the animal evidence, but the touting seems premature.

Second, if the supplement is a pure substance, but the evidence favoring it comes from assumptions derived from food data about what people eat in relation to health issues, be wary. Beta-carotene is our example here. It was long thought to be the substance responsible for the cancer-preventive, antioxidant properties of fruits and vegetables, until a large study demonstrated that the incidence of lung cancer actually *increased* in smokers who took beta-carotene supplements. Researchers then discovered that alpha-carotene, not beta-carotene, is probably the active carotene in fruits and vegetables protecting against cancer. Beta-carotene may in fact under certain circumstances act as a pro-oxidant, and may increase or activate a number of carcinogen-metabolizing enzymes.[2]

Third, the action and fate of the material within the body should be reasonably well understood according to traditional biochemical concepts, and at different dosages. Vitamin C is considered well understood as to its role in the bodily economy. It functions as a reducing agent in the metabolism of collagen and connective tissue, and is the most effective of the water-soluble dietary antioxidants, scavenging, among others, hydroxyl and superoxide radicals, reactive peroxide, and singlet oxygen, and it protects against peroxidation of LDL, the bad form of cholesterol.[3] That's broad-spectrum activity. Sounds good! However, at doses of over 500 milligrams per day in humans, it may possibly behave both as an antioxidant and a pro-oxidant, i.e., as a free radical scavenger and as a free radical.[4] The chemicals 8-oxoguanine and 8-oxoadenine are derived from DNA that has been damaged by free radicals. At vitamin C dosages of 500 milligrams per day, 8-oxoguanine was found to be decreased in the white blood cells of experimental human subjects (therefore, C was acting as an antioxidant), whereas 8-oxoadenine was increased (pro-oxidant activity). Because the body pool is saturated at doses of 100 to 200 milligrams of vitamin C per day as a supplement, the large dosages that many people take might be counterproductive, in any case unnecessary.

Fourth, the experiments upon which the conclusions regarding supplements or other items are based should have been confirmed by independent investigators. There are numerous reports in the scientific literature about promising experimental results that were nonrepeatable and therefore incorrect. This is particularly true in the literature of life extension. Our example here can be Brown-Sequard, the first hormone replacement therapist. In 1889, 72-year-old Edouard Brown-Sequard, who had taught at Harvard and was occupying one of the most prestigious professorships in France, reported at a meeting of the College of France that for three weeks he had been injecting himself with a watery extract of dog testicles, had "regained at least all the strength I possessed a good many years ago," and had even satisfied the amorous inclinations of his new young wife. Soon thousands of physicians were giving a similar extract to eager old Frenchmen. But alas, the experiment was nonrepeatable. One favorable report is not enough—no matter who it comes from.

Finally, testimonial and anecdotal evidence should be regarded as categorically unacceptable if that's all there is, and again—no matter who it comes from. It's reassuring to have such evidence if it comes from someone you know and represents their personal experience; but even then, it's insufficient unless backed up by the items specified above.

I hope you get the message. The right supplements in the right dosages are useful adjuncts to a health-promoting program, both to correct possible deficits of a restricted diet, and because in larger than RDA dosages, they may exert additional, so-called pharmacological effects that are beneficial. Indeed, as you have seen (See Figure 5.1), supplements are included in my food pyramid. But don't just gobble down pills from the health food store because the clerk gives you a spiel, or fall for glowing propaganda from those who have much to gain but not enough evidence to fulfill at least most of our criteria.

WHERE IS THE 45-MONTH-OLD MOUSE?

Take a look back at Figure 3.1. You will notice that the maximum life span of a genetically favored long-lived mouse strain on a normal diet extends to about 38 months, equivalent to 110 years in humans. By significantly retarding aging in mice, the CRON diet can stretch that out to 56 months, equivalent (assuming for the sake of my illustration, that one can make the translation from mouse to man) to 167 years in humans. I have not yet seen the product of even a 45-month-old mouse by any supplement, or any combination of supplements, or *any* hormone replacement therapy. So when someone hawks you their anti-aging wares, simply inquire, "Pray tell, where is your 45-month-old mouse?"

Prevention of disease by supplements is of course another matter. For this, good evidence exists, as we shall see presently. But that's not anti-aging, and prevention of all the major diseases would only extend average human life span by five or six years, and maximum life span probably not at all.

FUNDAMENTAL DIFFERENCE BETWEEN
PREVENTING DISEASE AND RETARDING AGING

In 1825, a demographer by the name of Benjamin Gompertz noted that in human populations the mortality rate—defined as the percent of the population at each age that dies during the following year—doubles every eight years (except at the extremes of life, i.e. early childhood and old age). This doubling time, this *rate of change*, is

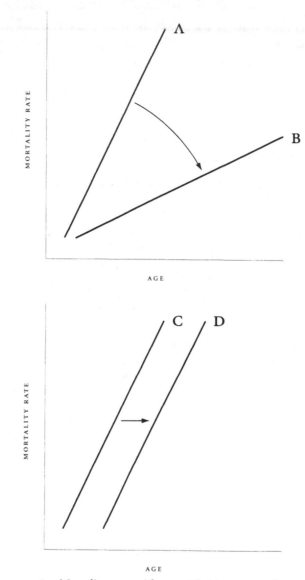

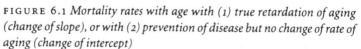

FIGURE 6.1 *Mortality rates with age with (1) true retardation of aging (change of slope), or with (2) prevention of disease but no change of rate of aging (change of intercept)*

characteristic for each species, and is regarded by specialists as the best measure of the rate of aging. It represents your *overall* vulnerability to any threats to your health; you become doubly vulnerable every eight years. Assuming that the CRON diet retards aging in humans, the mortality doubling time would change to, for example, every 12 years. This concept is illustrated in Figure 6.1 by the line A turning into B. You can see that the *slope* has changed, the age-related rate of increase in vulnerability has been slowed. *That* is anti-aging.

Curing or preventing disease, however, does not by itself necessarily change the doubling time, which is measured by the slope of the line. It may merely shift the line over a bit (C becomes D in Figure 6.1). If heart disease is wholly prevented, people will live a few years longer, but something else will get them if their rate of aging, their vulnerability, continues to double every eight years.

There is presently no convincing evidence that any supplement or combination of supplements or hormones accomplishes any more than a C to D shift. That's *not* anti-aging, and it will not produce a pronounced extension of maximum life span. A CRON diet, on the other hand will cause *both* an A to B *and* a C to D shift. The slope changes, and a shift occurs, the maximum life span is greatly extended, and the incidences of all major diseases of aging are decreased. This statement is supported by 60 years of research in numerous university laboratories.[5] It is unequivocally proven.

There is an important corollary to the above statements. People talk about certain diseases as showing "accelerated aging," such as progeria, Werner's syndrome, and others. I do so myself sometimes, and some of them certainly are, but it's easy to talk loosely on this subject. Diabetes is one example of a disease that causes so-called "accelerated aging." Diabetics have many symptoms and signs that would correspond to an older functional age than their chronologic age. They get arteriosclerosis at a younger age, have cataracts, hypertension, arthritis; but, so far as I am aware, their mortality rate doubling time remains eight years. In short, they show a fairly pronounced C to D but not an A to B shift. If this is true, then it is probably a mistake to think that diabetes truly accelerates aging, and that since it is caused by an out-of-control glucose/insulin metabolic system, if one could learn how to gain fundamental control of that metabolic system, one could not only prevent or cure diabetes but significantly retard the rate of aging and extend maximum life span. This mistake is not uncommon, even among professional gerontologists. Of course, preventing diabetes is highly desirable. But application of that knowledge will not necessarily give us a 167-year life span, or even 120 years.

LET'S LOOK AT THE FADDISTS AND COMMERCIALIZERS

Almost every bodily process changes with age. Among the vast, constantly outpouring medical literature, it's not hard to select an article or even series of articles that suggest that a particular vitamin, drug, chemical, or lifestyle will prevent or slow down a particular change. If you are not too critical about the evidence in these articles and if you neglect or underplay nonconfirming articles, you can build what sounds like a strong argument for any hot-topic product or procedure. But that's endless and often foolish, although you can bet it sells a lot of products! "Make-the-case-for" evidence can unroll forever, and be quite convincing! The popularity of antioxidants as potential anti-aging agents is built on plausible theory and fairly good inferential evidence. But if we insist on *hard evidence*—like the criteria I've outlined above—that the vitamin, drug, or procedure extends maximum life span in long-lived strains of animals (the only positive proof of an anti-aging effect)—we shall find that none of them have been shown to do so to any great extent in any mammals, including man. The boosters don't have a 45-month-old mouse.

AND NOW FOR THE ESTABLISHMENT PREJUDICES

In certain areas (aging and cancer are the best examples), and in reaction against junk advertising, the overenthusiasm of unqualified health nuts and charlatans, people with inadequate training, poor critical judgment, and no legal responsibility, orthodox medical and nutritional scientists stride too far in the opposite direction. With regard to anti-aging therapies, as a group they oppose, or at least say they oppose, anything that has not been positively proven by experimental evidence. "Orders of probability" are not even considered. This widens the gap between huckster and establishment, and the public is caught in the middle.

And not only the public! Three Nobel Prize winners in biology and medicine, Dr. Albert Szent-Györgyi, Dr. Linus Pauling, and Sir Peter Medawar,[6] all took vitamin C in excess of the RDA quantity. According to a report in the respected journal *Science*,[7] about 50 percent of nurses take multiple vitamin pills. So do many establishment doctors. And the National Research Council itself not very long ago specifically recommended a diet with "plenty of vitamin C containing material." In short, by the back-door route they seemed to be recommending more than their own official RDA of 60 milligrams per day. Even the naysayers are voting with their feet.

The simple fact is that in practice orthodox medicine has frequently and throughout its history recommended therapies on the basis merely of probable or inferential evidence—on educated guesswork. Orders of probability is not a new approach; the medical establishment just won't consider it for aging. Examples: during the period from 1930 to about 1960, medicine adopted a very conservative attitude toward any exercise more vigorous than walking: exercise was thought to cause the body to "wear out" more rapidly, or to undergo "stress." Medicine has now reversed itself, exercise is held to provide a needed stimulus for maintaining structural and functional integrity of a number of systems. For both these views, so firmly held during their times of influence, really hard evidence remained skimpy for a long time.[8]*

Vaccination against smallpox and the provision of clean water and drainage at times of cholera and typhus epidemics in nineteenth-century Europe were instituted without direct "proof" that they would work. Dr. I.P. Semmelweiss in obstetrics and Dr. Joseph Lister in surgery championed use of antiseptic techniques decades before the germ theory of disease was accepted. Many other ancient and modern examples could be cited. Today's official recommendations to decrease sodium and increase calcium intake in the diet are based on high probability rather than absolute evidence. Thus, there is plenty of precedent in medicine for acting on probabilities. But in certain areas, and anti-aging therapy is perhaps the chief area, because of the strange taboos about monkeying with "natural" aging (see Chapter 2 of my book *Maximum Life Span*), establishment medicine tends to insist on faultless evidence and to denounce vociferously any departure from an absolute proof-positive policy. It is well to be cautious, but not to be overcautious.[9]*

A side effect of this reactive overcautiousness is that any reports on toxicity of vitamin or other supplements are apt to be magnified out of proportion to their scientific worth. For example, it was widely believed in the medical fraternity, and often quoted in textbooks and review articles, that large doses of vitamin C might cause kidney stones. A 1984 article in *Nutrition Reviews*,[10] in stating that "vitamin C may be associated with the formation of oxalate stones" in the kidney, listed seven references. Six of these were in fact merely secondary sources, and everything ultimately referred back to a letter appearing in a 1979 issue of the British medical journal *Lancet*, which cautioned about "theoretically" harmful effects of vitamin C. The letter described a single patient who excreted large amounts of oxalate in his urine after taking 4 grams of vitamin C per day. But this patient did not actually have kidney stones. Other individuals taking the same amount of vitamin C did not excrete excess oxalate. There are in fact no cases reported in the medical literature of actual kidney stones due to oral intake of vitamin C in normal individuals. Yet the idea persisted until recently.[11]

These claims, and many others about possible adverse effects of vitamin C in doses well above the RDA, for example that it decreases absorption of vitamin B12, did not withstand final critical scrutiny.[12]* Thus, while the medical profession might have been correct in its position that the vitamin company claims for the health benefits of vitamin C were exaggerated, its own views about harmful effects were just as prejudiced.

As a second example, let's examine a report on the supposed toxicity of vitamin E published in 1981 in the *Journal of the American Medical Association*.[13] The author, a practicing physician, reported that during the previous ten years he had seen many patients with problems that seemed to have been caused by self-medication with large amounts of vitamin E. This article was often cited in medical circles as evidence that vitamin E might be harmful.

Let's look at the evidence in some detail. Among 50 patients who had thrombophlebitis (inflammation of the veins of the legs), the author was impressed that two had started taking vitamin E several months before the onset of the disease. And the symptoms improved following cessation of vitamin E and the beginning of conventional treatment.

Basically, that's the evidence, all the evidence. It's totally unconvincing. Why? Because many other interpretations are possible besides the one that large doses of vitamin E may cause thrombophlebitis: (1) The patients' illness may have prompted them to start taking vitamin E as it was at one time widely believed to benefit vascular problems in the legs.[14] (2) The report gave no data at all on what proportion of persons who took vitamin E out of all the large numbers who were doing so, developed thrombophlebitis, compared with the percentage of *non-*vitamin E takers who developed the disease. (3) Some of the patients improved when they stopped taking vitamin E but at the same time they stopped, conventional treatment was started. We cannot know which of these two factors was responsible for the improvement.

The article went on to discuss a number of other diseases (hypertension, gynecomastia, breast tumors) that the author had encountered in patients who took a lot of vitamin E. He cited published articles implicating excessive vitamin E intake in 15 additional clinical disorders. And he cited a letter to the *New England Journal of Medicine* that stated that 800 units of vitamin E appeared to cause severe fatigue in friends and patients of the author of the letter. He *failed* to cite another letter to the same journal stating that doses of vitamin E from 400 to 1,600 units given daily to hundreds of persons did not lead to a single case of weakness or fatigue.[15*] Of all the literature cited, only one could be considered a controlled study; that one involved only eight subjects, and the results were not statistically significant.

This was definitely *not* good scientific evidence. It was the clinical anecdote, the second worst form of evidence, as we learned in Chapter 1. Despite this, the report was widely cited as evidence for potential toxicity of vitamin E at doses that are not all that high.

At one time there was thought to be a significant risk of toxicity if you took vitamin D in excess of about 1,000 International Units or IU (25 milligrams); but a recent in depth review[16] maintains that you would have to take more than 40,000 IU—67 to 100 times the RDA—to induce the high blood calcium seen with vitamin D toxicity. The author states, "Throughout my preparation of this review, I was amazed at the lack of evidence supporting statements about the toxicity of moderate doses of vitamin D. Consistently, literature citations to support them have been either inappropriate or without substance."

Orthodox medicine, if it has assumed a particular position (in this case, that whatever the faddists claim must be vigorously combated), tends to treat second- or third-rate evidence as first-rate if it reinforces that assumed position. Although complicated and precise studies have been demanded to prove points about any benefits of supplementing the diet with more than RDA amounts, the medical profession hastens to accept merely anecdotal information if it points in the negative direction of their thinking.

This leaves us between unqualified, uncritical, overenthusiastic promotion on the one hand and obstinate reactive prejudice on the other. We must therefore make up our own minds. You must make up your own mind. I will take a strong position in advising you about the CRON diet. It will work! Definitely! But as for the health benefits of large amounts of certain supplements, except for C, E, and probably selenium, the evidence is merely of a moderate, not high, order of probability.

THE RECOMMENDED DAILY ALLOWANCES

Let's talk next about the famous Recommended Daily Allowances, the RDAs. Establishment medicine has tended to advise against vitamin and mineral supplements because it is dazzled by the authoritative backup behind these RDAs. More than the RDAs cannot possibly do any additional good! After all, the RDAs were set by the Committee on Dietary Allowances of the National Academy of Sciences. Anything the National Academy of Sciences gets behind becomes sacrosanct in science (most of the time for good reason— but not all the time).

The Committee decides upon the RDAs for vitamins and other

"essential" food substances by sifting together knowledge from a number of sources, then making a very educated and careful but nevertheless subjective guess as to what is needed by the body. The knowledge basis for this estimate involves six criteria: (1) the amount that apparently healthy people consume of the particular nutrient; (2) the amount needed to avoid a particular disease (example: pellagra was rampant in the southern United States until its relation to a deficiency in nicotinic acid was recognized; improvement rapidly followed inclusion in the diet of foods rich in this B vitamin); (3) the degree of tissue saturation, or the adequacy of physiological function in relation to the nutrient intake (example: if your vitamin C intake is too low, your capillary blood vessels will be fragile, and you will have bleeding problems; the RDA of vitamin C will correct this); (4) nutrient-balance studies that measure nutritional status in relation to intake (Analyze the amount of the nutrient in all food and all excreta of an individual for three to five days and find the maximum level of intake at which all is absorbed and none found in the excreta: that's the minimum requirement, or the point of zero balance);[17]* (5) studies of volunteers experimentally maintained on diets deficient in the nutrient, followed by correction of the clinical signs of deficiency when a certain amount of the nutrient is resupplied; and (6) extrapolation from animal experiments in which deficiencies have been produced by exclusion of a single nutrient from the diet.

All of the above are excellent criteria, but a seventh can be suggested, perhaps the best criterion of all for our purposes but one that the National Academy of Sciences Committee on Dietary Allowances has never considered. To quote the 1985 chairman of the Committee, Dr. Henry Kamin:[18] "I must admit that we do not have much information about the intake of specific nutrients and *remote* [my italics] rather than short-term effects."

Just recently the Food and Nutrition Board of the Institute of Medicine (part of the National Academy of Science) initiated an investigation to consider establishing a Dietary Reference Intake (DAR) for the carotenes, where DAR is defined as estimates of nutrient intake required not just to prevent clinical deficiency but to promote optimal health.[19] One hopes they will incorporate a seventh Criterion into their recommendations.

THE SEVENTH CRITERION

Suppose that separate groups of animals (and by implication humans) were fed the same basic, well-balanced diet but with increasing amounts of a particular supplement from small to mega-dose quantities. This is kept up throughout their whole lives. Records are kept on survival, cancer types and frequencies, and other diseases for all the animal groups. Now let's set the RDA at that dosage of the nutrient that is associated with the longest average or maximum survival, the lowest overall disease frequency, and evidence of improved function. This new RDA may be quite different and larger, indeed much larger, than the RDA established by the six standard criteria outlined above, the only ones actually used.[20]*

In considering the Seventh Criterion, we are pretty much restricted, in terms of longevity and disease information, to extrapolating from animal experiments, supported by studies of the effects of supplements on functional parameters in humans. The immune-response capacity in humans, presumably important in resistance to disease, can be enhanced by administration of more than RDA amounts of, for example, vitamins C[21] and E.[22] In addition, vitamins C plus selenium and the sulfur-containing amino acids (glutathione for example) may display antioxidant properties unrelated to their role in classical nutrition. This additional activity is probably beneficial.[23]

In the next chapter I will deal with the various individual antioxidants drugs, vitamins, and other chemicals with emphasis on the Seventh Criterion wherever possible. To what extent have these substances been shown in animal (or human) studies to extend average and/or maximum life span? Do they influence susceptibility to the major killer diseases? Do they improve any of the biomarkers of aging? What precisely is the place of supplementation in the CRON diet program for life extension?

Meantime, and to round out the present chapter in the light of what has been said, we may consider in a generic form certain preventive, supplementary or related treatment regimes now in vogue for the retardation of aging or prevention of disease, those that stand generally at the margin between traditional and borderline medicine.

THE CLASSES OF SUPPLEMENTS

ANTIOXIDANTS

The antioxidants are by all odds the most touted anti-aging chemical remedy. They are supposed to prevent or neutralize those damaging agents spontaneously produced in the body and called free radicals. Described as "great white sharks in the biochemical sea," free radicals are fragments of molecules that have become unstuck. Ordinary chemical molecules share one characteristic: their electrons (those minute electrical charges swirling around the nucleus of each atom) are paired.[24]* An ordinary chemical bond between two atoms involves two electrons. Each atom contributes one. When a chemical reaction takes place and the bond is broken, one fragment generally keeps both electrons.

Not so with free radicals! A bond can break so that each separate fragment retains one electron. At one time the fundamental laws of modern chemistry (the concepts of valence and molecular weight, if you please) seemed to forbid this. But in the 1930s, oil-industry scientists showed that even though free radicals might have a life span of a mere few thousandths of a second, their activity accounted for some spectacular chemical transformations—the rancification of fats and oils, for example. These discoveries gave birth to the development of the plastics and polymers industry.

In biology it took longer for free radicals to catch on. Enzymes were all the rage then, whereas free radicals looked spooky and forbidding. Free radicals are hyperactive. Once generated, they grab on to everything in reach. And once triggered, free radical reactions tend to be unstoppable, uncontrollable, irreversible, almost explosive. Bam! Like Sodom and Gomorrah! Turn you into a pillar of rancid fat!

To biologists, conditioned for half a century to the delicate interplay and self-regulating equilibrium of enzyme cycles, free-radical reactions seemed irrelevant to life. So it was a feat of considerable insight and perhaps even foolhardy daring for Dr. Denham Harman to propose as early as 1955, and on the basis of preliminary and in retrospect rather unconvincing experiments, that such a major biological process as aging itself might be caused by free radical attacks against the constituents of the body. He called his proposal the free radical theory of aging.

While I shall be talking at length about free radicals, I must emphasize that the free radical theory of aging is only one of at least six important theories of aging (See note 54, Chapter 3), and that some of the others are just as well founded, maybe more so. Indeed, we can explain almost all existing experiments about free radicals and health by supposing that they have much to do with disease (cancer especially) but very little to do with intrinsic aging. However, an equally strong opposing argument can be put forth.[25] The reason for this duality is that nearly all the evidence for an anti-aging effect is inferential. There is no 45-month-old mouse.

The impetus behind all the hoopla in pseudoscientific popular health books and magazines is that the free radical theory is at least very plausible. One can make an excellent case for it, and having done so, one can promote an almost unending bevy of products (antioxidants) that are supposed to neutralize the damaging free radicals. Some of these products are clearly beneficial, although rarely as much as claimed, but a real danger exists here. Overpromotion of antioxidants, vitamins, and various drugs tends to steer people away from what are far more important for both health and life extension: careful diet, exercise, and stress avoidance. I cannot give a better illustration than to quote from the June 1983 issue of *Whole Life Times* (hardly a pro-medical establishment magazine, but a part of the health food industry itself): "It is dangerously deceptive to think that a person who smokes and drinks heavily, eats a high-fat, low-fiber diet, drinks six cups of coffee a day and runs on stress and anxiety with unhealthy social relationships and an oppressive work situation, is going to somehow achieve optimal health and an extended life span simply by consuming the right nutrients and anti-aging substances. Yet this hardly exaggerates the position of [Durk] Pearson and [Sandy] Shaw, who represent one extreme in anti-aging thought."

Notwithstanding the hoopla and the lack so far of definitive proof, the free radical theory of aging and disease continues to receive the attention and support of many distinguished experimental scientists.[26]

The particular free radicals we are most concerned with are the products of oxygen metabolism taking place within the energy factories of the cell (the mitochondria). About 2 billion years ago, before oxygen became available in the atmosphere, organisms obtained energy from breaking down carbohydrates by a process called *glycolysis*. This is not very efficient, and life forms, struggling to multiply, developed the ability to use a new atmospheric constituent that was becoming available, oxygen. The by-products of this new source of energy were the free radicals. While certain free radicals are necessary in the evolving chemical reactions taking place within the body, any excess is bad. The damaging free radicals are thus the excess, unused by-products of the new high-energy metabolism, just as radioactive wastes are by-products of the increased energy we can get from the atom.

Both are detriments. We're not doing so well with our radioactive wastes, but the by-products of metabolism have been around for a longer time, and Nature has found ways to deal with them. Down the ages, cells have compartmentalized. The mitochondria, where many free radicals are generated, are separated from the rest of the cell by their own unique membranes. And within each cell, protective free radical neutralizer "scavengers," or to use the more popular term, *antioxidants*, are manufactured.[27]*

Where the Battle Takes Place Chief sites of attack are the cell membranes, both those inside cells (mitochondrial and nuclear membranes) and those forming the external walls of cells. Major components of these structures are lipids (fats), both saturated and unsaturated. (They are fatty acids really, but I'll use the simpler term.) A greater membrane concentration of unsaturated than saturated fats is essential to the pliability and elasticity the cell needs to move and flex its membranes. But—and here is the big problem—it is precisely these unsaturated fats that are most susceptible to attack by free radicals.

The radicals may also damage DNA, the hereditary blueprint for life within each cell. Indeed, many of the substances that cause or promote cancer may do so by stimulating cells to produce free radicals that then damage or alter the blueprint until the cell becomes cancerous.[28]

Evidence for the Free Radical Theory of Aging: It's Plausible The maximum life spans of different species are proportional to the levels of antioxidants that occur naturally in their blood. Longer-lived species have higher levels of antioxidants in relation to their *lifetime energy potential*, the amount of calories they burn up per pound of animal in a normal life span.[29]*

Some of the damage from free radical reactions increases with aging. A yellow-brown age pigment called lipofuscin accumulates in the cells of older animals. It is a breakdown product related to the action of free radicals upon cellular membranes. This waste is taken up by digestive vacuoles in the cells, but it's indigestible; so it piles up with age. In the human heart, for example, the pigment increases at the rate of about 0.06 percent per year. Eventually up to 5 percent of the total heart-muscle volume can be taken up by yellow-brown inert gunk.[30]* Many other experimental observations, which we need not review in detail, can be interpreted in the light of the free radical theory.[31, 32]

Effects of Antioxidants on Biomarkers of Aging Can one improve the biomarkers of aging by including antioxidants in the diet? The amount of age pigments in tissues can be substantially reduced by antioxidants such as vitamin E, methionine, BHT, or selenium,[33] or by ingestion of any of a number of brain-reactive chemicals that may have partial antioxidant properties (DMAE and centrophenoxine). However, the joke is that even though these agents retard the buildup of age pigment, the maximum life spans of animals are not increased—at least, not those of long-lived strains. So the evidence could be equally interpreted as *against* the free radical theory of aging in that you can decrease the production of one of the main products of free radical reactions without influencing maximum life span. Many other antioxidant experiments present such an equivocal aspect when viewed critically.[34]* We'll consider the evidence in more detail when we discuss selected individual antioxidants (vitamins C and E, selenium, and others) in the next chapter.

The free radical approach is a bit like the Bible. Once you are persuaded to believe in the Bible as the literal Word of God, or in this case the free radical theory as the Word of Nature, you can give a plausible explanation for many phenomena—in this case cell deterioration, a number of diseases, and aging. This ability to explain phenomena is a necessary first step for any scientific theory. But it's only a first step. The second is to use the theory to devise experiments or treatments that will alter the course of a phenomenon in a predictable way: for example, to retard aging, or prevent or cure disease.

Effects of Antioxidants on Life Span Certain dietary supplements, including antioxidants, will probably extend the average life spans of animals by decreasing disease susceptibility. If one is dealing with a short-lived strain of, say, mice—short-lived because it has a high incidence of disease—then the maximum life span of that strain may be extended if the antioxidant affects the disease; but this does not mean that aging has been retarded. Only if we can break the *species'* maximum life span barrier, not the *strain* barrier, can we say we have retarded aging. No vitamin, antioxidant, or other supplement has been shown to do that in higher animals such as mammals.[35]* If we look at actual survival curves for populations of mice and rats that have received relatively high doses of antioxidants throughout much of their lives, we find the results to be clearly marginal: sometimes a moderate extension is noted, sometimes not. No changes in the mortality rate doubling time have been reported. The modest extension of average life span is often accompanied by a lower average weight, so the effect could be attributed in some (not all) instances as much to reduced food intake (a mild CRON effect as the animals have possibly had their appetites suppressed by the food additives) as to free radical scavenging.[36] And most of the strains used were not particularly long-lived for their species.[37]*

Effects of Antioxidants on Disease Here there is fairly abundant evidence that certain antioxidant dietary supplements in excess of the RDA, or independent of the RDA because they are not even on the list, can influence susceptibility to a variety of diseases, including cancer, heart disease, and neurodegenerative diseases. The evidence is both experimental, involving both animals and humans, and epidemiological.

PHYTOCHEMICALS

These were more or less unknown, or at least had received little attention, when the first edition of this book was published in 1986, but are now even close to being given official sanction by a National Academy of Science panel of experts. That's a good illustration of why you should eat a careful well-rounded diet and not depend too much on supplements. You'll almost certainly be missing something that will find its way into later editions.

Epidemiological studies showed that consumption of certain foods is associated with lower incidences of various diseases, including heart disease and cancer. Most of the so-called *phytochemicals* (plant-derived chemicals) responsible for these effects have antioxidant activity, some have hormonal activity. These nonessential micronutrients encompass a vast group of unique organic phytochemicals that are not strictly required in the diet, but when present at sufficient levels are linked to the promotion of good health.

HORMONES AND HORMONE REPLACEMENT THERAPY

Brown-Sequard started it, but Daniel Rudman[38] gave it the big push. I refer to the idea that if the level of a certain hormone declines with age, and you bring that level back up by injecting the hormone, or by some other means, you may slow the rate of aging, even achieve some degree of rejuvenation.

Three hormonal systems show decreasing hormone concentrations during normal aging: (1) estrogen in women and testosterone in men, (2) DHEA and DHEA-S, and (3) the growth hormone/insulinlike growth factor axis. Some of the changes in aging are related to this decline in hormonal activity.

Rudman[39] reported in the *New England Journal of Medicine* in 1990 that of 12 men ages 61 to 81 whom he injected daily with rather high levels of synthetic human growth hormone, there was a 9 percent increase in lean body mass, a 14 percent loss in fatty tissue, and an enhanced sense of well-being. This paper started about as much of an avalanche as Brown-Sequard's announcement in the preceding century. HRT (hormone replacement therapy) became a big deal, and extended to include other hormones (testosterone, DHEA, to name two). There is no doubt about an increase in muscle mass, bone mineral content, and the fat redistribution following growth hormone administration,[40] but while many GH-recipients claim they feel better, objective double-blind tests (Rudman did not do these) for cognitive function and sense of well-being have shown no difference between test and control subjects. [41] This last study was conducted in elderly men ages 70 to 85. In one mouse study, beginning with middle-aged mice, a prolonged survival of GH-receiving mice was reported,[42] although the strain of mouse used was not particularly long-lived, plus the study was not run to the end of the survival curve, and it's dangerous to draw conclusions without doing that. By contrast, in another GH study (in rats)—a study much better orchestrated than the mouse experiment—there was no difference either in disease pattern or average (tenth decile) or maximum survival between test and control rodents.[43]

DHEA fares somewhat better. This material was introduced into gerontology by Dr. Arthur Schwartz in the early eighties, and has received a great deal of attention. As far as life extension is concerned, I have yet to see a 45-month-old mouse. However, two well-controlled studies in humans given DHEA in the dosage range of 50 to 100 milligrams per day for six months to a year induced an increase in perceived physical and psychological well-being, an increase in muscle strength and lean body mass, and increased IGF-1 concentrations,[44] with no significant adverse effects (blood glucose and insulin not increased). Possible risks of long-term usage, if any, are not yet identified.

There is good evidence that estrogen given to postmenopausal women has some protective quality against the development of Alzheimer's disease, and perhaps other forms of neurodegeneration, including memory loss.[45,46] Also, it may delay atherosclerosis, bone loss, and loss of cognitive function; but life expectancy is not altered, suggesting that the basic aging process is not altered. In a major study, during the first ten years of hormone use, the risk of death among hormone users was diminished by 40 to 50 percent, which was largely attributed to decreased risk of death from heart attacks.[47] On long-term use (over 10 years), however, such gains may be partially offset by an approximately 40 percent increase in breast cancer.[48] Since far more women die of heart disease than of breast cancer, the trade-off in risk would seem worth it. Disturbingly, however, recent studies seem to indicate that synthetic estrogen does not in fact protect against heart disease, but may actually increase it.[49] Abstracting from rodent data, the CRON diet should be highly protective against breast cancer, and women who wish to take estrogen but are concerned about breast cancer may wish to opt for the CRON program. Of course the CRON program protects mightily against heart disease as well.

Testosterone replacement in men is on equally controversial grounds.[50] Available data point to a positive effect on muscle mass and strength, cognition, and sense of well-being; but the effect on the size of the prostate and a possible growth stimulatory effect on in situ prostatic cancerous lesions are not yet well worked out. Nevertheless, it should be said that the reasons for concern about potentially harmful effects on the prostate now seem substantially less than formerly thought.

Can the literature of CRON give us any insight into HRT. Yes, I believe so. Growth hormone and its effector agent, the so-called insulin-derived growth factor (IGF-1), are *decreased* in CRON animals. In short the adaptation consequent to calorie restriction, the only procedure known to retard aging, *decreases* growth hormone. Does it make sense, therefore, to be trying to *increase* growth hormone by injecting it, in order to retard aging? Well, possibly it does, for roundabout reasons,[51*] but I would like to see the 45-month-old mouse. It is also worth mentioning here that a type of dwarf mouse deficient in growth hormone, prolactin, and TSH (thyroid-stimulating hormone) lives significantly longer than its normal siblings.[52]

CRON does slightly increase the level of glucocorticoid hormone, which has given rise to one theory as to how CRON works.[53] It also increases the level of androstenedione, including in humans.[54] Androstenedione might therefore be a candidate for HRT but of course more work needs to be done.

FATTY ACIDS

The primary omega-6 fat—linoleic acid—is an essential fatty acid, which is heart friendly as it lowers total cholesterol and LDLs; but too much of it in relation to another class of fatty acids, the omega-3s, may increase cancer risk. The other essential fat—linolenic acid—is an omega-3. It is reported to reduce blood clotting, prevent abnormal heart rhythms, improve immune function, and promote eye and brain development.[55]

The brain is about 60 percent fat, and one of the most important fatty acids in the brain is the omega-3 fatty acid, docosahexaenoic acid, or DHA. However, most people are deficient in this and other omega-3 fatty acids. Another fatty acid of importance is eicosapentaenoic acid, or EPA. People with psychiatric disorders, including depression, may have low levels of omega-3s, and may respond favorably to therapy with these compounds. The cardiac protective effects of the Mediterranean-style diet may be due to its high content of omega-3s.[56] It is estimated that about 3 grams per week of omega-3s are required to secure disease-prevention benefits.[57] More on these in the next chapter.

DRUGS AS SUPPLEMENTS

In this category we would include aspirin, well established as having preventive properties in relation to heart attacks, and the nonsteroidal anti-inflammatory agent, ibuprofen. It has been noted on epidimiologic studies that people taking ibuprofen over a long period— generally for arthritis—have a lower incidence of Alzheimer's disease.[58]

SUMMARY AND CONCLUSIONS

There seems little doubt that substances present normally in foods may have substantial health benefits, for disease prevention certainly, for aging retardation only dubiously, and that these benefits may be enhanced by taking more of the substances, in concentrated form as supplements, than can be obtained in any reasonable quantity of food. The cancer-preventive phytochemical lycopene is a good example. Several pounds of tomatoes are required to achieve a therapeutic dose, but academic nutritionists as a group have a near dogmatic obsession against supplements. They want you to obtain everything from food. They are mistaken, because in some instances (vitamin E is a good example) you cannot get enough from food to optimize the beneficial effect. But they do have a point. It may be only a guess as to what the component is from food that is giving the good effect, as was the case with beta-carotene.

These various problems will gradually clarify as the experiments unfold. Supplements are good to take if you don't go overboard. Individual supplements will be discussed in the next chapter. What in fact should you be taking, and how does one decide?

CHAPTER 7

PRACTICAL
SUPPLEMENTATION

INTRODUCTION

ALTHOUGH THIS IS A PRACTICAL CHAPTER, I SHALL ALLOW myself the indulgence of beginning with a couple of paradoxes. Evidence strongly suggests that CRON works to extend life span and prevent disease by harmoniously upregulating the multiple systems that protect the body from the various forms of stress: the stress of high temperature, of infection, of food shortage, of irradiation, of exposure to toxic compounds. Protection against high temperature was initially found by accident. In one researcher's animal quarters (Dr. Arlan Richardson's), the air conditioning failed over a very hot weekend. Nearly all of the control rodents died while most of the CRON animals survived.

If we could upregulate these protective systems still more, we might not age at all. There are indeed animals that show only negligible senescence, or perhaps do not age at all.[1] They may not live forever, but the slope of their mortality curve is nearly flat. They have already been sufficiently upregulated by Nature to take care of damage. So it's not a pipe dream to think of inducing such an upregulation by artificial means!

Perhaps there exists or can be concocted a magic potion we can take that will upregulate the necessary systems in ourselves! In essence, such is the hope of the supplement enthusiasts. Of course this hope was also one of the quests of the alchemists. They sought the *elixir of life*.

Going back still further, one finds the soma of the ancient Sanskrit writings. Soma was, mythology tells us, derived from a plant. One may well ask, "Was the secret ingredient therefore a *phytochemical?*" Well, if it existed at all, it was certainly a phytochemical. A place called Shangri-la did in fact exist! It was in the mountains of Bhutan. And the Olympian Gods of the Greeks, it's not true they were immortal. They lived about 5,000 years, so they *seemed* immortal to the Greeks.[2] They showed what Professor Caleb Finch of USC calls "negligible senescence."[3] And these Olympian Gods—they drank a kind of soma, a nectar passed round by the cupbearer, Ganymede.

So maybe it's still out there, the soma plant, waiting to be rediscovered. Unlike the ubiquitous vitamins and minerals, specific phytochemicals are often unique to certain plant species or genera.[4] And ecologists tell us that over 80 percent of the plant species on Earth still wait to be discovered—or rediscovered. But alas, with the decline in biodiversity caused by humankind's "conquest" of Nature, the soma plant is probably extinct. We are cast forth once more from the Garden of Eden before we have eaten of the Tree of Life, only this time not by the Lord on High, but by our reckless selves.

To date, the CRON diet is the only method able to retard the aging process and extend life span in mammalian species. But to avoid the possibility of chronic, borderline deficiency in any essential nutrients while you're following this low-calorie regimen, I recommend that you take as supplements half or full RDA amounts of most (not quite all, iron being the most notable exception) of the vitamins and minerals.

As a second but more controversial measure, I will recommend taking considerably larger than RDA amounts of vitamins E and C, plus modest increases in selenium, B6, folic acid, and B12. These nutrients are all naturally present in the diet anyway. They are innocuous if the added dose is not too high, and there is some evidence, albeit not conclusive, that they may extend average life span, in part by preventing disease. They have not, however, extended the species-specific maximum life span, at least in mammals. There is no 45-month-old mouse produced by supplementation. We have not yet found the soma of the ancient texts. But appropriate supplements may be health enhancing and help square whatever survival curve you would be on (your genetic potential) if *you* consisted of two hundred identical twins (or clones).

I will also briefly discuss the current status of a number of additional agents hailed as having anti-aging properties and/or health-enhancing

TABLE 7.1 *Recommended or "safe and adequate"*
daily allowances for essential nutrients, and recommendations
for supplementation (See text for details. RDAs are not given
for phosphorus, iodine, floride, molybdenum.)

NUTRIENT AND UNITS OF MEASUREMENT	RDA, OR "SAFE AND ADEQUATE"	UPPER SAFE LIMIT ON LONG-TERM USAGE	MY RECOMMENDATION FOR SUPPLEMENTATION	COMMENTS
vitamin A (fat soluble) units = IU	5,000 IU	10,000 IU (= 25 mg.)	None, or RDA amount	*Obtain from food sources*
vitamin D (fat soluble) units = IU	<50 yrs. old, 200 IU; > 50, 400 IU; >70, 600 IU	10,000 IU, but see Chapter 6, under Establishment Prejudices	800 IU–1,000 IU, including amount from milk or sunlight*	*Excess may yield high blood calcium, with deposits in arteries and kidneys (but see Chapter 6).*
vitamin E (fat soluble) units=IU	men: 10 IU women: 8 IU	2,000 IU	100–200 d-alpha; 100–200 d-gamma; 100 IU tocotrienol	*1 IU = 1 milligram in this case.*
vitamin K (fat soluble) units = micrograms	men: 70 mcg. women: 65 mcg.	none, or 30 mg.	400 mcg. total, including food sources	*½ cup cooked collards = 440 mcg.; ½ cup spinach = 360 mcg.; brussels sprouts = 235 mcg.; broccoli = 113 mcg.*
vitamin C units = milligrams	60 mg. both sexes	2–4 gm.	500–1,000 mg. in ester form	
thiamin (vitamin B1) units = milligrams	men: 1.2 mg. women: 1.1	50 mg.	RDA amount	
riboflavin (vitamin B2) units = milligrams	men: 1.3 mg. women: 1.1	200 mg.	RDA amount	
niacin units = milligrams	men: 16 mg. women: 14	great individual variation	100–300 mg.	*1 to 3 grams/day used to treat hyperlipidemia, may get liver toxicity at this dosage.*

TABLE 7.1 *(Continued)*

NUTRIENT AND UNITS OF MEASUREMENT	RDA, OR "SAFE AND ADEQUATE"	UPPER SAFE LIMIT ON LONG-TERM USAGE	MY RECOM- MENDATION FOR SUPPLE- MENTATION	COMMENTS
folacin units = micrograms	men: 200 mcg. women: 180 mcg.	2,000 mcg.	800 mcg.	*50% to 90% lost in food processing*
pyridoxine (vitamin B6) units = milligrams	1.5 mg., both sexes	200 mg.	50 mg.	*Folacin, B6, and B12, taken together, reduce the blood's homocysteine level.*
vitamin B12 units = micrograms	2.4 mcg., both sexes	3,000 mcg.	200 mcg.	*Folacin, B6, and B12, taken together, reduce the blood's homocysteine level.*
pantothenic acid units = milligrams	4–7mg., both sexes	3,000 mg.	500 mg.	
biotin units = micrograms	30–100 mcg., both sexes	2,500 mcg.	300 mcg.	
calcium units = milligrams	<50 yrs., 1,000 mg. >50 yrs., 1,200 mg.	2,500 mg.	Enough to bring total intake to the RDA level	
magnesium units = milligrams	men: 420 mg. women: 320 mg.	800–1,000 mg.	500 mg.	*Average U.S. diet contains approxi- mately 250 mg.*
selenium units = micrograms	men: 70 mcg. women: 55 mcg.	toxic at over 800 mcg. (nail & hair loss, nerve damage)	200 mcg. to achieve can- cer-inhibitory effects	*Take one or two Brazil nuts per day.*
iron units = milligrams	men: 10 mg. women: 15 mg.	none estab- lished as level of "iron over- load" varies with person	none	*Has pro-oxidant effects: do not take any unless told to do so by your physician.*

TABLE 7.1 *(Continued)*

NUTRIENT AND UNITS OF MEASUREMENT	RDA, OR "SAFE AND ADEQUATE"	UPPER SAFE LIMIT ON LONG-TERM USAGE	MY RECOM-MENDATION FOR SUPPLE-MENTATION	COMMENTS
zinc units = milligrams	men: 15 mg. women: 12 mg.	50 mg.	limit any supplement to no more than 30 mg.	*Bioavailability quite variable; too much zinc over long period ◊ copper deficiency. One steamed oyster = 12 mg.*
manganese units = milligrams	2–5 mg., both sexes	< 10 mg.	RDA amount	
chromium units = micrograms	50–200 mcg.	1,000 mcg.	50 mcg.	*Chromium picolinate may be mutagenic (?); the nicotinate and chloride are not.*
?alpha lipoic acid	none	none established	120 mg.	
?acetyl-L-carnitine	none	none established	500 mg.	
bio-flavonoids units = milligrams	none	none established	250 to 500 mg.	
CoQ10 (fat soluble) units = milligrams	none	none established	100 mg.	
?SAMe units = milligrams	none	none established	200–400 mg.	
n-3 fatty acids (omega-3) units = milligrams	1,500 mg., both sexes	none	500–700 mg. of mixed EPA and DHA	*Skip on days when eat fish.*

* Total body sun exposure for 20 to 30 minutes is equivalent to an oral dose of about 10,000 IU vitamin D. (Beyond that time, there is no further manufacturre of the vitamin by the skin.) If you spend much time in the sun with your shirt off, no need for vitamin D supplementation.

effects: coenzyme Q10 (CoQ10), acetyl-L-carnitine, the omega-6 and omega-3 fatty acids, and several other materials, including a variety of phytochemicals. Most of these appear sufficiently promising to add to a supplement program, if one is inclined in that direction.

Table 7.1 gives the official RDAs (or, where these are not firmly established, what are referred to as "safe and adequate" dosages) for vitamins, minerals, and trace elements, and recommends an upper limit that I recommend not be exceeded, although it is still below the "toxic" level. The table also sets forth my personal recommendations for anyone on the CRON diet, assuming a relatively conservative approach to supplementation. In many cases, I judge the evidence interesting but not yet wholly convincing, in which case I have added a question mark (?). You must make your own choices about these.

I am far less certain about the entire field of supplementation than I am about the basic tenets of the CRON diet. The literature on supplementation is vast and frequently contradictory. You will perceive that my recommendations have continued changing, from my first book *Maximum Life Span*, in 1983, to the first edition of the present book, in 1986, to the third book, *The Anti-Aging Plan*, to now. The field itself continues to shift. Do not therefore be persuaded by promotional advertising or pseudoexperts to keep adding larger and larger amounts and different products to your list ad infinitum, nor be swayed on the other hand by the frequent overcautiousness of the establishment nutrition community. Supplements may add a modest benefit to the CRON diet, but not a great deal more on current evidence, and no combination of supplements will even approach the benefits of a low-calorie nutrient-dense CRON diet. Let's review the evidence.

VEGETABLES AND FRUITS AND OTHER FOODS

Most of the primary evidence pointing towards benefits connected with supplements, particularly the phytochemicals, is epidemiological and stems from the repeatedly confirmed observation that a population whose diet is high in vegetables and fruits, or certain other foods—fish, for example, or tomato products and olive oil—enjoys less cancer of various types, less cardiovascular disease, less diabetes, and so on. For example, a ten-year follow-up study of 48,000 middle-aged men indicated that among those consuming five or more servings per week of cruciferous vegetables (like broccoli, cauliflower, kale, Brussels sprouts), there was a 50 percent drop in the incidence of bladder cancer, whereas yellow, green-leafy, and carotene-rich vegetables conferred no protection.[5]

Following such an observation, scientists look to see what substances in the diets might be exerting the beneficial effects. It can be difficult to decide. There are, for example, about 600 different phytochemicals in plants, among which about 50 would be found in a normal diet. One must make an educated guess. One then tests the guess by giving an animal population (usually rats or mice) high doses of the selected material and seeing whether the incidence of cancer or other disease is reduced. One generally selects an inbred strain of rodent that is afflicted with a high incidence of the disease, carcinoma of the breast, for example. If the incidence is greatly reduced, one may go to a so-called "prospective" human study—which means you give the material to a lot of people for a long period and record what percentage develop, for example, breast cancer, compared to a population given merely a placebo.

The problem with this progression has been that sometimes everything seems to be working. The animal studies give positive results, then one arrives at the prospective human studies and one study gives positive and another negative results. The studies are enormously expensive to conduct and may be long-term, so a debate ensues. Aware of this, we will do as best we can in what follows.

It should also be recognized that whereas most experimental work has been with single nutrients or antioxidants at a very high intake (greater than tenfold above the RDA amount), the protective effects of a diet high in fruits and vegetables occurs at an intake in the range of two to threefold of the RDA amount.[6] Besides their beneficial effects on cancer and heart disease, the phytochemicals present in antioxidant rich foods (specifically spinach, strawberries, blueberries) have shown promise both in preventing and even reversing the course of neuronal and behavioral aging.[7] The most recent study in this series,[8] performed with 19-month-old rats (relatively old for a rat), which measured motor activity as ability to navigate on stationery or rotating rods, and other complex motor tasks, and cognitive ability via maze performance, found that the addition of blueberries to the diet in amounts that in humans would be equivalent to one cup per day, partially reversed the aging decrement in these tests. Even some reversal of age-related changes in the brain were observed on microscopic evaluation. Should everyone rush to the market for blueberries? In fact I have noticed that since this report came out, the blueberry racks are often empty.

ANTIOXIDANTS

Many of the substances listed below have antioxidant activity, but in this section we shall be concerned only with three: vitamin E, vitamin C, and lipoic acid.

VITAMIN E

Vitamin E has been lauded as the cure for sterility, old age, menstrual disorders, heart disease, diabetes, skin disease, and muscular dystrophy. None of this is true, but vitamin E does possess potential therapeutic benefits centering around its antioxidant properties. Vitamin E activity depends upon an "antioxidant network" involving other antioxidants and enzymes, which maintain vitamin E in its unoxidized state, where it can function to scavenge free radicals.[9] The most important maintainers are vitamin C and glutathione.

Once free radicals are unleashed, they tend to form a self-generating, self-damaging chain reaction. Vitamin E breaks the chain. It is the most significant fat-soluble chain-breaking antioxidant in human blood.[10]*

How about the effect of vitamin E on average and maximum life spans? As ever, this is for us a critical question. In lower animals such as worms and flies, it has been reported that maximum life span can be extended by the addition of vitamin E to the diet;[11] however, the interpretation of this data is not clear-cut.[12]*

How about mammals? At least three studies, including one by Dr. Denham Harman, the father and strongest proponent of the free radical theory of aging, have failed to show any effect of vitamin E on either average or maximum life span in mice.[13]

Despite the failure to affect life span in mammals, inclusion of substantial amounts of vitamin E in the diet will greatly slow up the accumulation of yellow-brown age pigment in the cells of the brain, heart, liver, and testes, [14,15]* an indication of an antioxidant benefit.

Larger than RDA doses of vitamin E beef up the immune response in humans, and increase the resistance of chickens, turkeys, sheep, and mice to infection.[16] In one experiment, doses of 5 to 20 units per kilogram of body weight per day of vitamin E injected into mice (equivalent to 350 to 1,400 units in a normal sized human) proved optimal in stimulating immune functions, but 80 units were inhibitory, and 400 units caused a fatal degeneration of the liver. The authors of this study concluded that a twofold increase in the *blood level* of vitamin E would yield optimal results with regard to immune function. We know that a tenfold increase of vitamin E in the diet is required to double the amount in human blood.[17] To achieve a twofold blood level would require supplementing a human diet with about 300 units of vitamin E per day. Other studies in humans agree with this figure as yielding optimal immune stimulation in humans.[18,19]*

Vitamin E is known to exert some cancer-inhibiting effects in experimental mice;[20,21]* and while the subject remains somewhat controversial, evidence based on epidemiologic studies plus a few intervention experiments in humans suggests that supplementation with vitamin E in humans in doses considerably in excess of the RDAs may decrease the risk of developing cardiovascular disease,[22] cancer,[23] particularly prostate cancer,[24] and cataracts.[25]

Vitamin E supplementation can partially protect experimental animals from chemical agents such as silver, mercury lead, carbon tetrachloride, and benzene, and very probably ozone, nitrogen dioxide, and paraquat.[26] Most of these toxicants act by stimulating free radical reactions. One of them, ozone, is a particularly important component of air pollution (smog). Lung damage begins at levels of 0.2 to 0.3 parts per million. The Environmental Protection Agency's acceptable daily maximum level is 0.1 parts per million.

There is no compelling reason for believing that vitamin E will slow down the basic aging process; but amounts quite a bit larger than the RDAs may render you less susceptible to several diseases and to chemical pollutants, and may slightly improve your general health for whatever number of years you do have to live. The only potential contraindication for high doses I know of is hypertension. Vitamin E interferes with platelet aggregation and may slightly increase the chance of a stroke in individuals with high blood pressure.

Vitamin E occurs naturally in eight forms. Your supplement program should include three of these: 100 to 200 milligrams of d-alpha tocopherol (not the dl-form), 100 to 200 milligrams of d-gamma/ mixed tocopherols, and 100 milligrams of tocotrienols. Vitamin E has important functions besides being an antioxidant, and these vary considerably with the form of the vitamin.[27] The d-alpha form is involved in the regulation of muscle cell proliferation in blood vessels; the d-gamma form (which is eliminated quite rapidly from the body) may be involved in reactions with nitric oxide, preventing the formation of the damaging peroxynitrite molecule;[28] the tocotrienols help reduce the level of cholesterol in the blood, as well as serving as antioxidants. You cannot obtain optimal amounts of all the forms of vitamin E except by supplementation.

VITAMIN C

As early as 1740, James Lind, conducting nutrition experiments on sailors in the British Royal Navy, demonstrated that scurvy could be prevented by a daily ration of fresh lime, lemon, or orange juice. Although his results were published in 1753, it was not until 1795, after 42 years of Royal Navy red tape and the loss of about 100,000 sailors' lives due to scurvy, that Lind's simple preventive measure became an official regulation for "men of war" sailors. England was the first nation to have warships on long voyages with crews free of scurvy, and Britannia began to "rule the waves." In fact, the British Empire was floated on fruit juice. Even so, the news did not get around fast enough. In the American Civil War, 30,000 Americans died of scurvy.

In the early 1930s, Dr. Albert Szent-Györgyi isolated in pure form from vegetables and fruits a chemical substance capable of curing scurvy. He called it ascorbic acid or vitamin C, and in 1937 he received the Nobel Prize for his discovery.

The turnover (the amount used in metabolism, which therefore must be either regenerated in the body or supplied from the food) of vitamin C is about 3 percent of the existing body pool per day.[29] It displays a number of functions besides being the primary water-soluble antioxidant obtained from food. Important in the body's manufacture of the components of connective tissue and bone matrix (hence the scurvy connection), vitamin C is also involved in the synthesis of carnitine, in brain metabolism, in the synthesis of adrenal cortical hormones, and possibly in the absorption of iron from the intestines.[30] If taken with food, 200 milligrams of vitamin C per day may double the amount of iron absorbed from food. This is undesirable unless you have an actual iron deficiency (usually showing up as an anemia) or are pregnant. (So don't take vitamin C with your meals, at least if you are not anemic and not pregnant!)

As for its antioxidant functions, vitamin C is an effective scavenger of a number of different free radicals, and protects against LDL and lipid peroxidation by regenerating the spent form of vitamin E back to the active form.[31] It also regenerates active forms of other antioxidants, including glutathione and the flavinoids (see below). Thus it is one of the central players in the "antioxidant network." It also functions inside the cell to protect DNA from oxidative damage.[32*] As a free radical scavenger or antioxidant, vitamin C acts both early, tending to inhibit the "initiation phase" of free radical production, and also later on as a water-soluble chain-breaking antioxidant.[33] But under certain conditions it may also have pro-oxidant properties, acting as a free radical itself. (Vitamin E is thought to counteract these pro-oxidant properties.[34])

While epidemiological evidence abounds that a vitamin C-rich diet is associated with reduced risks of cancers of the mouth, stomach, pancreas, lung, and breast (but not of colon, bladder, or prostate),[35] and while evidence exists for protection against cancer in animal models,[36*] in the limited intervention studies in humans where vitamin C has been given in large doses, no reduction in cancer incidence has been found.[37] The nagging question therefore occurs once again, is it the vitamin C or something else—something else that would be naturally present in a vitamin C-rich diet—that produces the beneficial anticancer effects in the epidemiological studies?

With regard to prevention of cardiovascular disease, we are on somewhat firmer ground.[38] A study at UCLA involving 11,348 men showed that those who took 800 milligrams of vitamin C per day lived an average of six years longer than those taking the RDA of 60 milligrams per day, death from cardiovascular disease was reduced in the high-dose takers by 42 percent, and the influence on overall mortality was greater than that associated with either blood cholesterol or fat intake.[39] And in test tube studies, vitamin C inhibits the oxidation of plasma LDL. By contrast, in the large, prospective Nurses' Health study involving many thousands of women, there was no significant correlation between vitamin C intake and coronary heart disease.[40] However, in the UCLA study dosage was found to be important. You need to take 500 milligrams or more daily!

Vitamin C has been reported to stimulate the immune system, although negative reports also exist. Giving old people vitamin C by injection for one month in amounts of 500 milligrams daily led to a substantial improvement in their immune response capacity.[41] In quantities from 500 milligrams to 3 grams per day, it was found to invigorate the proliferative response of the protective white blood cells known as lymphocytes.[42,43]

Very little work has been accomplished with vitamin C in relation to maximal life extension. In one study,[44] mega-doses decreased the average life span of guinea pigs; however, there was no significant effect on maximum life span. Large doses also decreased the average life span of fruit flies by 5 to 8 percent when present throughout the lifetimes of the flies.[45] But in some of the fruit fly experiments, when vitamin C was present only during adulthood, the survival was 5 percent longer than that of the controls. In a study in mice, large doses of vitamin C increased average life span.[46] Thus the life-span situation is unsettled, but certainly nothing remarkable has been reported.

Again, with vitamin C as with vitamin E, we are dealing with a scientific and pseudoscientific literature so profuse that you can select and arrange and interpret the reports to support almost any point of view. A lot of judgment is called for. My analysis leads me to recommend 500 milligrams of vitamin C, per day, along with modest quantities of bioflavonoids. (See Flavonoids below.) The vitamin C should be in the ester form and taken between meals.

LIPOIC ACID

Alpha-lipoic acid is a unique antioxidant in that it is both water and fat soluble. It plays a central role in the recycling of other antioxidants, boosts glutathione levels, chelates (neutralizes) damaging transition metals such as certain iron compounds, and is a critical factor in glucose metabolism. It has been shown to reverse the age-related decline in several mitochondrial functions, lower oxidative stress, and improve ambulatory activity in old rats.[47] Oxidative damage to proteins in normal and diabetic human tissues was reduced by lipoic acid.[48] Feeding old rats lipoic acid plus acetyl-L-carnitine for a period of weeks restored mitochondrial function and ambulatory activity and lowered the level of oxidants.[49] In one human trial alpha-lipoic acid improved glucose disposal in patients with maturity-onset diabetes.[50]

PHYTOCHEMICALS

FLAVONOIDS

Dr. Albert Szent-Györgyi, of vitamin C fame, discovered flavonoids in extracts from red peppers and lemons, and presented evidence that they potentiate the action of vitamin C and improve the condition of the walls of tiny blood vessels. No known diseases are associated with their absence.

A large group (more than 500) of poorly soluble compounds found widely in plants, the flavonoids in many instances possess antioxidant properties that serve to protect vitamin C and other plant compounds from oxygenation.[51*] They have been shown to have anticancer activity in animal models, inhibit the growth of some varieties of cancer cells in the test tube, to some extent inhibit the action of chemicals that cause mutations in cells, and may have some effects against cardiovascular disease.[52,53] Among the flavonoids, quercetin has been the most studied. It is present in large quantities in red grapes, especially the seeds, in onions, oranges, tea, and broccoli.[54] Other flavonoids include pro- and anthocyanin (in grapes, cranberries, and red wine), and naringin (in citrus fruits). The seeds and skins of grapes are exceptionally rich in proanthocyanidins, which, when bound together and known as oligomeric proanthocyanidin complexes—the extract is known as Pycnogenol, which may also be found in pine bark—are particularly powerful antioxidants, even more so than vitamins C and E.

Flavonoids are everywhere in nature. They comprise the pigments present in fruits and vegetables: yellow in citrus fruits, red and blue in berries. They are present in the skins, peels, and outer layers of lemons, grapes, plums, grapefruit, and apricots. The white, soft, fleshy part inside lemons and oranges is rich in flavonoids (in contrast to the juice, which is not). Onions with colored skins are exceptionally rich. A typical mixed diet might contain up to one gram of flavonoids, of which probably only half would be absorbable. In a concentrated form (as propolis, the brownish waxy substance collected from tree buds by bees and used by them to caulk the hives), flavonoids have been much employed in folk medicine, but not much investigated by orthodox medicine. In the meantime, they are responsible in part for the colors of autumn foliage, of flowers, and the bark of trees. They want to be noticed!

Recent evidence suggests that the flavonoids in blueberries may have special effects.[55] In amounts in old rodents equivalent to one cup of blueberries per day in humans, the rodents performed better on a number of tests, including memory and physical function tests, and some reversal of age-related changes in the brain were observed on microscopic evaluation.

The amount of vitamin C you take as a supplement should be matched with about half as much flavonoids. There are no reported toxic effects; however, commercial forms of flavonoids are sometimes processed in such a way as to render them almost wholly unabsorbable. Unfortunately product information on absorbability is usually not available.

PHYTOESTROGENS

Phytoestrogens are plant substances that have a weak estrogenic effect. By getting there first, however, they may block the action of natural estrogen.

Isoflavones These are present particularly in soy products, either cooked or uncooked. Genistein and daidzein are two examples. The isoflavones are converted in the body into products that have weak estrogenic activity, and part of their effect is considered due to interference with binding to those parts of the cell membrane (the "estrogen receptors") that allow estrogen itself to exert its effect to the estrogen receptor(s) on cells. Abundant epidemiological and animal model evidence indicates that diets rich in soy are inhibitory to breast cancer development.[56] Evidence for inhibition of development of prostate and colon cancer as well as osteoporosis and heart disease (lowering of cholesterol and triglycerides) is weaker, but some does exist.[57, 58] High intake of soy protein may lead to lower plasma cholesterol and heart disease risk.[59] Genistein and soy products do exert beneficial effects in osteoporotic patients. However, several large prospective studies failed to confirm a protective effect against prostate cancer.[60, 61]

Sounds good, but quite a disquieting epidemiologic report involving 17,000 men followed for over 30 years in Hawaii presented evidence that regular consumption of tofu for many years in midlife adversely affects brain aging, as manifested by accelerated atrophy and decline in thinking ability.[62] At time of final testing, the subjects were 71 to 93 years old. I am reluctant to believe these results, but the study appears well done. If borne out, isoflavones may exert both beneficial and harmful effects, the situation would remind one of antagonistic pleiotropy (see note 56, Chapter 3).

Lignans These phytoestrogens behave similarly to the above and their richest source is flax seed. Whole-grain foods, berries, and certain root crop are also good sources of lignans.[63]

ISOTHIOCYANATES

Present mainly in cruciferous vegetables, the isothiocyanates have been shown in many animal studies to inhibit experimental cancer development, providing they are given at about the same time as the animal is exposed to the chemical carcinogen.[64] They act upon the metabolic pathways that "activate" or detoxify the carcinogen, and eliminate it. The best known isothiocyanate, sulforaphane, is present especially in broccoli, and is much more abundant in broccoli sprouts than in the mature plant.[65] Best to sprout your own, as those obtained in markets spoil much faster than other sprouts! Epidemiologically the isothiocyanates appear to exert a protective effect against cancers of the gastrointestinal and respiratory tracts in humans.[66]

DIALLYLSULFIDES

Members of the allium vegetable family, which include garlic, onion, leeks, and chives, show in most (but not all) epidemiological studies a protective effect against cancer of the stomach and colon. Cooking destroys the effect in onions, not in garlic. In animal studies, garlic alters the incidence of tumors caused by those chemical carcinogens that require "activation" by the enzymes of the body, and reduces nitrosamine carcinogenesis. The water-soluble components of garlic may inhibit initiation of tumors by chemicals, but have no effect against established tumors; however, oil-soluble garlic compounds (diallylsulfides) may actually reduce proliferation of cancer cells.[67]

THE CHEMICALS OF TEA

Convincing evidence exists in studies of experimental animals and of cells grown in flasks in the laboratory, that tea, especially the polyphenols of green tea, decreases susceptibility to cancer.[68] Epidemiologic studies in humans remain equivocal, possibly due to dosages, since over ten cups of tea per day may be required to manifest a significant effect in humans for cancer,[69] for cardiovascular and liver effects, for lowering of cholesterol and triglycerides, and for an increase in HDL.[70] Again, it is tempting but uncertain to go from epidemiology, i.e., from associations, to causality. Possibly the lifestyle, including other food patterns that go with tea-drinking cultures, are responsible for the observed phenomenon. The tea-drinking Japanese have a low incidence of certain diseases that the tea-drinking British are prone to develop. To put it another way, the tea-drinking Japanese have black hair and a low incidence of certain diseases, but we do not attribute the low incidence of hypertension among the Japanese to the black hair. Epidemiology is a good pointer, but insufficient by itself to prove a hypothesis.

Recent evidence does suggest a mechanism whereby tea might suppress tumor growth. *Angiogenesis* is a process of blood-vessel growth required for tumors to grow and spread to organs other than the organ primarily involved. One of the chemicals of green tea appears to suppress such growth.[71]

Catechins, of which there are six different kinds in green tea,[72] are the most potent of the phytochemicals present in green tea (green tea extract is 35 percent catechin; black tea is 6 percent), but many other compounds also contribute to the beneficial effects. Green tea appears to augment the antioxidant defenses of the body, inducing an increase in catalase, SOD, and glutathione enzymes, all of which are major antioxidants made in and by the body.

It is worth mentioning that steeping tea for three to four minutes minutes is enough to get all the antioxidants in the beverage. Prolonged steeping releases oxalates, a component in three-quarters of kidney stones.

CAROTENES

Does a bowl of carrots every day keep cancer away? Since the principal relationship is with lung cancer,[73] it was once thought (incorrectly, as we shall see) that what kept the inveterate pipe-smoking Popeye from developing that terrible malady was his high consumption of carotene-rich spinach. The dark yellow-to-red vegetables and fruits (but not citrus fruits or berries) and dark green, leafy vegetables are carotene-rich: carrots, spinach, mustard greens, collard greens, broccoli, squashes, apricots, kale, beets, cantaloupe, and (in Brazil and West Africa) red palm oil. Carrots were first cultivated in Afghanistan, where ancient cults who worshipped the sun thought orange foods brought virtue. Levels of some of the principal carotenes in different foods are shown in Table 7.2.

Just as bioflavonoids are responsible for the color of autumn foliage, carotenes are partly responsible for the colors of birds and flowers, and for the yellow tint to animal and human fat. They are hydrophobic (water hating), so interact with the lipid portions of the cell, i.e., the membrane and fat globules inside, where they serve (1) to quench the radical known as singlet oxygen, and (2) can be either antioxidant or pro-oxidant, but under physiologic conditions are mainly antioxidant.

Beta-carotene is the strongest available antioxidant for the free radical known as *singlet oxygen*,[74] a very damaging form, being both mutagenic and peroxidizing.[75] In fact, the carotenes are manufactured by plants to protect them against the singlet oxygen produced as a by-product of the interactions of light and chlorophyll. In food, they exist either as solutions in the oil of the food, or within the matrices of vegetables or fruits, and so are not very bioavailable unless the matrix has been disrupted by cooking. (The carotenes are heat stable.)

Of the 400 or so known carotenes, about 30 are found in human plasma, including most notably those shown in Table 7.2. The most common of the carotenes, beta-carotene is not a conventional antioxidant like vitamins E, C, and selenium. Although it may complement the action of vitamin E[76] it is in quite another class. It is present in highest amounts in carrots, sweet potatoes, cantaloupes, and pumpkins.[77] A portion of the ingested beta-carotene may be converted to vitamin A, but only upon demand. Too much vitamin A is known to be toxic, but beta-carotene itself is virtually nontoxic.[78] Only a few milligrams per day are consumed in the average diet, but an average 160-pound man can handle up to 3 grams safely.[79] Of course, if the intake is high enough, one's skin will acquire a definite orange tint, especially the palms of the hands; but this effect is harmless and will disappear if the carotene intake is reduced to normal for some weeks. Because we ate a huge amount of sweet potatoes inside Biosphere 2, we crew members came out at the end of two years tinted pale orange.

The carotenes have received attention for the possibility of reducing the risks of certain types of cancer, cardiovascular diseases, and macular degeneration of the eye (the most frequent cause of blindness in older persons).[80,81] While there is evidence for an inverse association between intake of beta-carotene plus other carotenes and the occurrence of lung cancer in nonsmokers, as well as the risks for prostate, breast, and head and neck cancers, for cardiovascular disease, and macular degeneration, there is also a rather indecipherable mixture of positive and negative reports on all these issues.[82]

Some epidemiological studies have shown an inverse ratio between intake and plasma levels of beta-carotene and lung cancer among nonsmokers; but in smokers, supplementation with beta-carotene actually *increases* the risk of lung cancer.[83,84] To complicate things, a prospective study of beta-carotene supplementation by 22,000 apparently healthy male physicians showed no protection against development of lung cancer or any other disease.[85,86]

Proceeding now to other carotene antioxidants (See Table 7.2), we note that alpha-carotene is contained in the highest amount in carrots and pumpkins.[87] It is considered the main contender as protector against lung carcinoma in nonsmokers. Lutein, the carotene that may inhibit macular degeneration, is present in highest amounts in collard greens, kale, and both raw and cooked spinach. Popeye would have had good eyes!

Our final carotene, lycopene, is found in highest concentration in cooked tomatoes, including tomato sauce and paste, although present in lesser amounts in pink grapefruit, watermelon, and raw tomatoes.[88] Lycopene comprises about one-half the carotenes in human plasma. Vitamin E is required to potentiate its effects, but it is a considerably stronger antioxidant than beta-carotene. The benefits of the Mediterranean diet could in fact be due to lycopene rather than, for example, olive oil and/or fish oil. There is epidemiological evidence for protection by lycopene against cancer of the prostate, lung, breast, and stomach.[89,90]

Having said the above, I must add that a recent and thorough review of the relation of the carotenes to disease prevention is that of D.A. Cooper,[91] which considers cancers of the prostate, breast, head and neck, and lung, as well as heart disease and macular degeneration. Except for the lungs, the review concludes that none of the associations hold up very well when the totality of the evidence is considered. Something looks good, but another study contradicts it. In short, the jury is still out.

TABLE 7.2 *Amounts of carotenoids in various carotene-rich foods (values are in milligrams) (Source: U.S. Dept. of Agriculture/NCI Carotinoid Database)*

FRUIT/ VEGETABLE	ALPHA CAROTENE (MG.)	BETA CAROTENE (MG.)	B-CRYPTO XANTHIN (MG.)	LUTEIN/ZEA XANTHIN (MG.)	LYCOPENE (MG.)
Apricot halves, 6 dried	0	3.7	0	0	0.2
Beet greens, ½ cup cooked	0	1.8	0	4.9	0
Broccoli, ½ cup cooked	0	1.0	0	1.4	0
Cantaloupe, 1 cup chunks	0.1	4.8	0	0	0
Carrot, 1 medium raw	2.6	5.7	0	0.2	0
Collard greens, ½ cup cooked	0	3.5	0	10.4	0
Grapefruit, pink, ½ medium	0	1.6	0	0	4.1
Kale, ½ cup cooked	0	3.1	0	14.2	0
Mango, 1 medium	0	2.7	0.1	0	0
Mustard greens, ½ cup cooked	0	2.0	0	7.4	0
Orange, 1 medium	0	0.1	0.2	0	0
Papaya, ½ medium	0	0.2	1.1	0	0
Pepper, red, ½ raw	0	0.8	0	2.5	0
Pumpkin, ½ cup cooked	4.7	3.8	0	1.8	0
Romaine lettuce, 1 cup	0	1.1	0	3.2	0
Spinach, ½ cup cooked	0	5.0	0	11.3	0
Spinach, ½ cup raw	0	2.3	0	5.7	0
Squash, butternut ½ cup	2.2	9.2	0	0	0
Sweet potato, ½ cup mashed	0	14.4	0	0	0
Tangerine, 1 medium	0	0	0.9	0	0
Tomato, 1 medium	0	0.6	0	0.1	3.8
Tomato paste, 5 tablespoons	0	1.0	0	0	2.3
Tomato sauce, ½ cup	0	1.2	0	0.2	7.7
Watermelon, 1 cup cubed	0	0.4	0	0	6.6

Should we be taking supplemental carotenes? As noted above, evidence for the many beneficial effects claimed remains indecisive, and the carotenes have never been tested for possible influences on life span, although beta-carotene blood levels are higher in the longer-living species.[92] But free radicals are very likely involved in the genesis of cancer, possibly in aging; the carotenes, including beta-carotene, fill a unique place among those antioxidants normally present in our food supply, and are so far as is known virtually nontoxic. You must make up your own mind as to carotene supplementation. For me, choices made from Table 7.2 provide enough carotenes that I do not supplement further.

SELENIUM

Named for the moon (*Selene* in Greek), selenium was discovered by a Swedish chemist in 1817 in the lead chamber deposits in a sulfuric acid-manufacturing plant. He could hardly have foreseen that one day scientists would be investigating Earth's seventieth most abundant element as a "trace mineral" in preventing disease.

In 1973 selenium was identified as a component of one of the body's major natural antioxidant enzymes, glutathione peroxidase,[93]* which breaks down hydrogen peroxide and the peroxides derived from fatty acids. These peroxides lead to free radical formation if not attended to. Selenium itself (that is, not in the enzyme combination) is also a metabolic antagonist to mercury, lead, cadmium, and arsenic. It combines with and is eliminated along with them.[94]

Still a third way that selenium acts in the body is to influence the so-called "p-450" enzyme systems. In daily contact with simple organic poisons such as gasoline, benzene, naphthol, and naturally occurring organic materials from the environment, the body manufactures the p-450 enzymes to transform these intruder chemicals into forms that can be readily excreted. [95]* (The immune system takes care of eliminating unwanted large complex organic molecules, whereas small organic molecules are handled by the p-450 enzymes.)

And finally, selenium acts to bolster the apoptosis of cancer cells. (*Apoptosis* is the fancy biological term for cell suicide.) One of the ways the body fights off cancer is to induce the abnormal cells to self-suicide. Selenium potentiates this.

While selenium is essential for mammals, plants are indifferent to it. If there is none in the soil, plants still grow tall and strong. If the soil is rich, they will soak it up, but generally not to a concentration above 30 parts per million. A few plants, milk vetch, woody aster, and golden weed, known as "selenium accumulators," can acquire concentrations of 1,000 to 10,000 parts per million. These accumulators are no direct threat to humans since we don't eat them, but they can cause the devastating "alkali disease" and "blind staggers" in foraging animals, which wander in circles, stumbling over objects, become emaciated, and finally die. Agricultural runoff water from selenium-rich soil, repeatedly discharged into the 66,000 acre Grasslands Conservation District of California, built up the selenium there and killed a great deal of the wildlife.

Although organ meats and seafood are rich sources of selenium (0.5 to 1.5 micrograms/grams), the amount of total selenium in our food supply can be small or moderate depending most particularly on the soil where the food is grown. Where the soil is selenium deficient, higher incidences of colonic, rectal, and mammary cancer, and (possibly) heart disease occur. On the other hand, we are not apt to eat excessive amounts of selenium, as we do not consume the plant accumulators. Among plants we do eat, potatoes, tomatoes, carrots, cabbage, and especially onions and garlic take up the most selenium from the soil, although it is much less than that in meats and seafoods. Of the things we eat, Brazil nuts are by far the richest source of selenium: one medium-sized nut contains 100 micrograms of selenium.

Half a loaf of bread made from grain grown in the United States could contain from 12 to as much as 200 micrograms of selenium. Examples of the differing selenium levels in plants and dairy and other animal products from high and low areas are shown in Table 7.3. Plants grown in South Dakota, Wyoming, New Mexico, or Utah are good sources. Texas, Oklahoma, Louisiana, Alabama, Nebraska, and Kansas are also selenium-rich states. Connecticut, Illinois, Ohio, Oregon, Massachusetts, Rhode Island, New York, Pennsylvania, Indiana, Delaware, and the District of Columbia tend to be low, as are the states of Washington and Oregon and parts of Montana. Of course in today's market, vegetables may come from afar, so it's hard to tell your local situation exactly.

Will a higher than normal selenium intake extend life span? A few studies in which the element was present along in the diet with other antioxidants showed prolongation of average, but only marginally of maximum, life span. Other studies have shown only a slight effect or none.[96,97]*

TABLE 7.3 (A) *Selenium content of various foods from areas where the soil is either poor (Maryland) or rich (South Dakota, Venezuela) in selenium; and* (B) *average selenium content of different food groups in an area where soil is poor in selenium (Maryland) (adapted from B. Liebman,* Nutrition Action, *December, 1983)*

A		SELENIUM (MCG)		B		
FOOD	AMNT.	POOR SOIL	RICH SOIL	FOOD	AMNT.	SELENIUM (MCG)
Carrots, raw	1	1.8 to	105.4	Vegetables	1 serving	1.6
Cabbage, shredded	½ cup	1.8 to	316.6	Fruit	2 servings	0.9
Onion, raw & chopped	½ cup	1.3 to	1,513	Grains & Cereals	1 serving	12.3
Potato, raw	1 large	1.0 to	235.0	Dairy & Eggs	1 serving	3.6
Tomato, raw	1 large	0.7 to	164.7	Sugar	1 tsp.	0.2
American cheese	1.5 oz.	3.8 to	17.9	Seafood	4 oz.	37.8
Swiss cheese	1.5 oz.	4.5 to	16.0	Beef, Pork,		
Egg	1 large	4.8 to	86.6	Lamb & Chicken	4 oz.	22.7
Milk, whole	1 cup	2.9 to	28.1	Organ meats	4 oz.	149.6
Chicken breast	4 oz.	13.1 to	79.3			
Pork chop	4 oz.	27.0 to	94.1			

While no anti-aging effect has been proved, the evidence for selenium's effect on cancer susceptibility is abundant and rather convincing. This may be more due to the apoptosis potentiation than the antioxidant activity. In any case, substantial selenium increases in the diets of animals do decrease the susceptibility to developing both spontaneous cancer and chemically induced cancers, including cancers of the liver, skin, mammary glands, pancreas, and colon.[98,99]

Because of the usual conflicts of different studies, we do not have unequivocal evidence for humans, but the inferential and population evidence is quite strong that high selenium intake leads to lower cancer susceptibility. Also, in a recent well-controlled prospective study of 1,400 persons, the administration of 200 micrograms of organic selenium (selenium-yeast) was associated with a 37 percent drop in total cancer incidence: 63 percent for the prostate, 58 percent for colorectal cancer, and 46 percent for lung.[100]

Figure 7.1 shows that when the populations of different countries are compared, high selenium intake correlates with low incidences of breast cancer. And in the United States itself, when the selenium in the blood of people from different regions is compared with the overall cancer death rates in those regions, the death rates are lower when the selenium content is higher.[101]*

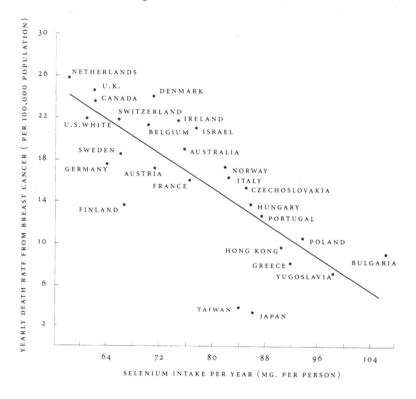

FIGURE 7.1 Relation between intake of selenium and death rate from cancer of the breast

What about dosages and possible toxicity at higher-than-average intakes? And which forms of selenium should one use, organic or inorganic?

There is no distinct RDA but the officially recommended "safe and adequate" range is given as 50 to 200 micrograms daily. If you are from a high-selenium state, you are probably getting well over 100 micrograms but not 200. If from a low-selenium state, you are probably getting less than 100 micrograms daily, which is suboptimal. One way to resolve the issue is to have your doctor test your blood selenium level. The normal value is 15 to 25 micrograms, and you're better off if you're on the high side. To maintain that level would in most cases require supplementing your diet with either 100 or 200 micrograms per day, depending on where you live. That's one or two Brazil nuts.

The officially recommended "maximum" intake is 400 micrograms per day. Japanese fishermen consume more than 500 micrograms per day without apparent detriment. Though the inhabitants of one county in China developed severe toxic symptoms after consuming 5,000 micrograms a day, the inhabitants of another Chinese county have consumed 750 micrograms a day for many years, and apparently remained healthy.[102] As you perceive, there is leeway, but not a great deal, between the amount for maximum potential benefit and possible toxicity. In the United States the toxic level is regarded as 800 micrograms per day. Better stay well below that, including dietary and supplement sources.

The organic form of selenium is generally considered both less toxic than at least one of the inorganic forms (selenite), and at the same time to yield a greater increase in blood selenium,[103] but there is conflicting evidence. Whereas in one study[104] two parts per million of selenite (equivalent to 1,200 micrograms per day in a human) proved extremely toxic to young rats, another study[105] in rodents found anticancer activity and no toxicity of selenite (an inorganic form) at a level as high as 6 parts per million. But that much inorganic selenium would cause severe liver damage. In view of this controversy, I recommend either an approximately one to one mixture of organic and inorganic selenium, the latter as either selenite or selanate or both,[106*] or else all in the form of so-called selenium-yeast.

B-VITAMINS: B5 (PANTOTHENIC ACID), B6 (PYRIDOXINE), FOLACIN, AND B12

Derived from the Greek word *panthothen*, which means *from every side*, pantothenic acid is found in many different foods, including whole grains, animal products, and vegetables. It is nontoxic in that as much as 10 to 20 grams daily (over a thousand times the ordinary intake) may cause only "occasional diarrhea and water retention." [107] Rich sources are liver, kidney, yeast, egg yolk, and broccoli (50 micro grams per gram), and royal bee jelly (500 micrograms per gram). About 50 percent is lost in cooking.

Pantothenic acid is central to the energy-yielding oxidation of glucose products via activities in the mitochondria, and in the synthesis of many essential molecules, including membrane lipids, methionine, and a host of others.

In the only recorded longevity experiment with pantothenic acid, mice of a basically long-lived strain were given 0.3 milligrams per day in their drinking water (equivalent to about 700 milligrams for an average human). While the control animals survived an average of 550 days, the pantothenic acid-fed mice, both males and females, lived 653 days, a 19 percent increase in average life span.[108] Maximum life spans were unfortunately not recorded. In these experiments the mouse strain was long-lived, but the laboratory conditions were not optimal; in my laboratory at UCLA, the average life span of mice of the same strain is well over 800 days.[109] Nevertheless, I would attach at least some significance to this early life-span study, although it ought to be repeated under modern conditions.

Large doses of pantothenic acid may augment the ability to withstand stress, as shown by seeing how long rats can swim in cold water (39 degrees Fahrenheit) before sinking. In one such experiment, rats on pantothenic acid lasted 62 minutes; those on a normal intake, 29 minutes.[110] Correspondingly, when men were immersed in cold water and their blood tested for certain chemical agents, those individuals who had been given large doses of pantothenic acid (10 grams daily) for six weeks prior to exposure showed improved adaptation to the stress. [111]

While little or no further work has been done on pantothenic acid in relation to aging since the above early studies, the fact that CRON may well produce its effects by upregulating all the anti-stress mechanisms of the body renders the early work on pantothenic acid worth our continued attention.

Increased serum levels of vitamin B6, folic acid, and vitamin B12 (all three) are associated with decreased levels of homocysteine, and a significantly reduced risk of coronary heart disease.[112,113] Homocysteine is now recognized as a risk factor in heart disease, probably more so than the better known blood lipids (cholesterol, LDL, HDL, triglycerides). You do not want a high homocysteine level! In the Nurses' Health Study, in which about 80,000 women were followed for 14 years, those with high folic acid levels had 47 percent less heart disease than those with the lowest, and every 200 microgram increase was associated with an 11 percent reduction.[114] Roughly similar percentages were observed for vitamin B6.

The concentration of vitamin B6 in the human body declines with age, and more than 20 percent of persons over 65 years of age may be vitamin B6 deficient. Chemical studies of the brains of senescent mice indicate a vitamin B6 deficiency.[115] In other gerontologic studies, vitamin B6 (pyridoxine) was found to increase the average life span of fruit flies.[116] Inclusion of vitamin B6 in the amount of 100 milligrams per killogram per day, in the drinking water of a long-lived strain of mice, and beginning at 18 months of age (mid- or late middle age for mice), increased their average life span by 11 percent. But this dosage would be quite a toxic level for humans. Finally, 20-month-old, vitamin B6 treated mice performed better than untreated mice of the same age in a test situation perceived by them as dangerous and requiring quick action.

A word of caution about vitamin B6! Severe toxic manifestations were seen in seven young adults after daily ingestion of 2 to 6 grams of vitamin B6 for 2 to 40 months: difficulty in walking, tingling sensations in the extremities, and other manifestations of central-nervous-system effects.[117] Of course these dosages were massive, but sensory nerve disease, ataxia (difficulty in walking), and liver injury may develop with vitamin B6 intakes greater than 500 milligrams per day. However, little or no toxic effects have been observed at doses up to 200 milligrams daily over periods of many months. Fifty to 100 milligrams should be the upper supplementation limit.

COQ10

Coenzyme Q10, or CoQ10, acts like a vitamin, although it can be manufactured by the body and does not have to be obtained from the diet. Essential in certain large enzyme complexes, it is itself a small molecule that carries electrons from the inside of membranes to the outside, where it releases them to another complex. This process is called *electron transport*, a sort of Flying Tigers airline in the cell. CoQ10 is an essential part of the membranes of the energy factories of the cell. Thus it plays a critical role in the respiratory chain providing energy for life. It also displays antioxidant activity.[118,119]

In 1981 Emile Bliznakov reported that when 17-month-old mice (equivalent to 50- to 60-year-old humans) were injected weekly with 50 micrograms of CoQ10, their average survival was another 11 months, compared to merely five months of the uninjected control mice.[120] This amounted to an 18 percent extension of average survival measured from time of birth, or 56 percent if figured from time when the injections began. Maximum life span for control mice was 26 months; for the injected mice, 36 months—an extension of 40 percent if considered from time of birth, or of 210 percent if from time of injection. However, we note again that, besides the smallness of the population size, the maximum life span of the mouse species was not exceeded. This often cited study, long overdue for confirmation, was finally re-examined (with both mice and rats) in the 1990s over a seven-year period of intense focus on the gerontologic aspects of CoQ10 by K. Linnrot.[121] A life-time of oral administration of CoQ10, while causing throughout life a two- to threefold increase in the plasma and liver concentrations, had no effect on average or maximum life spans of the rodents. Linnrot believes from an earlier publication of Bliznakov that he may have been using a CoQ10-deficient strain of mouse, which if so would invalidate the conclusions of the study. Linnrot also found that despite the elevated levels in blood and liver, levels in other organs, including heart and brain, were not increased in either rodents or humans (spinal fluid for humans), nor was there any prevention of the accumulation of the yellow-brown pigment (so-called "age pigment") in the heart and other tissues so characteristic of the aging process. The only apparently beneficial activity was an improvement in arterial tone in old rodents.[122*] The thorough and in-depth review of the literature—by Linnrot as part of his thesis study[123]—detailed a plethora of scientific publications dealing with use of CoQ10 to treat heart disease, hypertension, and other maladies . . . with conflicting results. But finally, the most recent studies—and by a very astute group of investigators[124]—suggest that CoQ10 may well be beneficial in prevention and treatment of neurodegenerative disease, and that levels in the brains of rats, and therefore presumably humans, can in fact be raised by oral administration.

CARNITINE AND ACETYL-L-CARNITINE

Carnitine is a transport chemical required for the passage of fatty acids across membranes of the cells' energy factories, the mitochondria. Mammals can generally synthesize their own, using the amino acids lysine and methionine present in a normal diet, but carnitine itself can be absorbed directly and used by the body. Meat and dairy products are the major sources. The redder the meat, the higher the carnitine content. Cereals, fruits, and vegetables contain very little. Acetyl-L-carnitine functions similarly to carnitine but is absorbed into the bloodstream more efficiently, passes more effectively through cell membranes, and is utilized more efficiently in the mitochondria of the cell, than carnitine itself.

About a 40 percent reduction in certain functions of heart mitochondria occurs with age in rats, corresponding to the 40 percent reduction in cardiolipin, a key (phospholipid) compound. Treatment with acetyl-L-carnitine restored the cardiolipin to the level of young rats, as well as the other mitochondrial functions.[125] In another study in rats, various aspects of mitochondrial function in old rats were improved by acetyl-L-carnitine;[126] however, the "efficiency" of electron transport was not improved. In still another study, acetyl-L-carnitine fed to old rats partially restored mitochondrial function and improved the ambulatory activity of the old rats (who generally just sit around), but seemed to increase free radical production per amount of oxygen consumed.[127] Thus, it appears to improve function but at the same time to increase oxidative stress, a bit like burning the candle at both ends. It is claimed, however, that the oxidative stress can be obviated by including lipoic acid along with the acetyl-L-carnitine supplementation.[128] All these studies are quite recent.

In older experiments, a variety of beneficial effects were claimed for carnitine in both animals and man—for example, an improved stress tolerance in damaged heart muscle in humans [129]—and antifatigue effects in healthy individuals who suffered lack of oxygen during prolonged muscle effort.[130] In an old and only briefly reported experiment, in rats given 50 milligrams of carnitine per kilogram per day beginning at 25 months of age, 70 percent of the treated animals but only 43 percent of the controls were still alive by 28 months.[131] In addition, the treated rats showed distinct improvement in a mental test and a significant increase in cardiac work ability. Of course this experiment needs confirmation.

FATTY ACIDS: THE N-6S (OMEGA-6S) AND N-3S (OMEGA-3S)

First a short lesson in organic chemistry about the nomenclature of the essential fatty acids. The commonest, called arachidonic acid, is written as $C20:4,n-6$. That means it has 20 carbon atoms (all in a row), for the most part with a single bond between them (written as C-C) except for four double bonds (C=C), and the first of these double bonds joins the sixth and seventh carbon atoms. That's what $C20:4,n-6$ means. The other three double bonds occur, for all the fatty acids in question, at every third carbon atom, so arachidonic acid could be written as $C20:4,n-6,9,12,15$; but since every third atom is characteristic for all the unsaturated fatty acids, we don't have to write their positions in, just for the first one. Now, since there is more than one double bond in the fatty acids we are discussing, they are called *polyunsaturated fatty acids*, commonly known as PUFAs, as opposed to MUFAs (monounsaturated fatty acids) such as olive oil and canola oil, or the saturated fatty acids like myristic and palmitic acid ($C14:0$ and $C16:0$), which will increase your cholesterol if you take too much of them (animal fat, butter, cheese). End of chemistry lesson!

The eicosanoids are members of a family of 20-carbon PUFAs derived largely from the oxygenation of the PUFAs we can designate as C20:3n-6, C20:4n-6, and C20:5n-3—each of which yields different eicosanoids. The oxygenation might continue as a "chain reaction," but vitamin E breaks the chain and saves the day. The most important PUFA is the C20:4n-6 fatty acid known as arachidonic acid.

The major eicosanoids contribute to a large range of physiologic functions. They are involved in cardiovascular, pulmonary, immune, reproductive, and secretory activities. They are important structural parts of cell membranes. But some of the later, down-the-line products of these eicosanoids, products like prostaglandin and thromboxane, are pro-inflammatory materials, useful in reacting to inflammatory agents but potentially harmful if in excess. Thus, overproduction of C20:4n-6-derived eicosanoids may potentiate the development of self-inflammatory and autoimmune diseases, like certain forms of arthritis, and lupus erythematosus.[132]

Eicosanoids made from n-3 PUFAs compete with those from the n-6 PUFAs in most or all of the above, but they are less active, particularly in the pro-inflammatory area. They tend to decrease any predilection for autoimmunity, lower blood cholesterol moderately and triglycerides markedly,[133,134] and help prevent heart disease, as well as some forms of hypertension (those forms associated with increase in the renin hormone). And at least in short-lived strains of mice, the combination of n-3 PUFAs and calorie restriction increases life span more than calorie restriction alone.[135]

The right ratio of n-6 to n-3 PUFAs is what you want in your diet. In the average American diet the ratio is about ten to one. A ratio of four to one is what is recommended for best health.[136,137] So you probably need more n-3s, and the best source is fish or—in terms of supplements—fish oil.[138] Vegetable oils may also contain PUFAs, but the ratio for many is not good; for example, in safflower oil it is 255 to 1. As for total quantities, 1 to 4 percent of your total calorie intake should be from n-6 PUFAs, and 0.3 to 1 percent from n-3 PUFAs. The rest of your fats should be mostly MUFAs, like olive or canola oil.

SAMe

SAMe is the accustomed shorthand for S-adenosyl-L-methionine. It is fundamentally important in reactions involed in nucleic acid and protein synthesis and to cell membrane fluidity and function. It is made in the body but can be absorbed and increased by oral administration. It prevents depletion of glutathione, one of the most important antioxidants in the body, which reduces the free radical activity of hydrogen peroxide and the organic peroxides and protects cells from oxidative damage. If you decide to take it, do so at the same time as the B vitamins listed above. Dosage would be 200 to 400 milligrams per day. (It is worth noting here that a CRON diet has been shown to increase glutathione in rodents.[139])

HORMONES: GROWTH HORMONE, DHEA, MELATONIN

I am not yet persuaded by the advocates of growth hormone. They must do their homework better. Body fat is redistributed, but the other claimed benefits have not been demonstrated to my satisfaction. It is direct and easy (but time consuming) to do animal studies, where mice or rats are given long-term growth treatment. The only two studies I am aware of in rodents (see Chapter 6) gave contrasting results, as have double-blind studies in humans. The evidence is not in my view sufficient to justify treatment with a powerful and potentially dangerous hormone. Growth hormone increases IGF-1, the so-called "insulinlike growth factor," which exerts multiple insulinlike metabolic effects, including increase in blood sugar, inhibition of lipolysis, and retardation of protein breakdown.[140] These effects seem undesireable. On current evidence one can argue either way, as illustrated by the article by Bartke et al.[141] entitled "Does growth hormone prevent or accelerate aging?"

It also troubles me that in the only age-retardation regime that really works, i.e., calorie restriction (everyone in gerontology agrees on this— it is indeed the only regime that works), growth hormone and IGF-1 are *decreased*. And of course glucose and insulin are also decreased.

DHEA, an adrenal gland hormone, reaches highest concentrations in human serum at about the time of puberty, then declines substantially with age so that by the seventh decade the levels are barely detectable. In calorie-restricted monkeys there is no change in DHEA for a long time, then gradually it becomes higher in the restricted ones than in the controls. However, this appears more of a biomarker effect than causal. DHEA has been reported to exert preventive activity against both breast cancer and chemically induced tumors in rodents,[142] and it may extend the life span of short-lived strains of mice.[143]* However, when DHEA is mixed into the diet of mice, they tend to eat less, and some of the reported effects may merely reflect a somewhat lower calorie intake compared to the controls. But my main reservation about DHEA is that it has been kicking around gerontology since the early 1980s, and I still have not seen a 45-month-old mouse. In the most recent and best-controlled study, administration of DHEAS to mice from middle age onward significantly increased blood levels of both DHEA and DHEAS but failed to influence either life span or cancer incidence.[144] Nevertheless, as outlined in the last chapter, in humans DHEA may induce an increase in physical and psychological well-being, an increase in lean body mass, in plasma androgen and in IGF-1 concentrations. Effect on life span and disease in humans has not been established.

In humans melatonin secretion from the pineal gland increases soon after darkness, peaks in the middle of the night and falls during the second half of the night.[145] No serious side effects or risks have been reported from the use of melatonin. Normal persons have been given as much as 80 milligrams, or concentrations mounting to 350 to 10,000 times normal. Dosages of 1 to 5 milligrams result in concentrations 10 to 100 times higher than the usual peak within one hour, followed by a decline to baseline within four to eight hours. Melatonin is a potent scavenger of the highly toxic hydroxyl radical and other oxygen-centered free radicals, and may thus give protection to macromolecules, especially DNA; however, high pharmacological doses in the order of 40 milligrams are required. Doses this high may also lower body temperature. They are impractical, as you will be groggy the next day. Current commercial melatonin products sometimes contain impurities. If you buy any, be sure of the company!

CONCLUSION

If you have read the first edition of this book, published in 1986, you will perceive that many substances that then looked promising enough, do not appear here: BHA, BHT, cysteine, thiazolidine-4-carboxylic acid (TC), thymic hormones, centrophenoxine, piracetum, DMAE, "active lipid." Although these looked auspicious at one time, and their touted beneficial effects have not in fact been disproved, they have more or less disappeared from modern gerontological research. Many (but not all!) of the current favorites will suffer a similar fate.

Table 7.1 shows the supplements I recommend to accompany the CRON diet. They are mainly at the RDA, or "safe and adequate," or ODA (optimal daily allowance) levels to avoid the possibility of malnutrition on a low-calorie intake, but some are in larger amounts. As for other supplements, many look promising. But when you apply the Seventh Criterion, subjecting the claim to the test of the survival curve(s) and using long-lived strains of experimental animals, the results are often disappointing—or there are no results at all beyond plausibility arguments at various levels of persuasion, because the experiments have not been done. Nevertheless, compounds not yet quite up to the mark but that look quite promising and in my view would at least cause no harm, I have labeled with a question mark. It's your choice.

Frankly, I find the stress of deciding from among all these supplement-contenders for the title of "champion soma pill of the moment," to be age generating in and of itself. In the one month spent writing this chapter, with malice towards none and charity for all—and notwithstanding my own calorie restriction— I have probably aged two months.

To Hell with it!

CHAPTER 8

EXERCISE, STRETCHING, AND THE MALADIES OF WEAR AND TEAR

INTRODUCTION

WHILE EXERCISE ITSELF WILL NOT RETARD THE RATE of aging, nor extend maximum life span beyond that characteristic for the species, it will nevertheless extend average life span—in other words, it will square the survival curve.[1] It accomplishes this largely by inhibiting the development of a number of diseases, most notably (in humans) cardiovascular disease. However, exercise has several potential downsides if not properly done.

On the CRON diet you are going to be inhabiting your body for a lot of additional years. There are circumstances that may be damaging to it, changes that are not secondary to "aging" but to the mere passage of time and the effects of constant use. You don't want to live to be 150 years old but suffer from severe traumatic arthritis for the last 50 from having engaged in hard-impact sports for 70 out of those first 100 years. While cancer, heart disease, diabetes, and other such illnesses will be much less prevalent in a long-living CRON society, or among a long-living cohort within a traditional society, other maladies will likely pop up if one simply lives a 150-year life span with an 80-year attitude. Let us give thought to these issues.

EXERCISE

Joggers, 20 million strong, an army of the fit, fanatically striving for perpetual youth and good health, along with hordes of tennis players, cross-country skiers, Nautilus pumpers, aerobic dancers, long-distance walkers, and swimmers: millions of Americans have for some time been pursuing one of the great lay religions of today—physical fitness. A whole generation of fitness fanatics has risen out of easy chairs in late youth or middle age and started exercising because they believe the gospel preached by Dr. Kenneth Cooper of Dallas (author of five books on the subject with 12.5 million copies sold and published in 29 languages) and other fitness gurus that by so doing they will live longer, more enjoyable lives.

There is good evidence to back up part of this faith. But like much else in the lay health field, the value of exercise and fitness has ballooned into a sky-high, free-for-all, no-questions-asked ride. Exercise makes you healthy and sexy, and the more you exercise, the healthier and sexier you grow. In the movie *Pumping Iron*, champion bodybuilder Arnold Schwarzenegger declares, "I'm *coming* all the time."

The value of exercise depends on what you want to optimize. Regular sports competition has nothing necessarily to do with health as a primary aim.[2*] But exercise can be fun; it generally makes you feel good; it helps relieve stress and depression, improves blood-sugar metabolism, and increases cardiovascular fitness.[3]

The goals of the CRON program include some of these but differences do exist. CRON goals are to optimize longevity, health, and freedom from disease. Does exercise actually promote all of these fully? What kinds of exercise? Is a certain amount helpful, and too much not helpful in relation to longevity? How do diet and exercise compare in importance? And what is the interplay between diet and exercise?

We know that dieters generally do better when they exercise fairly vigorously following or during weight reduction;[4] but let's look at the evidence in some detail. It derives from animal studies; from human-population studies; from studies of the effects of exercise on the biomarkers of aging in humans, on "risk factors for disease" in humans, on actual disease incidence, on human longevity; and from studies of the interplay between diet and exercise.

ANIMAL STUDIES

In old rats, the diaphragm muscle, which is actively used in breathing, shows little or no change with age in the number and diameter of its fibers. In contrast to the active diaphragm, the leg muscles of inactive (caged) rats deteriorate as they grow old. It's a "use it or lose it" physiology. In rodents, exercise begun in youth or middle age (12 months) and continued throughout life yields a 10 to 15 percent increase in average life span, but if it is not started until 24 months, an actual decrease occurs.[5] Lifelong exercise benefits cardiac function in rats as judged by enzyme patterns (they stay at a younger level.[6]) However, at a certain point in life (over 24 to 27 months in the rat, equivalent perhaps to 70 to 75 years in humans), a "threshold of age" appears. When previously sedentary 24- to 27-month-old rats are put on a vigorous exercise program, cardiac function may be damaged.[7]*

Aerobic exercise in mice and rats fails to decrease the accumulation of age pigment in their hearts, and such pigment is a biomarker of aging. In mice started on a running schedule at 14 and 24 months of age, no difference was noted in the amount of age pigment in their hearts compared with that of sedentary mice.[8] And in another study, a greater accumulation of age pigment occurred in the hearts of old exercised rats than in sedentary controls. By this particular biomarker, exercise does not do well.[9]

The overall animal data suggest that while exercise protects against certain diseases, such as arteriosclerosis,[10]* increasing average life span, it may fail to retard the basic process of aging. Certain kinds of exercise might even accelerate that process.

Both animal and human studies indicate that very strenuous physical exercise (exercise to exhaustion) leads to considerable oxidative stress (free radical generation) characterized by lipid peroxidation and DNA strand breakage. In humans at least, this can be inhibited or prevented by taking vitamin E (800 to 1200 milligrams daily) for three to 14 days before the exercise.[11] Persons engaged in marathons and other exhaustive sports might wish to consider this, although the main lesson here for life-extenders may be not to undertake this kind of sport at all . The data also suggest that starting exercise in youth or middle age and keeping it up throughout life is productive, but beginning vigorous exercise too late in life may be counterproductive. This is in line with the rodent data.

In a variety of occupational groups (indoor versus outdoor workers, skilled versus unskilled laborers, active compared with inactive post office workers), a greater incidence of heart disease has been found among the more sedentary. On a normal diet, sedentary persons run more than two times the risk of heart disease as active people.

That sounds straightforward, but in fact there are problems with such data as to its true significance. People in different occupational groups have different habits. Businessmen generally have more sedentary jobs than manual laborers, for example, but they also eat differently. They eat more fancy cheese, hollandaise sauce, and marbled red meat. And people of different physical types (genetically obese versus genetically slender) tend to enter different occupations in the first place, and maybe it's the physical type rather than the occupation itself that influences the disease susceptibility. So we cannot conclude much of anything from such human population studies. There are too many variables.

Effect of Exercise in Humans on Biomarkers and "Risk Factors for Disease"
Biomarkers and risk factors relating to heart function and susceptibility to arteriosclerosis are favorably influenced by aerobic exercise.[12] Exercise promotes a higher level of the beneficial HDL in the blood and lowers LDL as well as the total cholesterol-HDL/LDL ratio—one of the better indicators among the blood-fat factors of risk of cardiovascular disease.[13] Increase in blood HDL has been demonstrated in middle-aged male and female runners, young elite distance runners, Norwegian skiers, middle-aged Finnish runners and skiers, joggers, and male marathon runners.[14,15]* In both sexes, the beneficial effect on HDL levels is reached only when a person exercises until his pulse reaches 70 to 85 percent of its theoretical maximum rate (estimated very roughly by subtracting his or her age from 220) for at least 20 minutes three times a week.

Exercise increases the insulin sensitivity of the tissues and improves carbohydrate metabolism.[16] And the physically fit person has only about 60 percent as much chance of developing high blood pressure as a sedentary person.[17] It also increases the body's generation of so-called "heat-shock proteins."[18] These proteins are induced by most any kind of physical or metabolic stress, including those of hyperthermia and exercise, and they serve to repair other proteins injured by the stress, and to participate in new protein synthesis. They are important engines of maintenance and repair.

Exercise works against the slowdown in reaction time that occurs with age. Men in their sixties who have exercised vigorously for 20 or more years display reaction times equivalent to or better than those of inactive men in their twenties.[19] And in both young and older ages the more fit individuals have been reported to display a higher level of "fluid intelligence"—a term that refers to the ability to reason, to think things out, as opposed simply to memory.[20] Thus, very possibly the aging organism can postpone, by chronic exercise, the decline in oxidative capacity of the brain that usually occurs with aging.[21] A study was conducted recently to determine if aerobic exercise (walking) versus anaerobic exercise (stretching and toning) in 60- to 75-year-old adults would result in selective improvement in "executive control processes," including planning, scheduling, and working memory—all known to be supported by the frontal regions of the brain. Substantial improvement was noted in those who walked. Performances in other, nonexecutive control processes were not affected. The mental improvements following aerobic exercise may be selective, but they clearly do exist.[22]

The above results were derived mainly from studies of aerobic exercise, like running or swimming. What about resistance training, such as weight lifting or body building. Resistance training for 45 minutes three times per week has been found to lower cholesterol and LDL. Weight training can of course be done both aerobically and anaerobically in what is referred to as "circuit training" (little or no resting between the handling of the weights), and exert combined benefits.

Everything seems rosy, but to these encouraging data we must add a qualifier. We learned in Chapter 2 that maximum oxygen consumption, known as the VO2 max, declines rather steadily with age. This measurement of your "aerobic capacity" is one of the very best measurements of "physical fitness." [23,24]* The lowered VO2 max with age is due in part to diminished capacity of the tissues to extract oxygen quickly from the blood and partly to a lower maximal heart rate with age. Aerobic exercise will boost the VO2 max of a sedentary person to a substantially higher level. Some men in their sixties and seventies are able, for example to increase their VO2 max levels above those of healthy untrained younger men. However, we saw in Figure 2.2 that the rate of *decline* of the VO2 max with age may be steeper for trained than for untrained persons. One can thus argue that while exercise increases physical fitness and therefore resistance to certain types of disease (cardiac disease especially), it may actually slightly accelerate the rate of aging. The boosted VO2 max declines from a higher point, but does so more rapidly, and eventually reaches the same level as for an old, sedentary person. [25]*

EFFECT OF EXERCISE ON ACTUAL DISEASE INCIDENCE AND LONGEVITY

In a large follow-up study of 16,936 Harvard alumni from 1962 to 1978, it was found that habitual postcollege exercise—rather than amount of athletic participation as students—coincided with a lower death rate from heart disease. Sedentary alumni, *even former varsity athletes*, were at higher risk. [26] But while the death rates declined as the amount of exercise increased—from less than 500 to more than 3,500 calorie expenditure per week—beyond 3,500 the death rate *increased* slightly. In a more recent study, among 2,500 men aged 71 to 93, those who walked more than two miles a day had half the risk of heart disease as those who walked less than one mile. [27]

The Pritikin group have presented evidence that their program of diet and exercise inhibits the progression of peripheral vascular disease, coronary arteriosclerosis, and adult-onset diabetes. [28] But their studies do not differentiate clearly between the benefits of diet and those of exercise.

A common public fallacy about exercise and heart disease holds that exercise is more effective than diet in preventing an attack. That's decidedly not true. The idea that diet is rather irrelevant as long as you exercise strenuously is a myth. Jim Fix, author of the 1977 best-seller *The Complete Book of Running*, who transformed himself from a chubby 214-pound, two-pack-a-day smoker into a sleek 160-pound marathon runner, died at the age of 52 from a heart attack while pounding the road in Vermont. He paid dearly for his expressed belief that running all by itself would suffice to prevent heart disease.

Do not fall so deeply into the myth of exercise that you neglect other preventive health measures. Diet is the most important, even for heart disease, although exercise provides additional benefit. But there is no evidence in either animals or humans that exercise influences the incidence of cancer, the second major cause of death after cardiovascular disease, and we know that cancer is very heavily influenced by diet.

THE INTERPLAY BETWEEN DIET AND EXERCISE

Studies on this interplay in mice and rats have given confusing, indeed conflicting results where calorie restriction is concerned. At the time of my first edition in 1986, it seemed clear from reports by scientists at the National Institute of Aging, and confirmed by the eminent exercise physiologist, John Holloszy, that when fully fed, completely sedentary rodents were compared to similarly fed rodents allowed a wheel to run on, the latter lived longer; but that when calorie-restricted rodents were subjected to a similar comparison, the sedentary ones lived the longest. However, in later studies Holloszy seems to have reversed his position.[29] Wheel runners on a normal diet still enjoyed an average survival longer than sedentary rats on a normal diet, although their maximum life spans were the same; but when the restricted wheel runners were compared to restricted sedentaries of comparable body weights, the life spans and survival curves were identical, and both were substantially greater than those of the nonrestricted animals. It appears from these (and other) studies that once calorie restriction is instituted, the degree of restriction can be a little less if one is exercising—as long as the same degree of weight loss is maintained—and maximum life span extension to the same degree will occur.

I want to reiterate, however, that exercise alone, without calorie restriction, will not increase maximum life span.

It may therefore seem paradoxical that evidence reveals that being unfit confers an even greater risk of death than being obese, in that lean sedentary men (BMI < 25) showed twice the risk of mortality

from all causes than fit overweight men with BMIs > 28 [30]—but in neither case were these subjects on a calorie-reduced diet, in which a different metabolic set-up prevails. Similarly, the extent of decline with
age in respiratory chain function in the mitochondria is greater (50
percent) than anticipated from the low levels of mitochondrial DNA
mutations (1 percent) that occur with age, and reduced physical activity makes a major contribution to this decline, while physical activity
ameliorates and may even mask such mitochondrial "aging," at least in
muscle tissue.[31]

One careful study in humans compared the results of eight weeks
of calorie restriction (a 1,000-calorie reduction from an originally
2300-calorie intake) combined with resistance weight training (bench
press, biceps curl, triceps extension, leg press etc.—in all, eight exercises with three sets of ten repetitions each), to calorie restriction
alone, to weight training alone.[32] Calorie restriction alone was associated with decline in lean body mass, but addition thereto of weight
training prevented the decline; nevertheless, the same amount of
weight was lost—indicating that the combination led to fat loss but
not muscle loss. This is good news for those CRON dieters who want
to maintain their lithe and muscular California bodies.

RECOMMENDATIONS FOR EXERCISE

The overall evidence suggests that aerobic exercise considerably
increases cardiovascular fitness and substantially decreases the susceptibility to heart attack, and improves some features of carbohydrate
metabolism. At the same time—possibly owing to an increased generation of free radicals or a temporary increase in body temperature and
metabolic rate—it may slightly accelerate the basic rate of aging. Exercise definitely has a good effect and possibly a mildly bad effect.

The fitness effect increases rapidly up to a certain point as you exercise more and more, but beyond that point benefits may level off.
According to Dr. Kenneth Cooper, Dallas, running tops out its aerobic
benefits at fifteen miles a week. He says, "If you run more than that, it's
for something other than fitness." Others agree with this assessment. [33]

As the present book does not pretend to be an exercise manual and
I am not an authority on the subject, I will not lay out specific pro-

grams, but state simply what I myself do, and urge you to do the equivalent in whatever form you find most acceptable. Having been a gymnast in my youth, I find it simple and pleasant to spend four periods of one to one-and-a-half hours per week at a local gymnasium where I alternate aerobic workouts of 20 minutes each on a stair climb and two other types of aerobic exercise equipment, with circuit workouts on various types of Nautilus machines. In short, I engage in both aerobic and weight resistance exercise. If you wish to follow such a routine but don't know how, the gym owner or personal trainer will be glad to guide you.

STRETCHING

Flexibility exercises were not included in earlier editions of the above guidelines; but the College now recommends static stretches held ten to 30 seconds to the point of mild discomfort, repeating them four times per muscle group two to three times per week. The excellent book by Marilyn Moffat and Steve Vickery, reflecting the views of the American Physical Therapy Association on posture, gait, body mechanics, exercise, and flexibility is well worth consulting.[34]

On the subject of stretching, however, I have sought the input of my daughter, Lisa Walford, coauthor of The Anti-Aging Plan and a nationally recognized expert on restorative yoga. You will find a complete set of stretching routines plus other information on yoga on the Internet by clicking on Lisa's Section of the Walford web site, www.walford.com. An abbreviated treatment by Lisa, including eight stretches, is as follows:

In the last few years, Yoga has entered into our mainstream vocabulary, and is commercially successful in health clubs all over the country. According to a recent Roper poll, there are now approximately six million people practicing yoga in the United States.[35]

Hatha Yoga features movement and meditation to eliminate pain, reduce stress, encourage a full range of motion in the body while strengthening synergistic muscle groups, and improving coordination and balance, perfect for any anti-aging plan. Unfortunately, there is lit-

tle documented research on what, until recently, has been deemed eso-
teric. However, additional benefits to a Yoga practice include some prevention of osteoporosis; decrease in severity of symptoms related to
menopause; and other effects of the relaxation response on health.[36]

There is currently no uniform standard regulating Yoga instruc-
tors. Differences between styles and even between teachers varies
greatly. You should sample several classes and styles before you settle
in and then schedule several classes a week, at least for a while. Yoga
postures and movements are subtle, and you will profit greatly by taking a few good classes. (See Lisa's Section of the Walford web site for
web and journal sources to help you find classes.)

There are four main factors that may adversely influence your body
over time, which yoga specifically addresses: the effect of gravity on
the spine, posture, a sedentary lifestyle, and a poorly designed or
imbalanced exercise regime. By contrast, the stance of water bearers in
third world countries is light, long, composed, even as they balance
heavy loads on their heads. Through proper alignment of their skeleton they maintain a plumb line that gives them great strength with the
least amount of exertion and effort. This alignment is integral to Yoga.
It often implies a restructuring of the body's patterning and changing
postural habits.

In addition to posture, the wear and tear effects of any repetitive
motion, and particularly asymmetrical ones such as tennis, carrying a
baby on the same side of the body, getting in and out of a car, etc., lead
to such common complaints as bursitis, tendinitis, sacroiliac imbal-
ances, and general low-back pain. In fact, low-back pain is the fifth
most common complaint resulting in a visit to a physician; after
hypertension, pregnancy, general check-ups, and colds.

A well-balanced exercise program should increase the range of
motion in the hip joints and shoulder girdle (ball and socket joints);
and strengthen the corresponding and more vulnerable lumbar-
abdominal (lower back and abdomen) and thoracic-cervical (upper
back) component parts of the torso. In addition, it is imperative to
stretch the hamstring muscles, as they are, if tight, a major culprit in
weak lower backs. High impact exercise programs, often highly repetitive within a narrow range of motion, such as running, may more read-

ily result in joint problems if not accompanied by stretching exercises.

A basic anti-aging movement routine should have the following aims: to increase extension in the spine and lengthen the erector spinae muscles; strengthen the deep abdominal muscles to protect the integrity of the lower back; lengthen the iliospoas muscle to promote optimal support and length in the lower back; stretch the hamstrings to align the pelvis level with the ground; strengthen the upper back muscles (rhomboids, trapezius,) to prevent slumping; open and stretch the chest to reduce pressure on the neck and upper back; reverse the effect of gravity on circulation in the legs and abdomen. The following eight exercises touch briefly on these areas:

To stretch the hamstring and buttock muscles: (FIGURE 1A).

1) Lie on your back with your legs outstretched. Relax your shoulders down to the floor, so as to avoid tension in the neck and diaphragm. Bring one knee to your chest and wrap your arms around your shin. Firmly extend the straight leg, through the heel, so that you feel the entire length of your body elongate. Do not clench your stomach or push the lower back into the floor, as this will overextend the lower back muscles rather than target the hamstrings and buttocks. Hold the pose for six to seven breaths, and repeat several times.

Variation with belt: As above, only clasp your big toe and straighten the bent knee up toward the ceiling. Place a belt around the foot and hold on to the belt as you straighten the leg, so as to put tension on your hamstrings. Extend the floor leg as above, and hold the pose, keeping both sides of your torso long and free of distortion.

To stretch the lower and upper back: (FIGURE 1B)

2) Lie on your back and draw both knees up to the chest. Keep the diaphragm relaxed. Lower both legs to one side of your body. Gently hold the bent knees to the floor and twist away from the legs. As you inhale, lengthen the spine and the sides of your torso. As you exhale, as if you are wringing out a washcloth,

revolve your abdomen away from the bent knees. Continue to coordinate your movements with your breath, and allow time for your back muscles to release and to lengthen.

Variation: If you have strong stomach muscles and no back problems, you may practice this with straight legs. This will strengthen the oblique abdominal muscles and relieve tension in the shoulders and upper back. Begin from the bent knee position and extend your arms out to either side. Relax the shoulders away from your neck. Extend your legs up to the ceiling. Keep the torso long and your weight balanced on the lowest portion of the lower back, just above the tailbone. Lower the legs towards your hand on one side, and revolve your abdomen away from the weight of your legs. Initially, bend both knees to roll back onto your back before extending the legs vertically again. As you build strength in your stomach muscles and upper back, you may draw the legs back to vertical with straight knees.

To strengthen the buttocks, stretch the front thighs, and lengthen the lower back: (Figure 1C).

3) Lie on your back with your knees bent, feet flat on the floor, hip width apart, parallel to each other and close to your buttocks. Extend your arms overhead on the floor. If your arms do not reach the floor, and you feel any restriction in the neck or shoulders, then place a blanket underneath your forearms so you can lengthen your torso without straining your shoulders. Then, without tensing your stomach muscles, exhale, lengthen your lower back and lift your hips up off the floor. As if there were a leash attached to your tailbone, draw your tailbone up towards the ceiling, pressing your heels into the floor as you lift your hips. Hold this position for thirty seconds, then exhale and roll down vertebra by vertebra, lengthening your lower back.

To strengthen and lengthen the lower back: (Figure 1D)

4) Lie down on your stomach on a rug or mat. Place your hands on the rug underneath your shoulders. Lift your upper body up and pull with your hands as if you wanted to crawl forward. You should feel the shoulders rolling back and down away from your ears, and the spine in between the shoulders drawing in toward your chest. Look straight ahead. Keep your pubic bone on the floor and lift your chest further up off the floor. Hold the cobra pose for several deep breaths, and release down. Repeat several times, and then draw your buttocks to your heels into a fetal position with the arms extended out in front of you. Relax your back.

FIGURES 1A, 1B, 1C, AND 1D

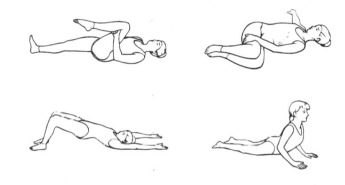

To stretch the chest, shoulders, and abdomen: (Figure 2A)

5) Get on your hands and knees, your feet hip-width apart and hands shoulder-width apart, then move your hands a few inches in front of your shoulders. Curl your toes under, exhale, lift your knees off the floor, and straighten your legs. Draw your weight off your hands and back onto your legs. Keep elbows and knees straight. Breath deeply, lengthening your back through your shoulders, waist, and hips. To release from the pose (called *downward-facing dog*), come back down onto your knees.

To stretch the deep hip flexors and front thigh muscles, and to lengthen the iliospoas muscle: (Figure 2B).

6) Facing a wall, place your legs very wide apart, one in front of the other as though you were taking a long stride. Inhale and extend your arms up overhead so that you feel the entire spinal column and torso lengthen. Square your hips and torso with the wall in front of you so that waist and rib cage are parallel to the wall. Press the back heel firmly down into the floor. Exhale, continue to stretch the pelvis up from the legs, and bend your front leg until your thigh is parallel to the floor. Your knee should be directly above your ankle. Keep your back leg straight as a rod, and realign your torso to parallel the wall once more. You should feel a big stretch on the front of your back leg and over the front of your pelvis. Stretch upwards! Hold this position for thirty seconds, and repeat on the other side. This pose is very helpful for those who sit, run, or stoop a lot. Repeat it several times.

To stretch the hamstrings, firm the side hips (women!), and relieve sacroiliac and sciatic tension: (Figure 2C).

7) Stand erect and place one foot up on a stool, countertop, or desk. The height depends on your flexibility. Keep your torso erect, and do not allow your pelvis to round in the direction of the lifted leg. Rather, press firmly into your standing foot and stretch your torso upwards. You may place your hands on the back of a chair beside you, to keep your balance if needed. Inhale and lengthen your torso more. Notice if your pelvis is parallel to the floor. If it is not, firm the outer thigh of your standing leg and drop the hip of your lifted leg until you feel that both sides of your lower back, waist, and pelvis are even. Elongate through the core of your body and both sides of the waist. It is this elongation that will stretch your lower back, so the details are important. Hold this pose for as long as you can. You may also practice this with the leg to the side. Begin as above but then turn your standing foot, your leg, and body at a 90 degree angle to its prior position. Align your pelvis as above.

Closing postures, to reverse the effect of gravity on circulation in the legs and abdomen, and relax: (Figure 2D)

8) Lying on your back, place your buttock against a wall and your legs up the wall, with a folded blanket underneath your hips and waist, and a small pillow underneath your neck and head. If your lower back rounds or comes off the floor, then your hamstrings are too tight, and you should move away from the wall slightly. Your legs will be at an obtuse angle to the wall, and your back released and relaxed. Release your arms out to the side, gently rolling the arms out, so that your chest opens. Your shoulders should be on the floor. Remain in this posture for at least five minutes.

FIGURES 2A, 2B, 2C, AND 2D

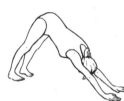

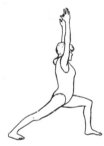

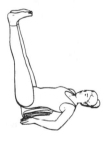

THE MALADIES OF WEAR AND TEAR

There are a number of potential medical problems whose incidence may increase with the mere passage of time, problems that even a thorough-going CRON diet may not protect you from, but that may be avoidable by other means. An easy example is your teeth. If they have to last 140 to 150 years instead of a mere 80 years, you should take good care of them.

While again not an expert on all the matters of wear and tear, I may at least serve good purpose by calling your attention to this area, and suggesting a few illustrative, preventive remedies.

In the maladies of wear and tear, of the back, neck, or joints of the extremities, the culprit is often merely the accumulated stress, strain, and abuse from years of poor posture and body mechanics, of not allowing minor injuries to heal before returning to active play. My intention is not to turn you into an overcautious wimp, but merely to call your attention to this area of concern, and to suggest, as a sort of symbolic dogma, the following: "Live dangerously if it pleases you, but with good posture and well-fitting shoes!"

Here's some advice:

(1) What appears to be "aging" of the skin is most often sun damage. Compare the skin of any older person's face or the skin on the back of their hands with that of their buttock, which one presumes has not seen much of the sun, and you'll prefer the relative smoothness of the latter. One hundred fifty years of unprotected, even casual sun exposure will leave you looking like Boris Karloff in *The Mummy*, regardless of the CRON diet. Always wear a hat and use sun screen if you intend to be hanging around for other purposes than multiple Halloweens.

(2) You will probably be spending a good many hours of your long life in chairs in front of desks, benches, or tables. If that is so, and because bad chairs lead to bad backs, go to an orthopedic chair store—every big city has these—and buy good chairs for wherever you will repeatedly be putting your sunless buttock

down. They are expensive ($500 to $1,000) but well worth the expense in preventive back maintenance.

(3) Ditto for shoes. Look into it, and buy the best for your precious 150-year feet!

CONCLUSION

The CRON diet will make you live long. Following the advice given in this chapter will substantially improve the quality, as measured by efficiency, accomplishments, and enjoyments, of that long life.

ADDENDUM

It's worth noting that evidence suggests that the protein intake for those involved in rigorous physical exercise of either aerobic or anaerobic varieties should be considerably higher (one and one-half to two times) than the official RDA.[37]

CHAPTER 9

THE WHOLE PROGRAM

INTRODUCTION

WHO SHOULD BE ON THE CRON DIET? FIRST OF ALL, anybody who wants to retard aging and extend not only *functional* but *chronological* life span—both, in short: add years to life *and* life to years. CRON is the only way at present widely acknowledged to do so. There are other reasons beyond this blanket "I wanna live longer" reason. There are very practical reasons, professional reasons, for being interested in slowing aging. Careers of modeling and acting in certain respects profit from retention of youth. Athletic careers are equally short-lived and would profit by extension of the youthful period. There is yet a third category of reason for opting for a CRON diet. I refer to those persons in whose families occurs a high incidence of some genetically determined or genetically influenced disease, and a disease that diet may substantially mitigate. A strong influence of CRON nutrition on the occurrence of most types of cancer—including prostate cancer and breast cancer—has been documented in rodents. In strains of mice in which breast cancer occurs with a frequency of 60 percent of all females, the CRON diet will reduce that frequency to 0 to 5 percent. If your family history reveals an increased incidence of diabetes, or of autoimmune diseases like lupus erythematosus, rheumatoid arthritis, and others, the CRON diet is a viable preventive option. Finally, most patients headed for cardiac surgery because of coronary disease should be given this option ahead of surgery, because a thoroughgoing CRON-diet regime will almost certainly not only largely prevent but actually reverse coronary disease. Ditto for high blood pressure!

Who is the CRON diet *not* for? It's not for people who are not having a good time in life and don't care about prolonging it. It's not for pregnant women nor for young persons who have not yet achieved full growth, nor for persons with advanced disease, or diseases clearly not affected by diet, nor for people who competent physicians say should not be on any sort of weight loss program.

On the basis of the evidence I've given you throughout this book, the present chapter will proceed to outline a program designed (1) to increase your resistance to the "diseases of aging" (cancer, heart disease, diabetes, arthritis, autoimmune disease, osteoporosis, Alzheimer's disease, etc.) by 50 percent or better—much better in most instances; and (2) extend your average life span, your maximum life span, and what can be referred to as your health span.

The degree of resistance and of extension of maximum life span will depend upon how old you are when you start the program and how well you follow it. If you start in your early midtwenties and adhere well to the plan, your maximum life span potential could well be 150 to 160 years. By this I mean that you would be on a new survival curve, one terminating at 150 to 160 years instead of the present one for humankind, which is 110 years. Of course, one cannot foretell when you might fall off that new curve. Even though, disregarding the very few outliers, the normal curve today crosses the finish line at 110 years, very few people actually live even that long. In fact, only three to five persons out of every 100,000 reach 100 years of age. But quite a few do live to be 80 to 90.

On an extended life span curve ending at, say, 150 to 160 years, only a few people will live to the end of the curve, but a large number will reach 120. So on the present plan, and starting as a young adult, you should be able to add 30 to 40 years to your life. And these will not simply be old years tacked onto the decrepit end of a normal span, but largely an extension of youth and middle age.

If you start later in life, the degree of extension would of course be less; but even as late as between the ages of 50 and 60, you should be able to enjoy an extension of 10 to 15 years, assuming that you do not already have cancer, moderately advanced heart disease, diabetes, or other such maladies. The program is preventive. I do not claim it to be curative.

In addition to the prospect of a longer life, and as more immediately recognizable benefits, you should feel a much greater sense of physical well-being, more vitality, and an enhanced "younger" intellectual and physical performance capacity, whatever your chronological age.

Why am I so convinced of the truth of the above statements? My conviction is based on translating from animals to man an enormous body of well controlled and many times repeated experiments, plus a modest amount of direct evidence from human populations, additional in-depth evidence from the Biosphere 2 experiments, and the documentation from the three monkey colonies on various types of CRON diets. Look at the data presented in the previous chapters, and decide whether it's worth the gamble. The stakes are high and the CRON diet is a fair amount of trouble, but all indications are positive that you are holding something like four aces in the poker game with Death. If those odds are not good enough, have another pork chop, jelly roll, Twinkie, soda pop, MacKingJackBoxBell burger—and see how soon Death wins the hand.

If you do opt for the program, carefully reread the evidence I've presented. You must hold the firm conviction that the human body can maintain its vigor and productivity to well beyond the present span of about 110 years maximum. And you must have the desire to make your life worthwhile—enjoyable and purposeful for all those added healthy years; otherwise, you won't stick to the regimen long enough to convince yourself of its benefits.

A major stumbling block to changing one's lifestyle enough to ensure that life lasts longer is the unfortunate acceptance of what we may call the "normal" goals for health, fitness, and life span. *Normal* means average or mediocre, and this is far from the best achievable. *Normal* means acceptance of premature disability and death, at age 75 to 80 or earlier, rather than freedom from degenerative diseases and an active life to well past the century mark.

You should also recognize that many of the reports and opinions coming from governmental agencies, accredited scientists, and august nongovernmental bodies such as Committees of the National Academy of Sciences, are prejudiced in several peculiar ways. They resist recommending anything in the way of nutritional change that in their judgment would not be "acceptable" to a large public, or that would constitute a fairly radical departure from what people are already doing or eating. There are several reasons for this attitude.

First: before recommending radical change, officials want the evidence to be absolutely 100 percent secure and overwhelming. Such an ultrahigh scientific posture is usually expressed by assertions that the data are inadequate, the conclusions premature, or there's need for more research. "Highly probable" will not do. In terms of *curative* medicine, that attitude is fine, but in terms of *prevention* it means that many people will not benefit from what we know today to have a very high order of probability of being true.

The second reason for the ultraconservative position is political. In 1979, for example, 14 congressional committees and 20 subcommittees were looking into national nutritional needs, each group with a slightly different ax to grind.[1] In 1983 a federal advisory panel of physicians, basic scientists, and nutritionists appointed by the secretary of Agriculture engaged in a politically charged controversy about changing the dietary guidelines previously published by the Carter Administration in 1980.[2] The most hotly contested of these "radical" guidelines advised Americans to "avoid too much fat, saturated fat, and cholesterol." This hardly extreme language was interpreted as anti-egg, anti-red meat, and anti-dairy products by the corresponding constituencies. The Midwest Egg Producers Association sent the secretary a letter of complaint containing the following language: "Midwest Egg Producers endorsed Ronald Reagan's campaign for the presidency primarily in response to the Carter administration's promotion of [these] dietary guidelines."

It's still like that today, and it's the same overseas. A government-appointed group of British nutritionists cooked up a dish of recommendations that also proved too hot for their nation's food industry. They recommended a reduction of fat from its existing level of 38 percent of total calories down to 30 percent; that sugar and salt intakes be cut in half; and that total energy intake should remain unchanged but that the calories replacing those due to butter and sugar should come from an increase in starches. Striking against publication of this recommendation, the British Nutrition Foundation, a food-industry spokesbody, drew attention to "worldwide economic implications" that would follow substantial reduction of sugar or butter consumption. Thus a posture of public concern was taken over theoretical financial losses involved in directing the population toward more healthful habits. Not quite so malevolent as the tobacco barons, but of the same ilk.

Still a third reason behind ultraslow-foot, hang-back dietary advice from accredited sources stems from the existence of two opposing schools of thought. One school, including the American Medical Association, brings a wholly clinical perspective to the issue. This group, whose bandwagon has been jumped on by livestock, egg, and dairy organizations, believes that dietary advice is best dispensed by physicians on an individual patient basis and cannot be prescribed effectively for the general population. The opposing school, represented by the American Heart Association and many nutritionists, believes that statistical and epidemiological surveys and laboratory evidence show that a large group of people can follow certain dietary practices without health risk, and in fact with great benefits.

With all these forces at work, and even if the scientific view were totally clear-cut, an official consensus opinion on dietary guidelines would be unlikely. You must, therefore, make up your own mind. You must know the evidence, and you must accept the responsibility of knowing how to evaluate the evidence.

A journey of 150 years starts with the first step. I will take four big steps with you. Then you're on your own.

STEP ONE: CHANGE OF FOOD HABITS

Assuming your food habits and preferences are not already nutritionally superb, you must first of all change them. That's not actually hard to do if you do it right. In any case, do that first. Before you try reducing calories or losing weight or exercising or getting your biomarkers checked, re-educate, and reprogram your dietary habits.

One good way to do that is to make the new food preferences delicious, and the experience fun. It will take a little preplanning, but let's get started. First off, you are going to prepare a huge, wholesome, delicious salad, one that Napoleon's army could travel on—even if that's all it had to eat. (One of his sayings was, "An army travels on its stomach.)"

Place the following into a big bowl: 2 cups of chopped Romaine lettuce, 2 cups of chopped spinach, ½ cup of chopped or grated yellow squash, ½ cup of chopped red bell pepper, ¼ to ½ cup of grated raw sweet potato, 1 cup of chopped raw broccoli (better still, 1 cup of broccoli sprouts if available), ½ cup of cooked long-grain brown rice with added chestnuts (see Readings and Resources about the chestnuts), 1 cup of cooked beans of your choice (not from a can, however—better if you prepare them from dried beans), 1 cup of chopped red cabbage, ½ cup of chopped red or yellow onions, and finally dump in one cup of fresh salsa (buy this at the market already prepared). Now for Napoleon's secret. It's in the vinegar and olive oil. Get a bottle of expensive balsamic vinegar (expensive means $30 to $50 per about 8 ounces—see Readings and Resources), and expensive extra-virgin olive oil (around $25). I know this sounds like an extravagance, but it's not all that much since the bottles will last some time. In any case, just do it. Go along with me and I will hook you into the system. Add the vinegar and olive oil to taste, sprinkle with popular seasonings, such as Vegit or Spike, and mix thoroughly.

The above is the basic salad. It's nutrient dense, calorie poor, and very good. The ingredients can be varied endlessly, so you can have variety. Instead of brown rice, or in addition, add wild rice, or other forms of grain (whole grain rye is excellent). The greens can be varied. You may add grated carrots, cauliflower, cucumber, mushrooms, celery, seaweed—it's up to you but it can be endlessly different, and easy to prepare. You may also add cooked, cold pasta in the form of elbows made from whole wheat.

The above salad is for lunches or part of dinner.

For breakfast, put the following into a blender: half to a whole banana (an overripe banana is better, as we discovered in Biosphere 2), a cube of tofu about one inch on a side, 1 cup of blueberries (fresh or frozen), and (depending on how thick you want it) either low-fat milk or skim butter milk. Blend! If this is not enough for breakfast, pour it over cooked oatmeal or cooked rice bran, or a mixture thereof, with added strawberries if you like. The oatmeal is both better tasting and more nutritious if it's whole oats (see Readings and Resources), by which I mean the whole grain (i.e., not "rolled" oats), which you cook by adding twice the volume of water and microwaving at one-half power for 12 to 15 minutes.

For dinner, and as an alternative to the salad, prepare steamed vegetables. Here you should favor cruciferous vegetables as the base: broccoli, Brussels sprouts, collard greens, kale, cauliflower, Chinese cabbage. Thereto add sliced carrots, squash, chopped onion, chopped regular or Elephant garlic, sweet or white potato. Steam for ten minutes, pour a can of tomato sauce or a ½ cup of pasta sauce over the mixture, and it's ready. Or you may add the gourmet balsamic vinegar instead of the sauce. Easy.

If you like meat or fish, add 3 ½ ounces to the dinner plate alongside either the salad or the steamed vegetables. Among red meats, ostrich, emu, or bison have the lowest saturated fat content. (See Readings and Resources for where to order these.) I suggest red meat once a week and fish twice.

If you like bread with the meals, get whole-grain or 100 percent stone-ground whole wheat (with no more than 100 calories per slice), and dip it into the good olive oil—not butter or margarine). If you don't mind being odorous, mesh several cloves of good garlic into 4 tablespoons of olive oil, let the mixture sit overnight, and dip your bread in that.

This is the basic start-up pattern. Eat as much of what I've described here as you like, adding items from the menus you'll find later on in this chapter, or at the back of this book if you wish—or just stick with variations of the above—for three to six months. There can be "off" days when you eat something else, something from your old habits, but these should gradually be decreased until only about every tenth day is an "off" day at home. When eating out, at this stage, do as you like. No fancy desserts, however, except, if you must, on the "off" day or when dining out.

If you cannot adapt to this diet, or something like it, give up. The life-extending CRON diet is not for you.

STEP TWO: GENERAL HEALTH MEASURES

Mild to moderate alcohol intake is considered health promoting in terms of heart disease, especially if in the form of red wine. One to two glasses per day, taken with meals, is fine. However, alcohol does equate to empty calories, with no accompanying nutritive value in terms of the RDAs, so be moderate if not abstemious. Table 9.1 gives the caloric content of common alcoholic beverages. Stick generally to red wine. (See the French Paradox, Chapter 10.) Naturally anyone on a health and longevity program should not smoke. If you are a smoker, there are already plenty of books, schools, and methods to help you stop. I won't attempt to add to these or to their exhortations.

TABLE 9.1 *Caloric content of alcoholic beverages*

CALORIES	BEVERAGE	APPROXIMATE MEASURE
114	Beer	8 oz. glass
73	Brandy	1 brandy glass (1 oz.)
67	Crème de menthe	1 cordial glass (⅔ oz.)
122	Daiquiri	1 cocktail glass (3 oz.)
105	Gin, dry	1 jigger (1 ½ oz.)
166	Highball	8 oz. glass
160	Martini	1 cocktail glass (4 oz.)
105	Rum	1 jigger (1 ½ oz.)
105	Whiskey, Scotch	1 jigger (1 ½ oz.)
84	California table wine	1 wineglass (4 oz.)
84	Champagne, domestic	1 wineglass (4 oz.)
84	Sherry, dry, domestic	1 wineglass (4 oz.)
180	Port or Muscatel	1 wineglass (4 oz.)
120	Vermouth, dry	1 wineglass (4 oz.)
190	Vermouth, sweet	1 wineglass (4 oz.)

There is no convincing evidence that stress in and of itself accelerates the basic aging process, although it may potentiate the development of arteriosclerosis, heart disease, and possibly even cancer (by its effect on the otherwise protective immune system). Stress experiments in mice performed years ago at Brookhaven National Laboratories by

Dr. Howard Curtis did not show any significant effects on survival curves. Stories that sudden fright may turn the hair white overnight are all based merely on testimonial evidence. Animal studies involving the "general adaptation syndrome" suggested at one time that certain forms of stress—those that put the animal into a "fight or flight" frame of mind—cause a sudden outpouring of adrenal hormones, and that too much of these hormones may accelerate some features of aging. But this appealing hyperadrenal-hormone concept, while it has very respectable adherents,[3] has not in fact been accepted as a good model of aging. The relation of stress to aging remains unsettled.

In terms of disease susceptibility, stress is another matter. You should try to avoid certain forms, not so much that of hard work, which is probably beneficial, but the stress of anxiety and/or frustration.[4] For some time it was thought that so-called "type A behavior," characterized by ambitiousness, competitiveness, and a sense of time urgency, predisposes one to increased risk of heart disease, but this idea has been questioned. A study of 2,320 men who had suffered a first heart attack was undertaken to evaluate risks for a second. The men were classified according to the amount of stress in their daily lives and the degree to which they were socially isolated. Second-attack rates in stressed, isolated persons were four times as frequent as in others, but there seemed to be little or no correlation with type A behavior or with the intensity of the personality.[5]

Fast cars and dangerous pastimes may shorten your life expectancy, but not by accelerating aging. Five percent of deaths are due to accidents, and it can be shown mathematically that if all diseases were eliminated and aging itself completely halted, but the accident rate remained at today's level, maximum life span would extend to about 600 years.[6] That's not too bad, and in any case your personal perils are your personal business, your own pleasure. Having hitchhiked and riverboated across Central Africa for my fifty-eighth birthday,[7] I won't tell you to sit carefully at home and avoid danger. But remember there are three factors operating upon the course of a normal survival curve, where "normal" means not subjected to wars, famine, earthquakes, etc. The factors are aging, disease, and accidents.

FIND A DOCTOR SYMPATHETIC TO LIFE EXTENSION

At the time of the first edition of this book, locating such a doctor was not so easy. Most regular MD's looked upon the possibility of retarding aging and extending life span as a fringe movement of marginal respectability. But this has changed substantially. If your present doctor believes you are serious, he will probably agree to monitor your situation and progress. If not, find someone else.

Locating a well-qualified physician is easier than you think. Most physicians are members of the county medical society, although some doctors who are full-time in medical schools may not bother to join. Call up the medical society in your vicinity. In Los Angeles, for example, you would find it listed as *Los Angeles County Medical Association*. Say you want to inquire about the availability and qualifications of physicians in your area of the city —Hollywood, for example. Tell them you are interested in finding a doctor in Hollywood who is a general practitioner, a specialist, or whatever it is you think you need. If you want an all-around doctor to give you an initial examination and supervise you in a preventive health program such as mine, you probably want either a general practitioner or a physician certified by the Board of Internal Medicine. Ask for recommendations in that category.

The county medical society will not recommend a specific person. Nor will they supply information on fees and such matters. But they will gladly give you a list of four or five practitioners located in your area and in good standing with the society. They will tell you where they went to school, where they served their internships and residencies, how long they have been a member of the county society, and their hospital or medical-school affiliations. If they are on the attending staff of a well-known hospital, Cedars-Sinai Hospital in Los Angeles, for example, that's a plus. Being a member of the recently formed American College of Gerontology would also be a plus.

Several organizations now publish lists of longevity doctors for different regions of the United States. Most of these are not very discriminating. Most include a mishmash of MDs, some good, some borderline, plus chiropractors, nutritionists, acupuncturists, and so on. There are good people in each of these categories, but you ought to know what type of basic credentials you are getting. For example, Dr. Robert Haas, author of the best-selling book *Eat to Win: The Sports Nutrition Bible*, is not a medical doctor at all. He is a Ph.D. from an unaccredited university. [8]* If that's okay with you, it's okay with me, but *know* what you are getting. Your county medical society is apt to have information on MD and non-MD alike. Seek out this information.

Having selected a short list of possible practitioners, call them up. Ask what their fees are, and (if you want to follow the CRON program) whether they are interested in preventive medicine, nutrition, and anti-aging remedies. Don't be bashful! If they don't want to talk frankly and freely, betake yourself elsewhere. Do not tolerate the damned authoritarian mystique that has grown up around and been fostered by traditional, organized medicine.

THE GENERAL STATUS EXAMINATION

If he has not done so already, your physician should do a history and physical examination, a urinalysis, a blood count, and whatever else he believes necessary. I would not personally recommend any X rays, blood chemistries, or electrocardiograms at this stage, except those included under your biomarker tests (to be outlined presently), unless something shows up on the history and physical examination. In addition to the biomarker tests, your physician should assist you in determining your BMI and percent body fat.

BODY MASS INDEX (BMI) AND PERCENT BODY FAT

The BMI is in most instances an acceptable indicator of the status of health from the standpoint of obesity (See TABLE 5.1); however, for athletes, in particular muscular ones, it may be misleading. At my gym I know a 220-pound man who is only about five feet, five inches tall, who is gigantically muscular, not much fat, and has a BMI of 38 (which ordinarily would correspond to extreme obesity). In his and any similar cases, the BMI may indicate obesity when there is in fact the opposite. But if you are an ordinary person in terms of body proportions, the BMI is quite sufficient to indicate your scale of obesity. You need not go further.

If on the other hand, you want a more accurate estimate of your percent of body fat, the simplest way (although not the most accurate) is by determining skin-fold thickness in certain parts of the body. Much of your fat lies right beneath the skin, and the thickness of this layer is a good indicator of your overall percentage of body fat. Many people whose actual weights are within normal limits are in fact carrying excess body fat (the opposite of the muscular athlete). By correlating body weight with subscapular (shoulder blade) skin-fold thickness in men, or with thigh and triceps (back of upper arm) skin-fold thickness in women, one can make a good estimate of body fat. The measurement requires special calipers, which your doctor should have. (See Readings and Resources.) Body fat (in kilograms) can be calculated from the following formulas:

FOR MEN: body fat (in lbs.) = 0.28 × body weight (in lbs.) + 28.5 × subscapular skin fold (in inches) − 36.

FOR WOMEN: body fat (in lbs.) = 0.49 × body weight (in lbs.) + 9 × thigh skin fold (in inches) − 22.7 × triceps skin fold (in inches) − 30.

You can then estimate your percentage of body fat by dividing your body fat by your total body weight and multiplying by 100. A thin man might have only 6 percent body fat; an average man, 12 percent; a plump man, 15 percent; a fat man, 20 percent or over. A thin woman might have 15 percent body fat; an average woman, 19 percent; a plump woman, 25 percent; a fat woman, 30 percent or over.

A more accurate way to estimate body fat is by the density method, whereby you are weighed while submerged in water. (See Chapter 5.) Your doctor can arrange this if you want it. It is also available at many of the sports and fitness clubs that have become popular around the country (at the Sports Connection in Los Angeles, for example, where part of the John Travolta/Jamie Lee Curtis film *Perfect* was made).

What percentage of body fat should you aim for on the CRON diet? The "set point" approach applies here just as it does to how much you should weigh. If you neither overeat nor diet, you will drift toward a set point characteristic for both body weight and percentage of body fat. Ultimately, on the CRON diet, your percentage of body fat should be about half that of your initial set point. But this may not apply if you are pregnant or are trying to become pregnant.[9]* And it should not be allowed to get below 5 percent for men and 10 to 15 percent for women.

STEP 3: YOUR BIOMARKER PROGRAM

The different biomarkers were discussed in detail in Chapter 2. Here I shall simply summarize what you should have done early in your program and again every one or five years. Remember that we have two types of biomarkers, those of aging (five years) and those of success (once a year).

BIOMARKERS OF AGING

The tests you can do by yourself or with a friend (see Chapter 2: skin elasticity, the falling-ruler test, static balance, and visual accommodation) are more toys than serious or definitive tests except for static balance, which is in fact quite a reliable marker.

Other suggested tests are those listed in Table 2.2. Repeat these every five years. More frequently is of no benefit (unless there is a health reason) as the age-related changes are not generally large enough to be detected on a one- or two-year basis. Two important tests your doctor can do are the Vital Capacity and the test for auto-antibodies in your blood. Both have predictive value for how much longer you may expect to live. A low Vital Capacity and/or the presence of auto-antibodies reactive with DNA, with thyroid gland tissue, with the rheumatoid factor, or any others are unfavorable signs for a long life. Fortunately, there is an excellent chance, on the basis of studies in my laboratory, that the CRON diet will diminish or entirely eliminate the auto-antibodies.[10] And that it will slow down the rate of loss in Vital Capacity with age, although it probably will not rejuvenate Vital Capacity to that of a younger age.

After being on the CRON diet for about two months, but before starting a new exercise program, your doctor may advise you to have your maximum oxygen consumption determined by means of the treadmill or stationary-bicycle test. An electrocardiogram is done concurrently with this—an added advantage because physical stress will tend to unmask slight or hidden cardiac abnormalities. Determining your maximum oxygen consumption, as you recall from Chapter 2, is more a test of cardiovascular fitness than of aging itself; but if yours is not high, you will want to increase it by changing your lifestyle.

BIOMARKERS OF SUCCESS

These are listed in Table 2.3, and at this stage are more important to have done than the biomarkers of aging. The changes to be expected if you are successfully on a CRON regime are also given in the table. Unless you are on quite a severe calorie-reduction program, do not expect as much as shown for the crew members of Biosphere 2, but the changes should be in the same direction. To these I would add a determination of blood homocysteine, now considered a definite cardiovascular risk factor,[11] but one which can be influenced by supplementation with vitamins B6, B12, and folic acid. You should also accurately determine your body temperature periodically upon arising in the morning, always at about the same time. Body temperature will and should gradually decrease by one or two degrees over six to twelve months on a proper CRON diet.

STEP FOUR: THE DIETARY PROGRAM

HOW MUCH WEIGHT SHOULD YOU LOSE?

Having adapted to the food choices during the initial three to six months of Step One (which did not involve eating less, but eating differently), and seen your doctor and undergone the initial biomarker tests, you should gradually reduce your total calorie intake, while maintaining the very high quality diet, losing weight gradually, over a period no shorter than from six or nine months to several years, until you are 10 to 25 percent below whatever your set point is for body weight (10 percent if your set point and BMI place you as already slender, 25 percent if obese), and/or about 50 percent below whatever it is for body fat, subject to the limitations given above. Reaching a BMI less than 20 is also desirable. (High fashion models' BMIs are generally about 18.) These are your general guidelines.

Set point, you will recall, is what you weigh when for a considerable period of time you neither overeat or undereat. It is probably about what you weighed for much of your life, but in particular during your young-adult years. For example, I weighed about 155 pounds in high school, college, and thereafter. When captain of the wrestling team at the University of Chicago, I trained down to 145 to 147, to make my weight class. And from ages 40 to about 55 I weighed around 150. So my set point is clearly in the range of 150 to 155 pounds. To translate the animal experiments to my own lifestyle, I should have lost from 15 to 37 pounds over one to three years. At the moment, at age 76 and on the program for about 12 years, my weight is about 130 pounds, and I am a vigorous exerciser. Inside Biosphere 2 it went down to 120 pounds. Many individuals on the Internet CR group have maintained themselves for long periods at a comparatively lower body weight than I.[12]

Suppose that to be 20 percent below your set point you need to lose 30 pounds. Buy yourself a good scale. (See Readings and Resources.) If you intend to embark upon a long-term project, it makes no sense to settle for a cheap, inaccurate bathroom-type scale. Now suppose you started at 150 pounds, and that losing 30 pounds over one to three years is your target. Of course you cannot do this perfectly smoothly; you do it in little lumps. Start with a goal of, say, 148. Weigh yourself when you get up in the morning. One morning it will be 147; another, 149 or even back to 150; another morning, 148. But hover around the 148 average point for a while, always on a high-quality diet, then drop your hover point another one or two pounds.

Different people have different strategies for losing weight and keeping it off. Some just eat less at all meals, some eat only once or twice a day instead of three times. I find personally that eating nothing for one day a week (a one-day fast), if I am above the hover point, works comfortably. It cuts the weekly calorie intake, and if one grows accustomed to a one-day-weekly fast, it cuts through the habit of scheduled eating. However, you must find your own preferred pattern.

Don't lose weight too fast, or you'll be putting lipophilic (fat soluble) pesticide residues into your blood faster than the body can detoxify them. That's one of the inadvertent lessons we learned from the Biosphere 2 experiment, as illustrated in Figure 4.1. Figure 4.1 also demonstrates, by the way, a compelling reason yo-yo dieting is bad. You are thereby flushing toxic residues in and out, and in and out, of your system, and maintaining them a long time in the blood stream. The body does not detoxify these residues very efficiently. It stores them in fat, where they are harmless. But if released from the fat—because the fat is melting away—they hang around for a long time in the blood. So yo-yo is a no-no! One theory why breast and prostate cancers are on the rise blames man-made chemicals that mimic the body's natural hormones.[13] These so-called hormone disrupters include pesticides, herbicides, insect repellents, and plastic byproducts. Hormone disrupters are stored in fat.

WHAT CALORIE LEVEL TO SETTLE ON

First of all, what to stay away from! In the 1970s, due to a fad diet called "The Last Chance Diet," which prescribed extremely low-calorie, liquid-protein intake of only about 300 to 400 calories per day, there were a number of sudden deaths due to heart failure in persons on the diet from two to eight months, and with weight loss of around 30 to 50 percent. So you don't want to go anywhere near that.[14]

The answer to the frequent question, on what calorie level should I settle, is, *There is no particular level*, it's different for each person. The daily food combinations in Appendix A vary from 1,100 to 1,500 calories. That's a basal level. You will most likely need to eat more or you'll lose weight too fast. But using the basal level as a guide, simply decrease your average caloric intake to whatever level allows you to lose weight gradually.

If you change from the typical American high-fat diet to the diet described in this book, you are apt to lose weight faster than planned. That's all right for the first three to six months; it will encourage you, but then you must slow down. Remember that animal studies indicate that crash diets leading to rapid weight loss are counterproductive: they *shorten* life span. People are drawn towards high-fat, high-protein, very low-carbohydrate diets (like the Atkin's diet) because weight loss is quite rapid; but it's an unhealthy alternative.

As you adapt to the CRON diet over a period of months, or after the first year, you will find that you tend to gain weight a bit more easily and on less intake than before. That's a good sign. It means that your metabolic efficiency has increased. Instead of burning off 70 percent of the ingested calories without benefit, and producing excess free radicals and other damaging by-products, your body is headed for the 50 percent mark of maximum metabolic efficiency.

If you are competent with the computer, it is extremely helpful to evaluate some or all of your daily meal plans with the aid of nutritional software. (See Readings and Resources.) Evaluate them not only for calorie content but for nutrient density.

AMOUNTS OF PROTEIN, FAT, CHOLESTEROL,
CARBOHYDRATE, AND FIBER

This has become a highly debatable subject, even among traditional dietary experts. Some now maintain that low-fat diets don't work well (the "fat-free" food craze) because if it's fat free or low in fat, people believe they can eat all they want, so they actually eat more in terms of total calories. Other experts and a number of nonexperts cashing in on the confusion, maintain that moderate fat intake (30 to 35 percent of calories from fat) is more satisfying in terms of not leaving you so hungry, and an increased fat intake is acceptable health-wise so long as the fat is not saturated—the best choices being MUFAs like olive or canola oil. But still other experts argue that for long-term sustained weight loss a moderately low-fat, high-vegetable, high-carbohydrate diet functions best.[15] I am myself of this latter opinion, but admit that the true situation is uncertain. You should find what works best for you in being able to sustain low-calorie intake, remembering that except for the essential fatty acids, fats—including olive oil—are nutrient poor.

I remain suspicious of diets too high in protein so far as aging is concerned. The levels of protein carbonyls (indicators of oxidative damage) in animals fed a low-protein diet are lower than in animals fed standard laboratory food, and treatment with irradiation induces a greater level of protein carbonyls in animals fed a high protein diet.[16] The official RDA for protein is 0.36 grams per pound of body weight per day, as set by the Dietary Allowances Committee of the National Academy of Sciences. New research has indicated that in persons over 60 it may be 0.50 grams per day. (Older persons don't use the protein as efficiently as younger ones.) Ordinary exercise doesn't increase the need, but endurance athletes may need 0.6 grams and a strength and power athlete 0.8 grams per pound of body weight per day.[17] More, however, you certainly don't need. A diet too high in protein over a long time may damage the filtration apparatus of the kidneys. In addition, the specific dynamic effect of excess protein (the need to produce energy to metabolize the excess) requires unnecessary energy expenditure, a kind of metabolic stress in itself. And diets too high in protein may exert a negative effect on calcium balance, with excessive excretion of calcium in the urine.

The CRON diet calls for about 40 to 80 grams of protein per day for the range of average-sized persons. This would correspond to deriving 11 to 22 percent of your calories from protein. If you consume 1,500 calories per day, no more than 20 to 25 percent of calories should come from fat, in my opinion, including all kinds of fat, but with emphasis on MUFAs, and on omega-3 fatty acids from fish or supplements. The rest of your calories should come from carbohydrates, preferably those of low glycemic indices (see Table 9.3 for examples). Your daily diet should include 40 grams or more of fiber—preferably up to about 60 grams, depending on your size. If you buy nutrition software, it will guide you in these allocations. If you don't have nutritional software, use the menus in this book and/or Appendix B. And you don't have to do everything at once. Take a step, and when it becomes easy and second nature, take the next.

A protein is "complete" if it contains the essential amino acids in the same proportions as given by the RDAs for those amino acids. If one or another amino acid is in short supply in the protein, that amino acid is said to be "limiting," which means that the other amino acids cannot be fully used for building the structures of the body. What cannot be used gets burned off in so called "futile cycles." (See Reaching for Metabolic Efficiency in Chapter 4.)

The completeness of a protein can be expressed as a score.[18] A perfectly balanced protein, as found in human milk or in whole eggs, merits a score of 100. Rice protein scores 75, soy flour 70, wheat flour 50. Two different protein sources may mutually supplement what each lacks, so the two together yield a high score. Beans and brown rice make a good twosome.

On a daily basis, your food selections should include material from at least the bottom two of the various food categories: from vegetables, fruits, legumes, and nuts as the first; from cereals, grains, and other low/medium-glycemic index carbohydrates as the second; then MUFA and fish; then dairy, eggs, poultry, and lean red meat products (see Food Pyramids, Figure 5.1). The last category may be omitted if you are a strict vegetarian. But it's a bit difficult to concoct fully adequate 1,500- to 2,000-calorie food combinations with no meat at all. Fish foremost and chicken or turkey next are preferable to red meats, in part because of the lower fat content or (for fish) differences in the type of fat. It's time the cattle industry began breeding for leanness rather than for marbling of the flesh it peddles. The fat content even of commercial chickens is substantially greater than it once was. However, low-fat tasty meats like bison, emu, and ostrich are becoming increasingly available from on-line and small-business sources. (See Readings and Resources.)

FOOD TYPES TO FAVOR

For beverages drink a mixture of green and black tea. The green has been the most studied; black tea inhibits the oxidation of LDLs. Tea is anticancer, anti-heart attack, a good source of fluoride, and of course a source of caffeine. Probably tea's potential benefits hold up even if you add milk to it, but there are differences of opinion on this point. Tea contains the flavonoids quercetin and a number of catechins.

Among meats, fish is best, containing both fairly complete proteins and the omega-3 fatty acids (EPA, or eicosapentaenoic acid, and DHA, or docosahexaenoic acid), which appear largely responsible for the low incidence of arteriosclerosis in Eskimos, despite their high-fat diet. The fattier fishes contain more omega-3 compounds (herring, mullet, anchovies, mackerel, freshwater trout, catfish, smelt, sardines, and salmon) as opposed to fishes of medium fat content (rockfish, sea trout, flounder, ocean perch, halibut, and swordfish) or low-fat fish (cod, haddock, lake perch, sole, whiting, red snapper, and pike). White-meat albacore tuna is of medium fat content and contains omega-3s, but in other kinds of canned tuna the fatty acids are apt to have been removed in processing. Shellfish are low in fat but relatively higher in omega-3 fatty acids than other low-fat "fishes." While for years shellfish were regarded as a forbidden food for people with high blood cholesterol, their cholesterol content is now known to be far lower than previous studies indicated; the early studies were picking up noncholesterol compounds along with cholesterol.[19] Table 9.2 displays the percent of calories from fat and the amount of omega-3 fatty acids in various fish.

If you are a vegetarian and don't eat fish, then green leafy vegetables such as spinach and mustard greens, wheat germ, walnuts, flaxseed, tofu, and soybean and canola oil contain linolenic acid, and other omega-3s that can be converted to EPA and DHA in the body. It isn't nearly as efficient a source as fish, however. Omega-6s make up 90 percent of the PUFAs (polyunsaturated fatty acids) we eat, and too high an omega-6/omega-3 ratio is not desirable. The omega-6s are higher in corn, sunflower, safflower, and soybean oils, and in foods made with them (mayonnaise, margarine, many prepared salad dressings).

Among vegetables and legumes the only fairly "complete" protein is that of soybeans. You can achieve protein completeness in a meal by combining legumes (low in the amino acids tryptophan and methionine, but high in lysine and isoleucine) with one of the grains or cereals (high in tryptophan and methionine, but low in lysine and isoleucine). Beans contain a great deal of folate, which helps reduced blood levels of homocysteine, a major risk factor for heart disease. They are also rich in soluble fibers (which lower cholesterol) and in insoluble fibers (which supposedly help prevent colon cancer, but recently doubts have arisen), and good sources of copper, magnesium, and iron. The iron is not very desirable (just enough to avoid anemia!), so do not take vitamin C along with a bean meal as the C potentiates iron absorption.

TABLE 9.2 *Percentage of calories from fat and amount of omega-3 fatty acids in different fishes*

Low-fat Dishes

SPECIES	% CALORIES FROM FAT	OMEGA-3 GM./4 OZ.
Haddock	7	0.2
Cod	8	0.3
Crab	7	0.3
Pike	9	0.2
Sole	0	0.3
Tuna, light, in water	10	0.2
Red snapper	11	0.4

Medium-fat Dishes

SPECIES	% CALORIES FROM FAT	OMEGA-3 GM./4 OZ.
Flounder	13	0.3
Rockfish	14	0.6
Tuna, white, albacore	14	0.5
Halibut (Atlantic)	20	1.0
Halibut (Pacific)	17	0.6
Ocean perch	23	0.3

High-fat Dishes

SPECIES	% CALORIES FROM FAT	OMEGA-3 GM./4 OZ.
Catfish	30	0.7
Sardines	55	> 1.0
Trout, rainbow	37	> 1.0
Shark	33	> 1.0
Salmon, pink, King, Coho	36	2.2
Salmon, sockeye, canned	36	1.8
Herring	43	1.3
Mackerel	52	2.5
Salmon, chinook	58	3.0

The cruciferous vegetables (broccoli, cauliflower, collard greens, kale, mustard greens, turnip greens, Brussels sprouts) are foods to be favored. They have been linked to cancer prevention in numerous studies, including bladder cancer, the sixth most common cancer, and one against which yellow, green-leafy, and carotenoid-rich veggies give no protection. Thus, cruciferous vegetables have unique phytochemicals. The other, so-called "cooking greens"—i.e., not cruciferous—include beet greens, dandelion greens, spinach, and Swiss chard. These have their own nutrient and phytochemical profiles.

Are raw foods more nutritious than cooked foods in terms of stability and bioavailability of nutrients? In general, yes, moderately so, so far as vitamins are concerned; but absorption of carotenoids including beta-carotene, lutein, and lycopene from raw foods is only about 4 percent, whereas from the same foods cooked it is 15 to 20 percent.[20] The distinction between raw and cooked (I do not mean "overcooked") foods is probably not worth making.

For many years it was assumed (without actual testing of the assumption) that complex carbohydrates or starches such as those contained in rice and potatoes were slowly digested and absorbed, causing only a small rise in blood sugar, whereas simple carbohydrates like table sugar were readily digested and rapidly absorbed, producing large and rapid increases in blood sugar and insulin levels. Upon experimentation, however, investigators found the situation to be quite variable.[21]

The idea of *complex carbohydrates* has evolved into the idea of *resistant starches*,[22] i.e., those that resist digestion. Among these are the high-amylose maize starches, which reduce both the insulin and glucose responses in the small intestine, and possibly improve bowel health by increasing fecal bulk. Different varieites and strains of grains such as rice or wheat vary in their content of resistant starch. These are being developed by selective breeding. At time of writing, the resistant starches are not readily available commercially; furthermore, their relation to the glycemic index is not clear. The long-grained rices are higher in amylose than the short-grained, and have lower glycemic indices. You should therefore favor the long-grained varieties in selection of rice.

The glycemic index[23] was devised to express the blood sugar response to individual foods. The index expresses the response for any particular food as a percentage of the response after the same weight of carbohydrate is taken in the form of pure sugar (glucose), or in some instances white bread. With glucose as the standard, the index of glucose would thus be 100 percent and the indices of other foods generally less. Surprisingly, the response does not closely correspond to whether a carbohydrate is simple or complex.[24]* The response of blood glucose (and blood insulin) to some starches (white potatoes, for example) is nearly as great as to refined sugars, whereas other starches (most grains, for example) give a low response. Pasta is lower than cereals. Many breads give a high response.

The glycemic indices for a number of foods are shown in Table 9.3. We see that carrots are rather high on the list and sweet potatoes low. The reasons for all these seemingly haphazard differences are not entirely known. Fiber content does not seem to be a factor in cereals, but fibers such as the guar and pectin found in fresh fruits and vegetables greatly influence the rate of carbohydrate absorption and subsequent blood-sugar responses. Legumes are digested less rapidly than other foods, so produce lower, flatter glucose responses. Chana dal, a split baby garbanzo bean, gives the lowest response, and cooks very rapidly (about 15 minutes), but is generally only available via online order. (See Readings and Resources.)

Other things being equal, for your CRON diet choices, select foods with the lower glycemic index. The list given in Table 9.3 is accurate and usable. One should not be led astray by listings that show that such items as potato chips and ice cream have low glycemic indices. They do indeed, but in these cases it's because the foods are high in fat, and fat delays emptying time of the stomach. A low glycemic index at the expense of a high-fat meal is a poor trade-off.

Fiber is also a favored substance in the CRON diet. As we recall from an earlier chapter, the term *fiber* refers to the indigestible portions of plants, the chemical substances usually present in the cell walls that give plants their structure and form. And different kinds of fiber exert different effects on the body. For an average-size person, fiber intake should reach 40 grams per day.[25]* Depending on your present intake, you may have to work up to 40 grams gradually to avoid temporary flatulence and bloating. But 40 grams is a minimal quantity, and most vegetarians consume a lot more. Sixty grams may be a quite reasonable amount. A word of caution: consuming very

TABLE 9.3 *Glycemic indices. The "glucose tolerance"*
response for each food is expressed as a percentage of the response
to the same amount of carbohydrate given as pure glucose.

100% OR MORE	80–90%	70–79%
Glucose (100) = the standard	Cornflakes	Beans, broad
Maltose (118)	Honey	Beets
Dates (110)	Parsnips	Bread, whole wheat
	Potato, baked	Bread, rye flour
	Watermelon	Bread, whole meal
	White bread	Millet
		Potatoes, white, steamed
		Raisins
		Rice, white

60–69%	50–59%	40–49%
Bananas	All bran	Beans, navy
Corn oatmeal	Bread, 100% stone ground whole wheat	Beans, pinto
Oatbran	Buckwheat	Bread, heavy mixed-grain
Rice, brown, short grain	Chocolate	Bread, pumpernickel
Rice, wild	Grapes	Oranges
Shredded wheat	Rice, basmati	Peas, dried
	Rice, brown, long grain	Porridge (oats)
	Spaghetti, white	Spaghetti, whole meal
	Yams	

30–39%	20–29%
Apples	Fructose
Beans, black	Lentils
Beans, garbanzos (chick peas)	Milk, whole
Butter beans	
Cowpeas (black-eyed peas)	**10–19%**
Grapefruit	Soybeans
Green beans	Peanuts
Lentils	Chana dal (beans)
Milk, nonfat	
Peach	
Pearled barley	
Rice bran	
Soy milk	
Yogurt	

large amounts of fiber between meals in the form of processed material like guar gum can cause sigmoid volvulus, a twisting and impaction of the colon.

The amount of fiber should be split more or less equally between cereal fibers, such as bran on the one hand, and the gums and pectins on the other, found especially in apples, pears, peaches, oranges, oats, and dried beans. Bran fiber does not influence cholesterol, but adds bulk and softness to the stool. Miller's bran can be added to your breakfast cereal; two tablespoonfuls weigh about 3 grams. The pectins and gums can reduce cholesterol levels, as will oat and rice bran.

A high-fiber diet will also help you control your weight. Fiber is filling but adds virtually no calories. Three apples contain about 24 grams of fiber, but their carbohydrates content equals that of only one fiberless candy bar.

Many cereal manufacturers and some bread makers include fiber information in their nutrition rundown on the back of the package. Look for the words *dietary fiber*, not just *crude fiber*. You want the former. Crude fiber dates back to 1887, and the test on which it is based doesn't pick up a number of materials now recognized as being fiber. In Table 5.4 I listed the fiber contents of representative portions of a number of common foods. Others are given in Appendix B.

DAILY MENUS THE EASY WAY

The goal is to devise each day's food intake so as to optimize nutrition and minimize calories. You want to approximate or exceed the RDA amounts of each essential nutrient, with protein, fat, cholesterol, carbohydrate, and fiber within the conditions outlined above. You want a sufficient caloric restriction to enable you to lose weight, but quite slowly. To fulfill all these requirements takes a fair amount of doing.

This *diet problem* is an example of a special *linear programming problem*, to use the mathematical term. The problem is usually expressed in economic terms applicable to the situation of Third World countries. A Third World inhabitant has dietary requirements like everyone else's: so much vitamin A, so much vitamin C, and so on. But he or she doesn't have much money. Hence, the selection of foods must be so that all nutrient requirements are met but the food cost should be as little as possible. (In our more fortunate case we minimize not cost but calories.)

In terms of economic planning, what is the minimum cost per person to feed a Third World population adequately? The first thorough consideration of this diet problem was undertaken in 1944 by the economist George Stigler, who considered nine nutritive requirements: calories, protein, calcium, iron, and vitamins A, B, B2, niacin, and C. He constructed a diet that satisfied these basic (but limited) requirements and cost only $39.93 a year per person (less than 11 cents a day) at 1939 prices. The diet consisted solely of wheat flour, cabbage, and dried navy beans. Of course, with the 31 items of the CRON diet, rather than merely nine, the problem becomes much more difficult; nevertheless, these are all programming problems.

Our CRON diet problem, of course, is to minimize calories rather than cost, and at the same time optimize nutrient value. But we are nevertheless still dealing with what is more popularly known in computer mathematics as a "bin-packing" problem: how to get all the essential nutrients into a bin that will not hold more than a certain number of calories, a certain number of grams of protein, with less than 20 to 25 percent of calories from fat, and so forth. In this more complicated case there is no general mathematical solution, but the problem can be solved for a number of special cases. For my book *Maximum Life Span*, I arranged for a mainframe computer to look randomly at an enormous number of combinations of food substances, eliminate those combinations that did not measure up, and print out the others. In computerese language, this is called solving the problem by "brute force." Many bin-packing problems can be solved only by brute force. Some of the food combinations and menus in the last section of this book were also arrived at by this technique. But there are other methods.

For those of you who own computers, I have put out a software package allowing an easy solution to the food selection problem. Called *Dr. Walford's Interactive Diet Planner*, it will permit the user to devise daily food combinations that, at any desired calorie level and with any other of the above restrictions, will approach or exceed RDA amounts of the essential nutrients. (See Readings and Resources for details.)

In addition, Appendix A of this book gives you representative complete food combinations for all three meals for 14 days, with a number of specific menus. The 14-day menu combination is quite enough to sustain you and allow for variety, but if you wish you can vary it further, utilizing the complete nutrient listings for 150 foods given in Appendix B. If you do own a computer, the easiest way to devise new daily combinations is to take any good popular diet book, such as any of Nathan Pritikin's books, or the Weight Watchers books, or *Jane Brody's Nutrition Book*, *The Omega Plan*, *The Glycemic Revolution*, or certain others, see what their menus may be deficient in by reference to my nutrition software or the information given in Appendix B, and do slight rearranging. The combinations in most popular diet books were put together without clear reference to the complete RDA list, and with fewer restrictions than we require. They almost never measure up to our full needs, but are often very excellent starts. And with that start, your rearrangement will almost inevitably be nutritionally better than anything else in the literature of cuisine.

If a 1,500- to 2,000-calorie complete daily diet leads to weight loss in less than nine months to several years, fill up with enough calories of just about any type (except saturated fat and certain obvious no-nos) to hold you to the gradual weight-loss rate.

WHEN EATING OUT, DINE

For the CRON dieter, eating out is not a major problem. It's the total weekly or monthly caloric intake that is important, as long as the quality is high. If you eat out often, you must be somewhat restrictive. But when dining out, concentrate mainly on the quality of the diet, rather than on simply its caloric content. Don't eat the white bread and butter most restaurants put on the table for you to nibble while you await the main course. Either don't choose a high-fat meal (roast duck, pork, or the like) or, with your doctor's permission (a prescription is necessary), 15 minutes before the meal take one packet of cholestyramine (brand-name, Questran) in a glass of water. Cholestyramine largely prevents the absorption of fats (see Table 5.3). It appears to be completely safe: it was used in the seven-year National Heart, Lung and Blood Institute study of the effect of lowering cholesterol on heart disease, and was taken by several thousand men at the rate of six packages per day without evident harm. Pectin has a similar but less powerful effect in hindering fat absorption.[26]

A number of good books contain suggestions about how to dine out without being too unhealthful. Pritikin's is one of the best, and again, *Jane Brody's Nutrition Book* has excellent suggestions. But if you are careful to stay on the CRON diet at home, you can be more liberal outside, provided that you insist on *quality*. In addition, look on the menu for items cooked without added fat: steamed, cooked in own juice, broiled, roasted, or poached would be okay. Avoid items sautèed, fried, braised, creamed, escalloped, pickled, or smoked.

You may also take advantage of the fact that some restaurants now offer low-calorie, low-fat meals, which in some instances are of gourmet quality. Marriott Hotels call this its "Good for You Program." It follows the guidelines set by the American Heart Association. The meals are on its regular menu but are marked with the American Heart Association seal. The seal is also on special meals served at Sheraton Hotel restaurants, and on American Airlines. Fairmont Hotels have a similar "Fairmont Fitness Menu." The entire chain of eighteen Four Seasons Hotels presents its low-calorie "Four Seasons Alternative" in which a three-course dinner totals no more than 650 calories. Hyatt Hotels have 600-calorie "Perfect Balance" meals on their menus. Holiday Inns have introduced a "Gourmet Health Menu" into its Asian chain. Sumptuous diet food is now the aim of many a resort from coast to coast: Gurney's Inn in Montauk, New York; Palm Aire in Pompano Beach, Florida; Sonoma Mission Inn in Sonoma, California. The trend was started some years ago with the "spa cuisine" of New York's Four Seasons restaurant. ("Spa cuisine" accounts for about 25 percent of the meals served there, and they're excellent.)

In adopting the CRON diet for health and longevity, first concentrate on switching toward the highest possible quality of food. You will find it far easier to limit your calories if the quality is high. And as you become accustomed to a perfectly balanced, high-quality intake, you will very likely begin spontaneously to lose weight, and it will be easy to keep this up by a gradual reduction in total calories.

SUPPLEMENTATION

But why not just eat tasty fast foods daily to the tune of 1,500 to 2,000 calories and take care of your deficiencies by ingesting RDA amounts of all the essential nutrients? That way you'd be losing weight, not have to be very careful about quality of food, and still get adequate nutrition! Right? Wrong.

There are a number of reasons why that won't work. First, there is still much we don't know about nutritional needs. Guinea pigs placed on a totally synthetic diet that contains ample amounts of *all the known essential nutrients* will not thrive at all. Not all essential nutrients have been identified. A CRON diet will probably include these unknowns; a fast-food/quick-pill or processed-food diet very likely will not.[27*] The nature of the problem is dramatically illustrated in Table 9.4, which shows the susceptibility of rats fed two different diets to the cancer-causing effects of three different chemical agents. Those on the semisynthetic diet were far more susceptible to the carcinogens than those on a natural whole-food diet. Now, this semisynthetic diet is analogous to a fast-food diet with vitamin supplements. Clearly that's not the best choice.

TABLE 9.4 *Effect of type of diet fed to rats on their susceptibility to cancers induced by different chemicals (adapted from P. M. Newberne and V. Suphakarn,* Nutrition and Cancer *5:107, 1983)*

| | | % OF RATS WITH TUMORS | |
CHEMICAL AGENT	LOCATION OF CANCER	SEMISYNTHETIC DIET	NATURAL WHOLE-FOOD DIET
AAF	breast	91	33
AAF	liver	67	29
DMH	colon	67	42
ethinyl estradiol	liver	96	48
ethinyl estradiol	ovary and uterus	67	11

Second, the form in which nutriments are taken is also important. While one can absorb essential amino acids either as pure amino acids or as complex peptides (amino acids strung together into one compound) or as protein in food, retention in the body of nitrogen derived from the peptides or proteins may be as much as 16 times that from amino acid mixtures. You cannot wholly depend on supplementation, even for *known* essentials.

A third reason for not settling for a poor but supplemented diet is that poor diets are bad for you not just because of what they lack, but because of what they contain: large amounts of saturated fat, for example, or *trans* fats.

While supplements cannot compensate for a poor diet, they can add to the quality of a good one, and I do recommend a selected list (Chapter 7) as part of the CRON program. But you do want top-quality supplements. Unfortunately, in the vitamin/mineral business there are no reliable industry standards for protecting the consumer, no national monitoring service with any power to inspect and enforce, and no governmental protection except for general laws on food purity, cleanliness, and false or misleading advertising. Because vitamins and minerals are defined legally as foods, legal standards are much more lenient than for drugs. In fact the industry is rife with rip-offs for the consumer. You must take care not to be hoodwinked into buying second- or third-rate products.

Because the processing equipment needed to extract or synthesize vitamins from raw materials costs millions of dollars, only a few big companies like Hoffmann-La Roche or Eastman Kodak actually *produce* the vitamins. These are then sold to either a vitamin company or a vitamin broker. The vitamin company compounds a final product (pill, powder, capsule, or liquid), packages it, and markets it either directly to retail stores or to distributors. However, if the vitamin made by the original big-company producer is bought by a vitamin broker, quite a different route may take place. He sells either to another vitamin broker (there may be a string of these) or to a contract manufacturer. The contract manufacturer then puts together a product designed for any marketing company that gives him an order. The marketing company then sells either to a distributor, to a retail store, or by mail order directly to the public. Thus, the route the product takes through a marketing company may be quite roundabout: more people involved, more time, more add-ons, less control. Exceptions there may be, but in most instances, products that come by this circuitous route are much less reliable. Look on the label. If it says "manufactured by," you are dealing probably with the shorter route through a vitamin company (Thompson, Solgar, or Plus, for example). If it says "manufactured for" or "produced for" or "distributed by," you are probably dealing with the longer route. The most hazardous procedure is to deal with a mail-order company. Such vitamins have taken the longest route of all, and while there are exceptions, these companies have the worst record for quality. I am not able to judge the online companies; they are too new.

Carefully inspect the label on the bottle. Do not be influenced by any promotional literature not part of the actual bottle or package. The label itself must conform to certain legal requirements that restrict false claims or misinformation, but accompanying literature can promise nearly anything the ad department decides is catchy. Even the label can at times be misleading. If you intend to take 500 milligrams of magnesium as a supplement and you buy a product whose label reads "100 milligrams of magnesium gluconate," you would have to take 56 tablets, because there are only 9 milligrams of magnesium in 100 milligrams of magnesium gluconate. The other 91 milligrams are the gluconate.

The word *natural* on any food product has no legal definition. It is so abused you should totally disregard it. Synthetic vitamins are neither worse nor better than those derived by direct isolation from foods, except for vitamin E. The food-derived vitamin E molecule, d-alpha tocopherol, differs in structure from the synthesized mixture of molecules d-alpha-tocopherol (a mixture of eight isomers). The d-alpha form is the more potent on a weight basis. On the other hand, the synthetic acetate or succinate form of vitamin E is effective and is not susceptible to becoming rancid, so might be preferred by some.

Look for the product that gives the most precise and specific wording on the label. Ideally, all labels should give batch number, date of production (the most important date), and date of expiration. So far as I am aware, not a single company provides all three of these. If you have the batch number, you can call the company and learn when the product was made and by whom. Recent rulings require that the amount of trans fats be listed on the label. Look for that when it comes.

Buy the freshest substances possible. Vitamin E should be no older than six months from date of production, and no other supplement should be older than 18 months.

It would be a great boon for the consumer if some of the larger, better vitamin companies banded together to finance a separate agency to set up standards for and certification of products. Something like the Good Housekeeping Seal of Approval, only better. In my opinion the Linus Pauling Institute or the Orthomolecular Society would be a good candidate to serve in this role.

Don't believe what the retailer in the store tells you about vitamin products. Most retailers know pathetically little about nutrition, and also they have big financial axes to grind. Don't go for "good deals" on vitamins. You will just get inferior quality. Expect to pay more for well-labeled, top-quality material. The good deal will be the health and quality of your life.

Glass bottles are better containers than most plastic. The polyethylene and polystyrene bottles used to package many supplements are not impervious to air. Their "oxygen barriers" are too low and the vitamins inside are subject to oxidation. The worst supplements you can buy are those packaged in little plastic, cellophane, or foil envelopes. Plastic bottles with the required properties can be made, but they require very costly equipment. Glass jars with nitrogen flushing would yield adequate protection, but no vitamin company offers this because of the expense.

Unfortunately, heavy advertising and promotion are greater keys to success in the vitamin/mineral business than quality of product. And because of intense competition there is pressure all along the line to minimize costs, which translates into inferior products. You must educate and protect yourself, and insist on more responsibility from this industry.

EXERCISE

My exercise program is aimed at balancing the positive effects of physical fitness on disease susceptibility against the potentially negative effects of exercise and increased energy turnover on the generation of free radicals.

The best exercise program is one that fits readily into your daily life, is varied and perceived as fun, emphasizes endurance and flexibility, does not depend too much on other people, and can be followed throughout your life. The multimethod type of training is recognized as superior for middle-level athletes, which is about the level we seek. Sticking to only one type of exercise, like swimming or jogging, is not best for your health. Deep adaptive shifts are undergone by the body for specialized performances. Heavy specialization is one of the reasons for the high performance records of Soviet athletes.[28] The elite athlete is thus quite different from the average athlete, but he is not necessarily healthier.

Studies performed at the Washington University School of Medicine give us a target range for exercise. Fourteen persons 65 years of age were followed through a 12-month, two-part exercise program. All started from a sedentary status. They first completed six months of low-intensity training, including moderately vigorous walking three times per week for a half-hour each time. During the second six months, they did high-intensity training, consisting of 30 to 45 minutes of endurance activity (cycling or jogging) at least three times per week. Maximum oxygen uptake, the best indicator of fitness, increased 12 percent during the low-intensity phase and 18 percent more during the high-intensity program. There was definite improvement in the blood fat and cholesterol levels and in the ability to metabolize glucose.

After you have passed a cardiovascular-fitness examination by your doctor, I recommend spending three or four 15- to 20-minute sessions each week at an aerobic exercise during which your heart rate is at 70 to 85 percent of its maximum. Your maximum heart rate can be determined as part of your initial fitness examination. Subtract your age from 220 and multiply that figure by 0.70 and 0.85 to obtain an estimate of the lower and upper limits of your target cardiac range.

The above should be coupled with a weight-resistance program (see Chapter 8). Bone will increase its content of calcium in response to short hard pulls more readily than to long sustained pulls. This means using Nautilus or Universal gym equipment or a regular weight lifters' gymnasium. Previously sedentary persons who do weight training three times a week for 45 to 60 minutes can expect a small drop in blood cholesterol within 12 weeks, and an increase in HDL.[29] Resistance weight training, or bodybuilding exercises, exerts a favorable influence on the blood-fat profiles, altering them in a way that reduces cardiovascular risk.[30] Blood sugar metabolism also improves.

There is a good chance that aerobic and resistance exercises in combination are additive in their benefits.

You now have an excellent all-around physical fitness routine, and except for the weight training, you will hardly notice any interference with your regular life. Tailor your own program, depending on your interest in sports. But remember that beyond the equivalent of about 15 to 20 miles of jogging per week, you won't gain proportionately in terms of increased cardiovascular fitness, and you may well lose something by the increase in metabolism and generation of free radicals induced by exercise. Don't overexercise unless you are doing it not primarily for health, but for enjoyment.

One more point: Once you are on an exercise program, you must stay on it or the cardiovascular benefits quickly disappear. The level of HDL in the blood, for example, drops rapidly (within about three weeks) if exercise is discontinued.

And part of your physical program should include stretching. While doing that, either via yoga postures or by other techniques, you might wish to contemplate what I'll discuss in the next chapter.

CHAPTER 10

FOODS AND TIPS FOR
A CRON-DIET CUISINE

INTRODUCTION

ALTHOUGH NEGLECTED BY HISTORIANS, FOOD HAS PLAYED a fascinating part in American history. By hunting and fishing, gathering nuts, wild seeds, berries, and herbs, and raising corn, squash, and beans, the Native Americans enjoyed a richer and more varied diet than anyone except the wealthiest Europeans. The Pilgrim settlers nearly starved their first winter, and had to kill and boil the great mastiffs they had brought with them from England for protection; but they planted seeds of cabbage, turnips, onions, and peas, and after their first harvest survived without mastiff stew. Thomas Jefferson served elaborate White House dinners prepared by an imported French chef. He considered food important in the art of diplomacy, and introduced macaroni to American cuisine—an innovation foreshadowed in the song "Yankee Doodle." Tom Jefferson stands as our Yankee Doodle par excellence.

Our more recent forebears, male and female, were not gourmets but gourmands of gargantuan capacity. Full-fleshed women, like the 200-pound Lillian Russell, were much admired in the early 1900s. A large belly was the sign of affluence in a man. William Howard Taft, "Diamond Jim" Brady, and Teddy Roosevelt exemplify the globular silhouette that was the period's popular look. These heroic trenchermen wore vests and watch chains and sat down to multicourse meals, starting off with a dozen oysters to "open the appetite." Indigestion and gout were widespread.

This same astonishing epoch and its aftermath saw the invention and development of modern food technology, another mixed blessing Americans gave to the world. Hot dogs hit the market in 1904, processed cheese in 1915, Wonder Bread in 1921, potato chips in 1925, Hostess Twinkies in 1930, Spam in 1937. The first McDonald's hamburger was sold in 1948, the first TV dinner in 1954.

We are now, one hopes, passing into a new era: from gourmet to gourmand to intelligent appraisal of the pluses and minuses. The influence of the environment, particularly diet, upon health, disease susceptibility, and longevity is being fully appreciated. People—at least some people—are beginning to refuse to eat themselves into mental deterioration, disease, accelerated aging, and early death.

This chapter, combined with the Appendices and the Readings and Resources, will provide you with further information and with menus to complement the basic start-up items of the last chapter, with food combinations and general advice on how to set up a varied, nutrient-dense diet that involves all the principles we have learned up to now. Your diet should be limited in calories. It should approach or exceed the RDAs for all important nutrients, with calories derived from fat not less than 8 percent and rarely more than 20 to 25 percent, with an unsaturated-to-saturated-fat ratio of much higher than one to one. Your diet should have ample omega-3 fatty acids, it should be high in fiber, with a total protein content generally between 60 and 90 grams per day. Most dishes should be uncomplicated to prepare, so you won't spend your 120 years in the kitchen.

I'll outline a 14-day menu program in Appendix A. When you wish to expand your choices beyond the startups of Chapter 9, eat your way through the 14-day program at least twice, alternating with the start-ups if you want to keep things simple. This should take about two months, and may require some effort, but the CRON diet is clearly the most important part of the program—much more important than supplements or even exercise, and you should give it your personal experimental best. Keep going for a total of three to six months, without trying to actually cut calories, and long enough to reinforce your change of food habits. That alone will enhance your sense of physical well-being, and pump up your energy. If you feel that good, you'll want to go for the 120 or more years. During these initial months, take no supplements beyond what you may now be taking. Don't change your habitual exercise pattern, whatever it is. I want you to experience the beneficial effects of the diet itself, and without wondering whether *part* of the good feelings might be due to a new exercise program, or to extra vitamins. One trick of vitamin/protein-drink, weight-loss faddists is to put people on a diet and also sell them pills. The people feel better because they lose weight, but the faddist sells them on the idea that it's because of the miraculous pills. Let's not play that huckster game. For the first three to six months just stay with the CRON food combinations. Don't change anything else in your lifestyle.

All the food combinations we'll be using were derived by computer techniques applied to extensive tables of food values (see Appendix B). You can check out the nutrient values of other published diets, or devise your own combinations, by means of my software program (*Dr. Walford's Interactive Diet Planner*—see Readings and Resources), or by plugging in the information given in the tables in Appendix B. For a long-term, low-calorie diet, it's not enough just to pick good-looking items from the various food groups, as many nutritionists seem content to advise.

As you start on the program, gradually stock your larder with the staple items to be used in the 14-day cycles. The herbs, spices, grains, cereals, and dry legumes should last for a long time. The produce should be bought fresh once a week, or more often if you prefer, and as needed for your meal plans for the week. Inquire where you shop as to what day of the week the produce is delivered. With supermarkets it's usually only once a week. Try to shop there on that day or the following day, to be sure of fresh produce. Or if there's a weekly farmers' market in your neighborhood, so much the better. Shop there!

STOCKING THE LARDER

Reserve a place on your shelves or in your refrigerator for the foods listed on the following pages. Buy one-quart canning jars with stick-on labels for the grains, cereals, legumes, nuts, seeds, and fresh herbs. Keep the fresh herbs in the refrigerator in canning jars with one-half inch of water in the bottom (except for ginger, which should be stored dry). Oils, nuts, seeds, and of course vegetables, meats, and dairy products should also be refrigerated.

EQUIPMENT

Besides the standard equipment like knives, long-handled cooking spoons, saucepans (two- and four-quart), plastic food containers and freezer bags, oven cooking bags, a wooden cutting board and salad bowl, and measuring spoons and cups, you should have the following:

Blender and/or food processor

Double boiler

Frying pan, nonstick: I highly recommend the new TFAL ware.

Kitchen weighing scale: None of the scales in the usual stores are very good, as they are very inaccurate in the low weight range. Go to a biological- or chemical-supply house, where you will find a large selection. I recommend the Ohaus #720, which is a balance scale with a large removable scoop.[1]* It is hard to break, easy to use, and accurate to 1 gram or less over the entire range of 1 to 500 grams. Price about $90. Contrast this with the top-of-the-line Soehnle Computer Kitchen Scale, accurate only to within about 8 grams and at a cost of close to $85.

Labels and a marking pen: to label foods on your shelves or in your freezer.

Soup pot, eight-quart

Vegetable steamer

Microwave oven: While not necessary and not integrated into the menu instructions for this book, a microwave oven will save you a lot of time. Microwave cooking is also less destructive of the nutritive values of foods than fire cooking. However, microwaved foods do not crisp or brown, and do not always cook evenly. They may require stirring or turning during the heating process, and tough cuts of meat may not become as tender as with slow-fire cooking. Microwave cooking is really an art in itself. Taking a short instructional course is better than just bumbling into it.

NUTRIENT-DENSE MENUS

For our menu data bases we require daily food combinations approaching full RDAs for 31 major nutrients, but with less than 1,500 calories. The list of 31 includes the essential amino acids, vitamins, minerals, and trace elements plus biotin, which is not established as "essential". It does not include essential fatty acids, sodium, and phosphorus, as it is almost impossible not to get enough of the latter two except on the most artificial type of diet, and the fatty acids are a special case (see Fatty Acids, Chapter 7).

If you are of average size, limiting yourself to less than 1,500 calories will induce a considerable weight loss over a six- to nine-month period—perhaps 10 to 20 percent of your body weight. That's too rapid. So for the more desirable slow weight-loss program, you can eat more, and within limits (not too much fat) whatever you want, since at the planned 1500 calorie level, you're already over the RDAs.

Full food values for 150 of the highest-quality foods are given in Appendix B. Selected foods that contain substantial amounts of two or three or more essential nutrients were featured in Table 4.3. Table 10.1 shows the foods highest in each individual category. By using these various tables, you can build additional, basic, nutrient-dense, low-calorie daily food combinations. Start with what you like, and then add what you need to bring the combination up to par for the day. It can be done simply with my computer software (see Readings and Resources), or with some effort by hand, using Tables 4.3 and 10.1 and the nutrient values given in Appendix B.

Appendix A provides 14 days of combinations and menus at less than 1,500 calories per day. You will be surprised at how much you can actually eat if you select nutrient-dense foods. To these daily menus you may add black coffee or better still tea (green tea preferred) or whatever is calorie free or low calorie, as you prefer. After the standard fare of the last chapter (Chapter 9, Step 1), and two or three 14-day periods, your eating patterns will have changed. It's okay to eat out occasionally during this period, again following the advice of Chapter 9. Remember, the CRON diet is not intended as a 20-day quick-

TABLE 10.1 *Best food sources for vitamins and minerals according to food categories; (1) meat, (2) fish, (3) dairy, cheese, eggs, (4) bread, cereals, grains, (5) vegetables, (6) legumes, (7) fruit, (8) nuts and seeds, (9) oils, (10) seaweed, (11) miscellaneous (+ means top quality, sometimes approaching 100% of RDA per ordinary portion. ○ means second best, but still good per ordinary portion)*

VITAMINS	QUALITY	SOURCES
A	+	(1) liver, (2) shark, (5) sweet potato, kale, turnip greens, chard, carrots, beet greens, (10) nori
	○	(2) swordfish, crab, (5) broccoli, spinach, Romaine lettuce
D	+	(2) sardines, mackerel, (10) kombu, nori, wakami
	○	(1) veal, (2) salmon, oysters, herring, tuna, shrimp
K	+	(1) liver, (4) wheat germ, (5) Romaine lettuce, tomatoes, cabbage, Brussels sprouts, broccoli, turnip greens, cauliflower, carrots, asparagus, (6) soybeans
	○	(1) ham, pork, (3) Ricotta cheese, cottage cheese, (4) wheat bran, (5) celery root, spinach, (7) strawberries
C	+	(5) kale, broccoli, Brussels sprouts, turnip greens, red peppers, (7) cantaloupe, papaya, oranges, strawberries
	○	(1) liver, (5) cauliflower, chard, cabbage, asparagus, (7) grapefruit, persimmon, lemon, watermelon, banana
E	+	(5) kale, sweet potato, (4) buckwheat, (6) soybeans, (8) sunflower seeds, almonds, (9) safflower oil
	○	(2) shrimp, (5) turnip greens, asparagus, celery root, (7) avocado, apple, (8) peanuts, (9) corn oil, olive oil
B-1 (Thiamin)	+	(1) pork, (2) catfish, (6) soybeans, cowpeas, (11) yeast
	○	(1) ham, lamb, veal, (2) snapper, salmon, (4) brown rice, bulgur wheat, (6) lima beans, lentils, split peas, garbanzos
B-2 (Riboflavin)	+	(1) liver
	○	(2) mackerel, catfish, (3) yogurt, milk, (4) wild rice, millet, (5) turnip greens, mushrooms, kale, broccoli, (6) soybeans, (7) banana, (11) yeast
B-6	+	(10) kombu, nori
	○	(1) liver, chicken (light meat) , turkey, rabbit, pork, beef, (2) salmon, mackerel, halibut, catfish, (4) millet, brown rice, (5) kale, turnip greens, cabbage, (6) soybeans, lima beans, lentils, garbanzos, (11) yeast

TABLE 10.1 *(Continued)*

VITAMINS	QUALITY	SOURCES
B-12	+	(2) oysters, salmon, mackerel, herring, sardines, crab, clams, catfish, (10) seaweed
	O	(1) liver, turkey, rabbit, pork, beef, (3) yogurt, eggs
Niacin	+	(1) rabbit, liver, chicken, (10) wakami
	O	(1) turkey, capon, veal, lamb, (2) halibut, mackerel, swordfish, salmon, shark, tuna, catfish, (4) brown rice, wild rice, bulgur wheat, whole wheat pasta, (5) mushrooms, (8) peanuts, (11) yeast
Folic Acid	+	(1) liver, (11) yeast
	O	(5) Romaine lettuce, turnip greens, beet greens, Brussels sprouts, (6) garbanzos, soybeans, pinto beans, lima beans
Pantothenic Acid	+	(1) liver, (5) mushrooms
	O	turkey (dark), chicken (dark), veal, pork, (2) salmon, (3) yogurt, eggs, (5) broccoli, kale, sweet potato, (6) soybeans, lentils, garbanzos, lima beans, (7) avocado, (11) yeast
Biotin	+	(1) liver, (6) soybeans
	O	chicken, (2) mackerel, salmon, sardines, (3) eggs, (4) barley, (6) cowpeas, garbanzos, (7) cantaloupe, banana, watermelon, (8) peanuts, (11) yeast
MINERALS		
Calcium	+	(3) milk, yogurt, cheese, (5) turnip greens
	O	(10) kombu, nori, wakami, (2) salmon, (5) kale, chard, broccoli, (6) soybeans, garbanzos
Magnesium	+	(6) soybeans, lima beans, cowpeas, (10) kombu, nori, wakami
	O	(4) buckwheat, wild rice, brown rice, millet, whole wheat pasta, (5) beet greens, chard, turnip greens, corn, (6) garbanzos, lentils, split peas, (8) cashews, almonds
Copper	+	(1) liver, (2) squid, oysters
	O	rabbit, (2) cod, lobster, (4) wheat bran, millet, brown rice, barley, (6) garbanzos, lentils, split peas, (8) sunflower seeds, cashews, (11) yeast
Zinc	+	(2) oysters, cod
	O	(1) beef, liver, hamburger, turkey (dark), veal, lamb, (4) wild rice, (5) turnip greens, (6) soybeans, split peas, lentils, garbanzos, lima beans, cowpeas, (8) sunflower seeds, (11) yeast

TABLE 10.1 *(Continued)*

VITAMINS	QUALITY	SOURCES
Chromium	+	(1) liver, (3) American cheese, (6) lima beans, green beans
	O	(1) beef, chicken, turkey, lamb, veal, pork, (2) sole, salmon, haddock, shrimp, tuna, crab, oysters, (3) nonfat milk, buttermilk, Swiss cheese, eggs, (4) rye and whole wheat bread, (5) white and sweet potatoes, broccoli, corn, Brussels sprouts, lettuce, (8) peanuts, (11) yeast
Potassium	+	(1) liver, (10) kombu, nori, wakami
	O	(1) beef, veal, hamburger, ham, pork, (2) clams, oysters, scallops, (5) chard, kale, turnip greens, mushrooms, (6) soybeans, lima beans, split peas, garbanzos, lentils, (8) pumpkin seeds
Iron	+	(1) liver, (2) clams, oysters, (5) soybeans, lima beans, split peas, (10) hijiki, nori, wakami, (11) yeast
	O	(1) beef, veal, ham, pork, turkey, rabbit, lamb, chicken, (2) tuna, scallops, (4) millet, (5) chard, beet greens, (6) garbanzos, lentils, cowpeas, (8) pumpkin seeds
Manganese	+	(5) beet greens, turnip greens, (6) soybeans, (8) chestnuts, (10) nori
	O	(4) wheat bran, wheat germ, millet, brown rice, barley, rolled oats, buckwheat, (5) beets, chard, kale, sweet potatoes, (6) garbanzos, lima beans, (7) pineapple, grapes, raspberries, (8) peanuts
Selenium	+	(1) liver, beef, (2) tuna, herring, ocean perch, mackerel, cod, sardines, (4) barley, whole wheat bread and pasta, (6) soybeans
	O	(1) pork, lamb, chicken, (2) oysters, lobster, shrimp, (4) brown rice, (5) Brussels sprouts, (6) lentils, (7) lemon, (8) sunflower seeds, (11) yeast

weight-loss program, although you can easily misuse it to that end. The first goal is a reprogramming of food habits. After the introductory period, you must choose your own direction, following the precepts I've laid down to whatever degree you're able, and depending on how healthy and long-lived you want to be and how much gluttony you want to sacrifice for enhanced physical well-being. Habit and social pressure will be more of a problem than hunger.

DRESSINGS

A comparison of a number of popular commercial dressings is shown in table 10.2. Since my earlier edition in 1986 there has been noticeable improvement in health qualities of commercial dressing in calorie, fat, and sodium content. Labeling, however, remains inadequate, e.g., levels of trans-fatty acids are not given. The fat-free dressings, at least, would not contain these undesirables.

A number of recipes follow for low-fat, low-calorie dressings (including mayonnaise and "cream cheese"), sauces, and broths. Most of these (including the four sauces for vegetables) can be thickened by the addition of a solution of gums. Guar gum, gum arabic, and gum tragacanth are the most common. You may wish to substitute Worcestershire sauce for soy sauce or tamari in your cooking. Worcestershire has 55 to 95 milligrams sodium per teaspoon (depending on the brand), whereas soy sauce characteristically contains 330 milligrams.

TABLE 10.2 *Calorie, fat, and sodium content (per tablespoon) of some leading commercial Italian dressings (adapted from* Nutrition Action, *October 1981)*

DRESSING	CALORIES	FAT GRAMS	SATURATED FAT	SODIUM MG
REGULAR				
Kraft	80	8	1	240
Wish-Bone	80	8	1	284
Seven Seas	70	7	1	400
REDUCED CALORIE				
Kraft	6	0	0	220
Wish-Bone	30	3	0	192
Walden Farms	9	1	0	300
NO-OIL				
Kraft	4	0	0	220
Herb Magic	4	0	0	NA
Aristocrat	6	0	0	2

LOW-CALORIE MAYONNAISE

Blend the following until smooth: 1 raw egg, whites of 2 hard-boiled eggs, 2 shallots, ½ clove pressed garlic, 1 teaspoon lemon juice, 1 teaspoon dry mustard. Pour into dish and fold in ½ cup nonfat yogurt. Store in covered jar or plastic container.

TOFU MAYONNAISE

Blend the following until smooth: ½ cup nonfat yogurt, 200 grams (7 ounces) tofu, ½ clove pressed garlic, 2 tablespoons cider or balsamic vinegar, 1 tablespoon lemon juice, 2 teaspoons safflower oil, 3 teaspoons Worcestershire sauce.

TOFU CREAM CHEESE

Blend the following until smooth: 1 cup (200 grams) tofu, 1 teaspoon umeboshi paste (Japanese salted plum paste), ¼ teaspoon tahini (sesame-seed paste). Add 1 tablespoon finely chopped scallions, ¼ stalk finely chopped celery, 1 teaspoon finely chopped parsley, and ¼ grated medium carrot, and stir into mixture.

LOW-CALORIE, LOW-FAT VINAIGRETTE

Add ½ cube vegetable bouillon and 1 tablespoon Worcestershire sauce to ½ cup boiling water and stir until bouillon is dissolved. Allow to cool, then add 2 tablespoons lemon juice, 4 tablespoons vinegar, 1 clove of pressed garlic, ½ teaspoon dry mustard, ¼ teaspoon each of dried marjoram and tarragon, 3 teaspoons chopped fresh herbs (either dill or basil), and 2 tablespoons safflower oil. Mix in blender and store in glass jar in refrigerator. For a still lower fat vinaigrette, substitute ½ cup low-fat or nonfat yogurt for the safflower oil.

BUTTERMILK DRESSING

Stir or blend together 1 cup buttermilk, 1 tablespoon prepared mustard, 2 tablespoons finely chopped scallions, ¼ cup grated cucumber, ¼ teaspoon dill weed, 2 teaspoons lemon juice, and ¼ teaspoon black pepper.

YOGURT-BALSAMIC DRESSING (MY FAVORITE!)

Stir or blend together 1 cup low-fat or nonfat yogurt, ½ cup top-grade balsamic vinegar, ½ cup buttermilk, 2 teaspoons extra-virgin olive oil (the oil can be omitted), and ½ of a peeled, finely chopped lemon.

COTTAGE CHEESE DRESSING

Process the following in a blender until smooth: ½ cup buttermilk, ½ cup low-fat cottage cheese, ¼ cup balsamic or other vinegar, 1 teaspoon Worcestershire sauce, 4 small red radishes, 2 to 3 chopped green onions.

YOGURT MIDDLE EASTERN DRESSING

Blend 1 cup yogurt, 1 tablespoon olive oil, 1 tablespoon fresh lemon juice, 1 small clove pressed garlic, 1 tablespoon fresh chopped mint.

YOGURT GREEN GODDESS DRESSING

Blend the following until smooth and very green (about 23 minutes): 3/4 cup yogurt, ¼ cup Low-Calorie Mayonnaise (see above), 2 teaspoons vinegar, 1 teaspoon dried or 1 tablespoon fresh tarragon, 2 tablespoons chopped green onions or chives.

SAUCES

MOCK SOUR CREAM

Blend until smooth: 2 tablespoons low-fat or skim milk, 1 tablespoon lemon juice, 1 cup low-fat cottage cheese.

MOCK CREAM CHEESE

Blend powdered milk or whey protein into the above to thicken to the desired consistency.

TOFU CREAM SAUCE

Blend until completely smooth: ½ pound tofu, ½ cup nonfat yogurt, 1 tablespoon each of sesame tahini, miso, and lemon juice.

CREOLE SAUCE

Cook 2 tablespoon chopped onion, 2 tablespoon chopped green pepper, and ¼ cup sliced mushrooms in nonstick skillet over low heat for 5 minutes. Add 2 cups stewed tomatoes with juice, ¼ teaspoon pepper, and ½ teaspoon basil. Simmer until sauce is thick, about 30 minutes.

BEAN SAUCE

Blend 1 cup low-fat or nonfat yogurt, ½ cup mashed, cooked beans, ¼ cup chopped chives, 2 tablespoons green chili salsa.

SALSA

Chop the drained tomatoes from a small can of salt-free peeled tomatoes. Add ½ stalk of finely chopped celery, ½ of a finely chopped green pepper, 1 jalapeno or yellow pepper seeded and finely chopped, ⅓ cup of lemon juice or apple-cider vinegar, 1 teaspoon cumin, ½ teaspoon chili powder, 2 tablespoons chopped cilantro (optional), and some freshly ground pepper. Mix well.

TOFU WHITE SAUCE

Blend the following until completely smooth: ½ package (7 ounces = 200 grams) tofu, ½ cup low-fat or nonfat yogurt, ¼ cup water, 2 teaspoons miso, 2 teaspoons tamari, 1 ½ teaspoons grated ginger, 2 tablespoons sherry, ¼ of a peeled lemon, and ½ of a freshly grated nutmeg.

FRUIT SAUCE

Finely dice 1 apple, 1 pear, 4–5 plums, 1 peach (can leave out any one of these but not the plums). Place in a saucepan; add 1 cup water, ¼ cup good-quality cider vinegar, 1 teaspoon sugar, 2 teaspoons tamari (or Worchestershire sauce), 1 clove of pressed garlic. Bring to boil and simmer on low flame for ½ hour.

GARLIC POTATO SAUCE (ANOTHER FAVORITE)

Boil two average-size white potatoes, skin them, and place in a blender. Add 6 cloves pressed or minced garlic, 1 teaspoon tamari, a cup of cider or ½ cup wine vinegar (whichever you like), and ½ cup low-fat or nonfat yogurt. Blend until smooth.

TOMATO VEGETABLE (TV) SAUCE

Finely chop 1 bunch of scallions, 2 garlic cloves, and ¼ cup of parsley. Poach in water to cover the bottom of a large frying pan, while stirring, until the onions are golden or very wilted (about 10 minutes). Add water if necessary during this time. Meanwhile chop 6 ripe fresh tomatoes (or use a 28-ounce can of tomatoes, drained). Add the tomatoes to the onion mixture and mix until the tomatoes are heated through. Add 1 tablespoon oregano, 1 tablespoon fresh, crushed mint (or a dash of dried mint), 2 bay leaves, and ½ cup of sherry. Simmer for 15 to 20 minutes only.

BROTHS

CHICKEN BROTH

Place a 3- to 4-pound chicken, mostly bony parts like backs and necks, with most of the skin removed in a large pot with 1 large quartered onion, 1 sliced stalk of celery, 2 small or 1 large sliced carrots, 4 parsley sprigs, 1 leek divided into 2-inch slices, 1 bay leaf, 2 cloves of sliced garlic, 8 peppercorns, and 4 quarts of water. Bring to boil and simmer for 2–3 hours. Remove chicken bones. Strain and chill broth. Allow fat to rise to top and remove. Boil down further to concentrate the broth. Freeze in ice-cube trays, then store the cubes in a plastic bag. Each cube may be used like a bouillon cube and can be diluted with water.

BOUILLON BROTH

Place 4 cups water, 3 vegetable-bouillon cubes, 2 cloves pressed garlic, and ¼ cup Worcestershire sauce in a pot. Bring to boil, and simmer until bouillon dissolves. Freeze in ice-cube trays and store cubes in a plastic bag.

BITES AND TIDBITS

These are alphabetically arranged notes on healthful foods (or unhealthful foods) and food related terms. For example, an apple a day can help keep the doctor away, but eating a Red Delicious every day could get boring. Did you know, however, that over 100 varieties of apples are still in cultivation, ranging from dark red to pale yellow, from sweet to tart, with all consistencies of firmness? Many varieties do not travel well in bulk, so only three or four types appear in the supermarkets. But in the proper season, you can have any of the others, or a selection of them, mail ordered to your home.

Apples: For variety in apples, write to Applesource, Tom Vorbeck, Route 1, Chapin, Illinois 62628, or for internet sources, see Readings and Resources.

Berries: Berries are a rich source of various antioxidants. As outlined in the Flavonoid section in Chapter 7, blueberries may have special, health-enhancing, even reparative properties.

Bioavailability: The term *bioavailability* refers to how much of the nutriment in a food can actually be absorbed, and also to the materials present in this or other foods that may interfere with its absorption. The bioavailability of zinc, for example, varies widely. Meat and seafood zinc is more readily available than that from vegetables. Indeed, one can develop actual clinical zinc deficiency on a completely vegetarian diet when the theoretical amount of zinc in the diet is far in excess of the RDAs. Iron can be a problem too. The body absorbs twice to four times as much of the iron present in meat, fish, and poultry as it does of the iron in plant foods. Vitamin C facilitates iron absorption. When drunk with or within an hour *after* a meal, tea may interfere with iron absorption by as much as 85 percent, and coffee by 40 percent. If it is drunk an hour before the meal, this does not occur. In multivitamin preparations, the presence of calcium carbonate and/or magnesium oxide may interfere with the absorption of iron in the same preparation. Too much bran in a meal, or a large amount of calcium, may bind certain elements like iron, copper, and zinc into insoluble complexes and prevent their full assimilation. As I have said, however, more iron than you actually require eases oxidative stress, so the above impediments to absorption may have benefits if not overdone.

The phytic acid present in cereals and nuts (in the bran and germ) seriously interferes with absorption of dietary calcium. In the presence of calcium it will also inhibit absorption of zinc and iron. When the cereal is soaked for 15 to 30 minutes before it's brought to a boil, the enzyme phytase renders the phytic acid less active. Spinach is high in calcium but contains substances that interfere with calcium absorption.

Absorption of iron (which, however, should not be taken unless prescribed by your doctor) from mineral supplements may be much less if the supplements are taken with meals. My advice: take major calcium and magnesium supplements separate from trace elements (iron, zinc, copper, chromium, selenium) and take both between meals.

Bread: Pita, sometimes called pocket or Bible bread, is correctly made of whole wheat flour, water, yeast, and salt. Avoid the white flour version in supermarkets, and indeed avoid all white bread. A basic loaf of good bread might contain only whole wheat flour, water, and yeast, but other materials are usually added: oils, molasses, honey, and salt, and/or other grains. Avoid any kind of white flour, enriched or not. Avoid anything labeled merely "wheat flour," as that could just mean ordinary white flour. Tortillas and chapattis are simply whole wheat flour and water. Or you may get corn tortillas, in which case they should be made from whole-grain cornmeal (most store-bought varieties are not so made). These and sprout bread (sprouted wheat berries put through a coarse grinder and baked), have no oil and are low in calories. If you must eat crackers, be guided by the data in Table 10.3 to select those low in both fat and sodium. I was surprised to learn how much fat Wheat Thins contain, and how loaded with sodium they are. Stoned Wheat Thins, even though manufactured by a company with the reassuring name of Health Valley, are hardly better.

TABLE 10.3 *Comparison of selected crackers,*
showing calories, fat, and sodium per ounce of cracker
(adapted from Nutrition Action, *April 1983)*

CRACKER NAME	BRAND	CALORIES	FAT (G)	SODIUM (MG)
Whole Wheat Matzo	*Manischewitz*	110	0	3
Whole Grain No Salt Flatbread	*Ideal*	72	0	18
Ry-Krisp Natural	*Ralston*	100	0	220
Golden Rye Krisp Bread	*Wasa*	98	0	312
Dark Caraway Rye Wafers	*Finn Crisp*	100	0	
Wheat Melba Toast Unsalted	*Devonsheer*	112	0	7
Bran Wafers No Salt	*Venus*	100	2	4
Stoned Wheat Thins	*Interbake*	128	2	111
Ry-Krisp Sesame	*Ralston*	120	3	302
Wheat Wafers	*Sunshine*	119	3	
Harvest Wheats	*Keebler*	140	4	
Herb Wheat Crackers No Salt	*Health Valley*	134	5	101
Triscuits	*Nabisco*	140	5	210
Stoned Wheat Crackers	*Health Valley*	134	6	189
Wheat Thins	*Nabisco*	140	6	240
Toasted Wheat Crackers	*Keebler*	144	7	
Wheat Goldfish Thins	*Pepperidge Farm*	140	8	260
Ritz Crackers	*Nabisco*	150	8	270
Sesame Wheats	*Nabisco*	150	9	281

Caffeine: Sir T. H. Herbert wrote about coffee in 1626, "It is said to be healthy when drunk hot. It destroys melancholy, dries the tears, softens anger and produces joyful feelings." Tradition has it that it was invented by Gabriel to restore the sinking Mohammed. That's the positive report. Each year Americans brew 2 ½ billion pounds of coffee, and eight out of ten persons drink an average of three to five cups per day. A typical cup of coffee contains 100 milligrams of caffeine; of tea, 20 to 50; the colas 30 to 45; and Dr. Pepper has 60 milligrams per 12-ounce can.

Whether caffeine is bad for you, and if so, how bad, remains debatable. A study from Finland reported that one to four cups of coffee per day would increase blood cholesterol by 5 percent, and nine cups by 14 percent; but three of five other studies did not confirm this. It might be important how the coffee is prepared, or what it is drunk with. The large-scale Framingham study found no association between coffee consumption and the risk of heart disease. In laboratory tests, caffeine appears somewhat mutagenic (potential cancer-causing), but there is no evidence of such an effect in human coffee-drinking populations. Coffee may contain residues of toxic insecticides banned in the United States but sold to coffee-producing countries.

Tea is certainly preferable to coffee as a source of caffeine. (Just brew it stronger!) It has positive health values from its content of phytochemicals (see Chapter 7).

Cereals (See also Grains): "Shredded" cereals are probably the closest to "wholeness" in a mildly processed cereal. Many of the highly processed mainstays of Kellogg, Post, General Mills, and General Foods are high in sugar content, up to 30 percent. Those low in sugar include Kellogg's Special K, Nutri-Grain Corn, Nutri-Grain Shredded Wheat, Puffed Rice, Puffed Wheat, Corn Flakes, Corn Chex, Rice Chex, and Grape-Nuts.[2] Processed cereals both low in sugar and best in nutritional quality include Cheerios, Grape-Nuts, Shredded Wheat, Instant Cream of Wheat, Instant Quaker Oatmeal, and Maypo 30-Second Oatmeal.[3]

Grape-Nuts is among the most nutritious of the processed cereals. Like many of the others, it is "fortified." According to studies by *Consumer Reports*, however, a serious question exists about the actual bioavailability of the added materials in fortified cereals.[4] For this reason, plus the fact that you don't know the source of the fortification substances, it's better to obtain supplements from a reliable company than from fortified foods.

Whole cereals and grains, such as whole grain oats, whole wheat berries, buckwheat, with as little processing as possible, are best. Whole oats cook up just as fast as rolled oats, just six to eight minutes in the microwave. Flakes are next best and retain a fair amount of their original nutritive values—as examples, wheat flakes, rye flakes, barley flakes, triticale flakes, and soy and oat flakes, which are also referred to as rolled oats, rolled rye, and so on. Creams vary widely in nutritive value. They are good if made from freshly ground 100-percent-whole-grain flour, but poor if made from processed flour. In puffed cereals, nutritional losses are substantial, so avoid them. "Hulled" millet, which cooks up in 15 to 20 minutes, is a good "whole grain," only the outer hull having been removed. One of the most nourishing of grains, hulled millet makes an excellent breakfast porridge. As much a grain as a cereal, amaranth seed can be eaten in pancakes and porridge. It was a basic food in America before Columbus arrived, and is just becoming popular again. Amaranth protein is closer to a complete protein than that of any other cereal or grain, having more lysine, in which the others tend to be poor. The leaves of amaranth are also highly nutritious.

Cereals (as well as soy-based foods) contain inositol phosphates, which by reacting with copper and iron ions prevent the latter from participating in reactions producing the destructive hydroxyl radicals. Thus, cereals contain several phytonutrients not present in fruits and vegetables,[5]* a point to be remembered by those who are so gung-ho for ultralow carbohydrate diets.

To cook most whole cereals, simmer one part of cereal with two parts of water for about 15 minutes, until the water is absorbed, or microwave for eight minutes at half power. If you need to save time in the morning, soak the cereal in cold water overnight and it will cook in just three to four minutes. Wheat germ has been overpublicized as a health food. It is a concentrated source of protein and contains a lot of vitamin E, but its major component is oil, and it becomes rancid easily. The best form is that delivered to health-food stores from local mills on the same day each week, the day it is made. Buy it that day, refrigerate it, and use it up in the next few days.

Complementarity: There are eight amino acids essential for adult humans. When these are present in the ratios represented in the RDA amounts, *all* of the protein can be used in making the building blocks of the body. If the supply of one is deficient, a proportionate amount of the others is merely converted into energy, i.e. burned off. If a single one is in great excess, the excess also is simply burned off.

Achieving complementarity has been in and out of favor among nutritionists. The position now is that as long as you are above the RDAs in all eight, an excess amount of one, two, or three is irrelevant.

But that's probably not true for anti-aging regimens. "Burning off" an excess intake of any kind may create additional free radicals, and/or use up your lifetime caloric allotment (the so-called *lifetime energy potential*).[6] So complementarity is in fact important, at least for us. Eggs and milk afford the most complete protein followed by red meat, then fish. Soy products are fairly complete. Rice is deficient in isoleucine and lysine, but can be complemented with broccoli, cauliflower, spinach, or beans. Millet and corn are deficient in lysine: add tofu, pumpkin seeds, nuts, soy products, brussels sprouts, broccoli, spinach, or mustard greens. Beans tend to be low in methionine and tryptophan. Most nutritionists take the position that rice, millet, and the cereals, for example, can be complemented by addition of a small quantity of dairy products or meats. That does indeed bring everything above the RDAs, but still leaves an imbalance, and the excess will have to be burned off. For anti-aging purposes, we want as close to a real *balance* as can be achieved without a big fuss. This can be done best by computer techniques.

Dairy products and eggs: Milk, cheese, yogurt, and eggs are all sources of complete protein, vitamin A, calcium, and essential fatty acids. Unfortunately, some also supply saturated fats and cholesterol. Whole eggs contain a considerable amount of cholesterol, although in the Framingham study there was no close relation between egg intake and either blood cholesterol or coronary-artery disease. If eggs are eaten along with a source of vitamin C—for example, with a glass of orange juice—one may observe an increase in HDL without an increase in LDL.[7] Total fat intake, especially saturated fat, is much more important than dietary cholesterol intake in controlling blood cholesterol levels.[8] In fact the amount of cholesterol in the diet is now thought to have only a minor influence on blood levels of cholesterol.

Oxidized cholesterol in the diet is another matter. Improperly stored cholesterol may contain up to 32 auto-oxidation products, some of which exert a toxic effect on arterial cells and lead to arteriosclerosis. The oxidized forms may be found in dehydrated or powdered eggs (as present in many noodles) and in cooked meats stored unfrozen for an appreciable time before being eaten.[9] A fresh raw egg is free of oxidation products. Fried or hard-boiled eggs produce about 12 times, scrambled eggs six times, and raw or soft-boiled eggs only three to four times the levels of oxidized cholesterol as controls. So if you eat eggs, eat them with the yolks as soft as possible. A recent study following 38,000 men and 80,000 women, ages 40 to 75, for 8 to 14 years found that people who ate an egg or more daily were no more likely to develop heart disease or stroke than those limiting themselves to less than one egg per week.[10] Eggs are now available from chickens fed diets high in grains and flax seed, and these contain considerably higher than the usual levels of omega-3 fatty acids. I recommend them if you like eggs.

Regular cheese like cheddar, Swiss, and other "natural" cheeses derives about 65 percent of its calories from fat, and some cheeses much more (cream cheese, 90 percent; blue cheese, 74 percent). Even so-called low-fat or part-skim cheese still derives 50 percent of its calories from fat. Thus, with a few exceptions, low fat cheese is not really low in fat. The one exception among regular natural cheese may be St. Otho's, which is reputed to be only 5 percent fat. Unfortunately, St. Otho's, while quite delicious, is hard to find. I only found it once, after a long search in New York. Regular cottage cheese and part-skim mozzarella (Kraft) derive about 35 percent of their calories from fat. Dorman's makes a low-fat skim Edam cheese that derives about 25 percent of its calories from fat. On the other hand, low sodium cheese is truly low in sodium. Unless you buy the no-salt-added kind, cottage cheese may be quite high in sodium; also, unlike other dairy products, it is not a good source of calcium. Low-fat cottage cheese derives only 10 to 25 percent of its calories from fat. At 180 calories a cup, it can be used in recipes to replace ricotta cheese (430 calories per cup). Pot or farmer cheese is low in fat and can replace cream cheese at ¼ the calorie count. Sapsago cheese is fat free and excellent grated on spaghetti, but hard and rather biting by itself. No-fat cheeses made from tofu protein are also available.

Whole milk is 3.3 percent fat by total weight, which doesn't sound bad, but 50 percent of the calories in whole milk are derived from fat; 36 percent of the calories in 2 percent, or "low-fat," milk in fact comes from fat; skim milk, or "nonfat" milk, derives 10 percent of its calories from fat. Use skim milk when possible, with added vitamins A and D. (And of course sunlight is a major source of vitamin D.)

Many non-Caucasian adults and even a few Caucasians are troubled by cramps, gas, and diarrhea when they drink milk. These problems develop because of genetically determined low levels of the intestinal enzyme lactase in many adults. Present in all children of every race, lactase is low or absent in the intestines of 30 percent of adult non-Caucasians and 10 percent of adult Caucasians. Lactase is necessary to digest lactose, the sugar in milk. If milk disagrees with you in this fashion, try Lact-Aid, which can be added to milk to predigest the lactose. Sweet acidophilus may also be tolerated, and mild evidence exists that it has a beneficial effect on colon cancer and blood cholesterol levels.[11] Since there are few dietary sources of vitamin D besides milk, people who consume no milk should consider a vitamin D supplement.

Through the ages, a good deal of folklore has grown up about yogurt. According to a Persian tale, an angel taught Abraham how to make it. Well tolerated by lactase-deficient people, it has all the nutritional content of milk, except that low-fat and nonfat yogurt are usually not fortified with vitamins A and D. Regular yogurt contains 150 to 210 calories per eight-ounce serving; low-fat yogurt, 140 to 160 calories; nonfat yogurt, 90 to 110. Most flavored yogurts contain about 6 teaspoon of sugar per cup (or enough to make up 25 to 50 percent of the total calories in Dannon fruit yogurt, for example). Avoid these. Yogurt is good food, but not with a lot of added sugar.

Fiber: Water-soluble fibers such as pectin and the various gums will lower cholesterol. These "soluble fibers" are found in dried beans and peas, fresh peas, corn, sweet potatoes, pears, prunes, and oat bran. Pectins are found mainly in the white rind of citrus fruits, and in bananas, carrots, and apples; gums can be found in beans and oatmeal and oat bran. Fibers in Chinese vegetables such as pea pods, bamboo shoots, and Chinese lettuce are especially good cholesterol binders. Water-insoluble fibers such as those in wheat bran help normalize bowel function and (now in some doubt) help prevent bowel cancer and diverticulosis.[12] Another soluble fiber, galactomanin, acting against both diabetes and elevated cholesterol, is found in fenugreek seeds. Supplements of ground fenugreek seeds have been shown to lower blood glucose levels in both healthy persons and diabetics,[13] and, by tying up bile acids, lead to lower cholesterol levels.

Large quantities of fiber may inhibit absorption of iron, calcium, zinc, and other minerals because the phytates in them tend to combine with the minerals, rendering them insoluble. In ways not well understood, fiber contributes to satiety and prolongs the time before you are hungry again.[14] Diets should contain 30 or more grams of dietary fiber for every 1,000 calories. The average American consumes, in his 3,000+ calorie diet, only about 20 grams total—much too little. If you want to increase your fiber intake with wheat or oat bran or other additives, do it slowly, as a rapid increase may cause intestinal discomfort. Fiber contents of a number of foods were given in Table 5.4. Wheat bran, incidentally, is not merely inert roughage, as many assume. It contains substantial amounts of manganese, magnesium, niacin, and vitamin K per 15-gram portion. Rice bran is in fact among the most nutritious of the grains.

Fish: Most fishes afford relatively complete protein and either are low in fat (cod, haddock, halibut, lake perch, whitefish) or contain the kind of fatty acid that inhibits the development of arteriosclerosis. White-meat albacore tuna, mackerel, and pink salmon, followed by freshwater trout, herring, anchovies, and catfish, all contain eicosapentaenoic acid (EPA) and docosahexaenoic acid (DHA). Whitefish and bass are both low in total fat and fairly high in EPA and DHA. Unfortunately, some seafoods from some locations are contaminated: mercury in tuna and swordfish, and insecticides and other chemical residues in other fish, especially the fatty ones. Residues such as the PCBs tend to accumulate in fatty tissues, and may be high in fish that live all or part of their lives in shallow estuaries (bluefish, striped bass, Atlantic sturgeon, white perch, and white catfish, depending on where they come from, and Chinook salmon from the Great Lakes). Santa Monica Bay off Los Angeles, San Francisco Bay, New York Bay, and Chesapeake Bay have been hot spots of contamination, as well as the whole East Coast from Chesapeake Bay to Boston. Eighty to 90 percent of the tomcod population over two years old from the Hudson River have liver tumors due to pollutants. The contaminant danger is not great enough that it should scare you off fish, but be wary. The safest fish are small white-fleshed ocean varieties plus a few others including snapper, sea bass, sole, cod, flounder, mackerel, perch, herring, and sardines. Proper cleaning and cooking can eliminate 25 to 50 percent of the toxins in fish. Two fish dishes per week will help prevent heart disease.

Stick to fresh fish or to frozen plain varieties. To freeze a fillet, drop it into cold water, place on foil, and freeze 20 minutes, then transfer to a plastic bag and seal. Such a fillet can be cooked directly from the frozen state; simply add 50 percent to the usual cooking time. Avoid supermarket prepared fish. For example, Van de Kamp's Light and Crispy fish fillets contain 68 percent of calories derived from fat. Fast-food fish are no better; Carl's Jr.'s Fillet of Fish Sandwich contains 43 percent of calories from fat, and McDonald's Fillet-O-Fish, 52 percent.

Garlic and onions: Some years ago at a hearing of the House Committee on Aging, the late Representative Claude Pepper asked a number of octogenarians to what they attributed their longevity. The commonest claim among the oldsters was eating a lot of onions. Of course, that's only testimonial evidence—the very worst kind.

Onions and garlic (especially garlic) do have a long folkloric history. Egyptian pharaohs were entombed with carvings of garlic and onions to ensure that the meals in their afterlife would be well seasoned. Roman nobles fed garlic to their soldiers to make them brave, and to their women to make them strong. Elizabethans hailed garlic as an aphrodisiac. It was used against the plague in the eighteenth century and was the main ingredient of the "Vinegar of Four Thieves," a concoction invented by four thieves that enabled them to burglarize the houses of the dead and dying in plague-ridden Marseille without catching the plague themselves. Garlic does have antibacterial action. And of course it wards off vampires! Useful stuff, besides being a great seasoning.

The oils of onions and garlic appear to inhibit tumor promotion by certain cancer-causing agents,[15] although how many onions and garlic cloves one would have to eat to produce a measurable effect is not certain. Onion oil contains at least 55 components. Which of the components are the tumor inhibitors is not established at present. Gangshan County in China has the lowest gastric-cancer death rate of all of Shandong Province, and Quixia the highest. Gangshanites regularly eat up to 20 grams of garlic daily (about five cloves), Quixiites little or none.

A number of animal and human studies have indicated that garlic and garlic oils may lower blood cholesterol and fat levels.[16,17] In one study in humans, the consumption of 0.5 millileters of fresh garlic juice per kilogram of body weight per day over a two-month period led to an average fall in serum cholesterol of about 28 percent. Well-controlled studies of the Jain sect in India indicate that populations eating more garlic and onions have lower blood cholesterol levels. In a Moslem community in Udaipur those who ate about ten cloves of garlic per day per person enjoyed a very low incidence of hypertension, heart disease, and cancer compared to neighboring groups.[18,19]*

There are many varieties of garlic, in fact over 200. The small red-skinned variety is the strongest, and keeps the longest. Purple or violet garlic is medium in strength, and the familiar white variety the mildest. Elephant garlic has very large white-skinned cloves and is quite mild in flavor, but it is not a true garlic. Varieties of garlic can be obtained (seasonally) from a number of suppliers (see References and Resources). Buy from one of these in summer or fall, to obtain fresher, better garlic and of a wider variety than you can find in supermarkets. If you like garlic, buy six to eight varieties at a time, mince them in a little olive oil, and taste on a small piece of bread. You will soon become a garlic gourmet. A few sprigs of parsley after each tasting will cleanse your breath.

Do not store garlic in the refrigerator as the moist air will cause spoilage; rather, store the bulbs in a cool dry place, and in the dark to slow down sprouting. An easy way to prepare garlic as a seasoning is to let ten to twelve heads stand for five to ten minutes in hot water, which softens them and makes them peel more easily, then peel them and make into a smooth paste via a food mill or processor, add a little olive oil, mix and keep in a small jar in the refrigerator. The preparation is good for several weeks. In preparing onions and/or garlic for sauces and dressings, one may also sautè them in a small amount of oil. Elephant garlic is good steamed. Commercially produced garlic powders and salts are in general not recommended. Garlic salt is usually 90 percent plain salt.

Grains (See also Cereals): We are here concerned with barley, buck-wheat, corn, millet, rice, wild rice, rye, and wheat. Wash thoroughly before cooking. Generally a dry grain expands to 2 ½ times its volume when cooked. Cooked grains will keep up to three to four days in the refrigerator, so make enough for two meals if you wish. Cooking times and amounts of water to be added per cup of different grains are shown in Table 10.4.

TABLE 10.4 *Cooking times and water required*
per cup of different grains

GRAIN	COOKING TIME (MINUTES)	AMOUNT (CUPS)	WATER (CUPS)	COOKED AMOUNT (CUPS)
Buckwheat	20	1	5	3
Bulgur	15	1	2	2½
Brown Rice	35–40	1	2	2½
Short-Grain Rice	35–40	1	2½	2½
Long-Grain Rice	60	1	4	2⅔
Triticale	60	1	4	2½
Wheat Berries	60	1	4	2½

A few minutes before the grain is wholly cooked, you can add cinnamon or cloves for a sweet flavor, basil or oregano for an Italian flavor, finely chopped fresh ginger, coriander, or cumin for an Indonesian flavor, saffron or curry power for Indian. Of all the grains, rye (and amaranth—see Cereals) has the highest percentage of the essential amino acid lysine. Rice, wheat, and bulgur are deficient in isoleucine and lysine. Rice is also low in riboflavin, although wheat is not. Use hulled or, even better, unhulled barley, not pearl barley. Pearl barley is too far along the big-food-company chain; it's a polished product lacking in insoleucine and lysine. Nutritionally one of the best grains, millet is the staple of the Hunzas of India, an allegedly long-lived population. Millet has one of the most complete proteins of all the grains. Although listed here, buckwheat is not a grain at all; it is related to rhubarb. Groats are buckwheat with the hull removed, and when these are roasted, constitute kasha. Buckwheat has two and one-half times as much of the B vitamins as whole wheat, and lots of potassium, phosphorus, and biotin. Among the grains, rice bran is one of the most favored. It's rich in vitamin B6, thiamine, and niacin, and it has a glycemic index of only about 26 (see Table 9.3).

Heat, effect on nutrients: Cooking has positive and negative effects on the nutrients in foods. It decreases some nutrients, increases the availability of others, and also destroys some contaminants. The pesticide EDB, which causes cancer and genetic mutations, is about 80 percent destroyed by cooking. The B vitamin folacin is easily destroyed by heat, so when using dark green leafy vegetables, eat them only slightly cooked (steamed). Some of the phytochemicals, lycopene for example, are released from binding by heat, and made more available for absorption.

HDL levels: It's desirable to raise your HDL levels. How? Moderate intake of alcohol will raise HDL but not LDL, which is good so far as it goes. Chocolate is composed primarily of stearic acid, a saturated fatty acid that may raise HDL; and, incidentally and along with red wine, chocolate contains flavonoids which inhibit the oxidation of LDL cholesterol.[20,21] Fish will raise HDLs. MUFAs like olive oil and canola oil when substituted for other cooking oils, will raise HDL but not LDL, giving an improved ratio. PUFAs like corn oil and safflower oil will lower both HDL and LDL. Finally, exercise is almost certainly the best way to increase HDL.

Herbs: The possible health benefits of various herbs is too extensive a subject for discussion here, but an excellent introductory article and guide is the review by K. Mcnutt in *Nutrition Today*.[22]

Internet, the use of: Here of course we witness a veritable explosion of opportunity since my first edition in 1986. The internet may even help reverse the terrible ongoing loss of the various varieties of domestic produce, since it allows relatively small farmers to do business online. Take apples. There are, or at least were, more than a hundred varieties, but agribusiness, which dominates the supermarket business, only deals with a few, and 12 years ago it was quite difficult to get anything else. Now simply go to Yahoo or other search engines, and type in apples, or garlic or whatever you fancy, and you'll find biodiversity.

Labels: *Organic, natural, raw, uncooked, unfiltered, low-calorie, sugarless, sugar-free, enriched, fortified*: don't fall for these prohealth buzzwords! Some of them are meaningful, others not.*Organic* is understood to mean grown without artificial chemical fertilizers, herbicides, or pesticides, but in fact the word means nothing unless the grower has been certified by an organic growers' association. Look for this certification on the package. However, true organic food is better if you can get it, to avoid pesticide residues. During the past 40 years pesticide use has increased by over 1,000 percent. Speaking of pesticides, genetic modification of plants is dandy if it's done to increase the nutrient value of the foods, or to stimulate the generation of a special and useful product; but when it's done to render the food-plant more resistant to an herbicide or pesticide, so that these agents can be used in *increased* quantity in the field, further contaminating the environment as well as ourselves—that in my view is a corporate crime, committed in part to increase sales of herbicides and pesticides.

In setting acceptable residue limits, the U.S. Department of Agriculture assumes a person eats no more than one-half pound *per year* of avocados, artichokes, Brussels sprouts, cantaloupe, eggplant, melons, mushrooms, radishes, and summer and winter squash.[23] That one-half pound may be the yearly American average, but it's not the level in a good diet; hence the allowable residue limits are simply too high.

It is incorrect to think that all the pesticide residue is only on the outside of the produce. About half the total may be in the flesh, albeit at a lower concentration gram per gram than the skin. Furthermore, fat-soluble pesticide residues and industrial toxicants accumulate in fat (see Figure 4.1). Animal fats, particularly animals fed on animal products, like on fish meal, are a source of these. First babies may get a big dose from many years accumulation when fat is mobilized as part of their mother's milk. When it comes to imported fruits and vegetables, pesticides are a common concern. Those banned in the U.S. can legally be exported for use by other countries, and can then find their way back via imports, since the FDA tests only about 2 percent of imported products.

Food products that are claimed to be *natural* often contain lots of sugar as well as unbleached wheat flour. In fact, when I see the word *natural* on a product, I regard it as a phony label, an attempt to fool the customer, and I'm apt not to buy that product. For example, Ragu's Home-style spaghetti sauce contains, for each 74 calories, 2 grams of fat, 470 milligrams of sodium, and no added sweeteners, whereas Ragu's 100 percent Natural spaghetti sauce has 3 grams of fat, 770 milligrams of sodium, plus added sweeteners. But does either of these terms make any nutritional sense? None whatever.

The terms *raw*, *uncooked*, and *unfiltered* also have no legal definition, so they mean very little on a label. Legally, *enriched* means that thiamine, riboflavin, niacin, and iron have been put back into refined cereals or breads to the level they had before processing. *Fortified* is used interchangeably with *enriched*. Neither of these terms means you are getting any more nutrients than in the simple unprocessed food. *Sugar-free* and *sugarless* just mean no sucrose (table sugar); the material may still have large amounts of fructose, glucose, sorbitol, mannitol—all just variants of table sugar. *Reduced calorie* legally means one-third or more fewer calories than the regular product, but if there were a lot to start with, one-third fewer is still a lot. *Low calorie* is the only meaningful term in all this misleading verbiage. Legally, foods whose labels say "low calorie" must contain no more than 40 calories per normal serving.

Whatever you are buying should bear a complete list of ingredients on the label, in descending order of quantity. Read this and pay no attention at all to words like *natural*. *The most important thing a health-conscious public can demand is full and proper labeling.* We are certainly not getting it.

Legumes (Beans and Peas): Legumes are plants in which the seeds develop in pods. Besides what we usually think of as beans, alfalfa, clover, and peanuts fall into this category. Except for lentils, split peas, and adzukis, beans need to be soaked for several hours or overnight before cooking. The soak water should be discarded. A small amount of nutrients will be lost, but well-soaked beans cause much less flatulence. Two of the carbohydrates in beans, stachyrose and raffinose, which can be partially removed by soaking, are indigestible by the enzymes of the small intestine and are passed along to be digested by bacteria in the colon, with the formation of gas. Cook lentils, split peas, fresh black-eyed peas, and adzuki beans for one hour, the other beans for one and one-half to three hours. Beans are fiber-rich, contain no cholesterol, and are low in fat (except for soybeans, which derive 40 percent of their calories from fat). Adzuki beans have an exceptionally low-fat content for a bean, and do not need to be presoaked. Legumes have a significant iron content, but their bioavailability is low. Chana dal beans, which are split baby garbanzo beans, have one of the lowest glycemic indices among foods (see Table 9.3).

Mediterranean diet: There are several variants, but the common components are high MUFA/saturated fat ratios; moderate consumption of alcohol, mostly red wine; high consumption of legumes, fruits, vegetables, and grains; moderate consumption of dairy products; and low consumption of red meat products.[24] Risk of heart disease is much less and remaining life expectancy at age 45 is two to three years longer in Mediterranean countries than in the U.S. or Great Britain. A good, brief review of the Mediterranean diet as well as the Lyon Diet Heart Study version of it is given in the Notes and References at the end of the book.[25] Much ado has been made of the Mediterranean diet, but the CRON diet promises far more than a mere two to three years longer average life span.

Mushrooms: They come in many varieties. For a good sampler of chanterelles, French morels, Italian porcini, and French cepes, with recipes, write to Key Gourmet, Box 3691, Beverly Hills, California 90212. Look also on the internet.

Nuts: Nuts are an ancient food. Pistachios date back to the Stone Age 9,000 years ago. Ground nut powder, especially from almonds, was used to thicken sauces by the Romans, Persians, and Arabs. The Greeks made the first travelers' trail snack, called Hais, with pounded nuts and dried fruits rolled into balls and dusted with powdered sugar.

Nutritious but tending to be very high in fat content, nuts have lots of calories. One cup of peanuts contains as many calories as four and one-half cups of brown rice or eight baked potatoes. You could hardly eat that much rice or potatoes, but could easily munch away a cup of peanuts. Brazil nuts, macadamias, filberts, and pecans are especially high in fat (93 percent of calories); pecan pie is perhaps the world's highest-calorie dessert! Pistachios derive 88 percent of their calories from fat, and walnuts, 81 percent. However, the high fat content is mostly PUFAs and MUFAs (see Figure 10.5), rather than saturated fat, and walnuts in particular have a high content of omega-3 fatty acids. So-called low-fat nuts include cashews (45 percent fat), almonds, and peanuts. But hail to the chestnut! Quite unlike any other of the common nuts, it is high in carbohydrates, low in fat, and low in calories. You can obtain vacuum-packed chestnuts from Williams-Sonoma, Mail Order Dept., P.O. Box 7456, San Francisco, California 94120-7456.

Despite the fat content, nuts qualify as being nutrient-dense. The FDA uses a so-called Index of Nutrient Quality (INQ) as an index of nutrient-density. For any nutrient, the INQ is the ratio of the percent of the RDA of the nutrient in 2,000 calories of the food.[26] If 100 percent of the RDA is contained in the 2,000 calories, then the index is one. If we look at nuts in this way, they come out quite well. Peanuts are the most nutrient-dense of the nuts, with INQs of one or more for nine nutrients: fiber, vitamin E, thiamin, niacin, folate, phosphorus, magnesium, copper, and manganese. Almonds, cashews, and Brazil nuts are nutrient dense in seven nutrients, walnuts in four. Brazil nuts contain very large amounts of selenium, with an INQ of about 100. All nuts contain INQ amounts of copper and manganese.

These are good reasons for the daily consumption of a handful of nuts.

Because of their high, largely unsaturated oil content, nuts do tend to become rancid. If you want them to keep longer, buy only unshelled nuts, and shell them yourself before use; or at least buy unbroken nuts, and store them in a closed jar in the refrigerator—not on a shelf.

Oil: Oil and fat are really equivalent, since fats are simply oils that are naturally solid at room temperature. The structure of fats and oils consists of a glycerol backbone to which three fatty acids are attached. The differences between various oils reflect which among many different fatty acids are actually present. Some of the carbon atoms in these fatty acids are joined by what are called *double bonds* and some by *single bonds*. The double bonds designate *unsaturated* and the single bonds designate *saturated* sites. The unsaturated sites or bonds tend to protect against arteriosclerosis, but they are subject to oxidation and the generation of free radicals. Diets high in polyunsaturated fats are associated with decreased cardiovascular disease compared to diets high in saturated fats; however, auto-oxidation of the polyunsaturated fats, initiated by heating, causes them to combine with oxygen to produce peroxidized free radicals, strong oxidizing agents that may increase the incidence of cancer. Olive oil and canola oil are the best oils for general usage. They have only one double bond, hence are monounsaturated. Attention should also be given to the omega-3 and omega-6 fatty acids.

In general, the lower the fat content of your diet the better, whether the bonds be unsaturated or saturated, although a minimum essential amount is required (equivalent to about 6 percent of calories from fat per 2,500 calories, depending on the type of fat or oil). It's almost impossible not to consume the bare minimum of essential fatty acids (unless you stick to highly processed oils), and dangerously easy to get too much of the saturated variety. A fat intake amounting to about 20 to 25 percent of total calories seems comfortable as to beneficial effects and taste. However, the average American takes in over 21 pounds of salad oil and cooking oil per year, whereas for a tablespoon's worth of corn oil from the natural source, you would have to eat 14 ears of corn. Furthermore, regular commercial corn oil has probably been heated to about 400 degrees Celsius and in animal experiments heated corn oil is more prone than unheated oil to cause arteriosclerosis. It is possible that margarine, which is apt to be highly processed and hydrogenated, is in fact worse for your arteries than butter. High-quality corn oil does happen to be one of the better polyunsaturated oils. High in vitamin E, it is less apt to go rancid than, say, safflower oil, which is highly polyunsaturated and not especially high in vitamin E.

Processed or highly refined oils are not recommended. These categories include both hydrogenated and partially hydrogenated oils or fats. Natural fatty acid is the so-called *cis* form, whereas in processed oils as much as 60 percent may have been converted to the *trans* form. Crisco and Spry are partially hydrogenated. Avoid them. Avoid anything that is simply labeled vegetable oil. It is apt to be highly processed. The FDA has recently proposed that foods listing saturated fat content must also list the amount of trans fat in that total. Let us hope this gets approved.

TABLE 10.5 *Percentages of non-stearic saturated fats, of stearic acid,*
monounsaturated and polyunsaturated fatty acid in various oils and nuts.
(Nuts average 84% of their total calories from fat, except for chestnuts,
which only get eight percent of their calories from fat.)

| | Type of oil or fat | | | | |
Source of oil or fat	SATURATED (NON-STEARIC)	STEARIC ACID	MONOUNSATURATED	POLYUNSATURATED	OTHER FATTY SUBSTANCES
Olive oil	11	2	74	9	4
Canola oil	4	1	62	28	5
Safflower oil	7	2	12	75	4
Corn oil	11	2	24	59	4
Soybean oil	11	4	23	58	4
Cottonseed oil	23	2	18	52	4
Chicken fat	24	6	45	21	6
Lard (Pork fat)	25	14	45	11	4
Chocolate (cocoa butter)	27	33	33	3	4
Beef fat (tallow)	31	19	42	4	4
Butter fat	50	12	29	4	5
Palm oil	45	4	37	9	5
Coconut oil	84	3	6	2	5
oil in Hazelnuts	6	2	79	9	4
oil in Pecans	6	2	62	21	4
oil in Almonds	8	2	65	21	4
oil in Walnuts	8	2	23	63	4
oil in Peanuts	12	2	49	33	4
oil in Cashews	13	7	59	17	4
oil in Brazil nuts	15	9	35	36	5
oil in Chestnuts	16	1	35	40	6

While saturated fats should generally be avoided (butter, margarine, palm oil), stearic acid is one saturated fat that seems to have no ill effects on serum lipid concentrations.[27] Myristic acid seems the worst of the saturated fats, stearic acid the least damaging. Table 10.5 shows the percentages of saturated and unsaturated fats in various oils and nuts.

You may be surprised to learn that pork fat is probably better for you (or less harmful) than beef fat, since the former contains mainly oleic and linoleic fatty acids (linoleic is an "essential," unsaturated fatty acid), whereas beef fat contains mainly palmitic and stearic fatty acids, both fully saturated. Furthermore, the pork industry has been breeding hogs that are 50 percent leaner than 30 years ago, and lean cuts of pork have the same cholesterol content as beef (60 to 80 milligrams per one-quarter-pound serving). Remember that wild and free-roaming, grass-eating animals have far lower fat contents than the fatted calves and steers most of the cattle industry is serving up to us. However, among red meats, bison, ostrich, and emu are much lower in saturated fat content than beef, pork, lamb, or chicken. (See References and Resources for where to obtain these.)

As I indicated, monounsaturated oils, such as olive oil and canola oil, are the all-around best bet. Italian olive oil is government regulated, and the better qualities are by law designated *virgin, superfine virgin,* and *extra virgin*. Obtained by manual pressing of the olives between cold stone wheels, extra virgin is tops. After pressing, it may be filtered through cheesecloth to be clarified. If unfiltered, it is cloudy, dense, and called mosto. While of the highest quality, extra virgin is subject to oxidation, so should be used over a period of weeks to months, not years. Highest-quality Italian brands are Badic, Coltibuono, and Colavita from Tuscany, and Il Castelluzza from Umbria. Olive oil and peanut oil are monounsaturated, and chemically stand between saturated and polyunsaturated oils, but biologically they may be just as anti-arteriosclerotic as the polyunsaturated oils or even more so.[28] They all lower LDL and cholesterol, but the polyunsaturated oils may also lower HDL, while the monounsaturated oils do not. (Remember that you want low cholesterol, low LDL, and high HDL.) Olive oil is the best oil to use on a low-fat diet, if you use any at all. The term *pure* olive oil means oil extracted from the second pressing, at a higher temperature and pressure, followed by the use of hot-water treatment or solvent extraction. It is not at all of the quality of extra virgin! Olive oil, as well as any other oils, should be refrigerated once opened, to avoid oxidation or rancidity. Put a drop on your wrist, rub it in, and smell it: if it smells good, it's probably okay. A few oils are packaged with nitrogen flushing, which cuts down on the oxidation. The label should tell you this.

The term *cold pressed* on many domestic oils means little—another health-food buzzword. There may be no such thing as a truly cold-pressed large-scale commercial American oil; any that you buy have been mechanically pressed, involving temperatures up to 150 degrees. The term *100 percent virgin* on an American oil is the top designation, and indicates the first pressing of the olives, no additives, and that it is unrefined. The Marsala and Sciabica oils carry this designation, and are among the best domestic oils. The word *prepressed*, while somewhat misleading, indicates a better product than cold pressed. *Unrefined* as applied to oils means no refining, bleaching, or deodorizing, but it does not exclude extraction with hexane (instead of pressing) followed by distillation to get rid of water. Unrefined oils smoke more when cooked, become rancid faster, and tend to be darker with sediment, which should be shaken into the oil before using.

Pasta: At the Chamber of Commerce in Bologna there is a solid-gold noodle, one millimeter thick and 6 millimeters wide—the standard dimension of the perfect raw tagliatelle noodle. Pasta is made from the flour of durum wheat, whose starch is too hard for making bread but ideal for pasta, which must stay together while being boiled, baked, or steamed. Good pasta is nutritious, but you should use only pasta made from "whole durum wheat flour," *not from semolina*, which is refined for the sake of color and variety. Other grain and vegetable powders are sometimes added to the basic durum wheat flour: spinach, artichoke, soy, buckwheat, amaranth. Take advantage also of pasta's endless shapes and textures. Shells or fusilli catch the sauce better than long slim shapes.

To cook pasta, add a teaspoon of olive oil to boiling water to prevent sticking, and drop in the pasta. Cook until firm and slightly chewy but not starchy, usually about ten minutes. If you can easily bite all the way through a noodle, it is done. Drain in a colander and toss with sauce in a bowl to coat and separate the noodles. Do not rinse with cold water! It renders pasta soft and gummy. If you use cheese, the best Parmesan is Reggiano; the best Romano, Peccorino. Use only freshly grated cheese. The fat-free Sapsago cheese is also good grated on pasta.

Poultry: The fat content of commercial chickens has tripled in the last 25 years. In 1960 it was 5 grams per 100 grams; now it is 15 grams. This increase has been due to selection for larger size and more rapid growth rate and use of less expensive feeds. It's the same unhealthful commercial pattern we have already seen in the cattle industry. (As fish farming becomes big business, there also we shall probably see the lean turned into fat.) In chickens, the skin and the fat pad between the skin and the meat contain about 85 percent of the fat. To a considerable extent these can be separated off and discarded. Chicken breast without skin derives 19 percent of its calories from fat; chicken thigh without skin, 47 percent.

Seasonings: Important as they are nutritionally, many foods such as grains and legumes are rather bland. Vegit and Jensen's Broth & Seasoning are excellent general-purpose seasonings for rice or beans. It's more interesting to use pure seasonings, bought fresh weekly when possible. Among liquid seasoning, beware of the sodium content. Examples: regular soy sauce and tamari contain about 1,200 milligrams of sodium per tablespoon—-much too much. Worcestershire sauce is similar in flavor and much lower in sodium. Miso has excellent food value but is high in sodium. Sugarless ketchup, to be preferred on a CRON diet, must by law be labeled as "imitation ketchup." By quirks of the law like this one, some things that must be labeled "imitation" are in fact more healthful than the real thing. Mayonnaise is another example.

To clue into the different seasonings, to find out what tastes best to you, divide the dish into two or three equal portions and flavor each differently. Suggested combinations might be as follows:

Cabbage:	oregano, savory, tarragon
Carrots:	mint, thyme
Eggplant:	basil, marjoram, sage
Green beans:	dill weed, marjoram, savory
Lentils:	oregano, sage, cumin
Lima beans:	oregano, sage

White potatoes:	dill weed, mint, oregano, rosemary, thyme
Rice:	cumin, coriander, thyme, cinnamon, all spice, mint
Spinach:	marjoram, mint, rosemary

Having tested these separately, mix them together for the combined effect.

Seaweeds: These plants are becoming popular in the United States, and with good reason. They are highly nutritious, and particularly rich (for a nonmeat source) in iron, as well as calcium, vitamin B6, possibly vitamins B12 and D—there is some dispute about the presence of these last two—and other nutrients. To North American tastes, dulce is the most palatable of the seaweeds. But unlike other seaweeds, it contains a fair amount of fat. It requires only gentle boiling. Become familiar also with nori (which is used to wrap sushi, but can be cut up and added directly to salads), with sweet kombu, wakame (needs moderate boiling), and single-bladed and finger kombu (both require rather long boiling). Kombu will reduce the starchiness of beans, shorten the cooking time, and eliminate the flatulence. It's one of the highest nonmeat sources of iron. Best (freshest) kombu brands are Erewhon and Westbrae. High in calcium, iron, and possibly vitamin B, the seaweed wakame (Alaria) contains a lot of alginic acid, which precipitates heavy metals such as mercury, lead, and cadmium if they have contaminated the food source.

Seeds: Like nuts, seeds are nutritious but high in fat, mostly unsaturated. However, they are more nutrient dense than nuts and so are the wiser choice. Pumpkin seeds (pepitas) are quite high in iron and zinc. Zinc is the element most often deficient in the American diet. If possible, buy only mechanically hulled sesame seeds, as the common variety has had the hulls removed by chemical solvents (usually lye), which may diminish the nutrient value. Seeds, like nuts, can go rancid as a result of their high fat content. Store them in the refrigerator.

Soy: The types of protein and the isoflavones in soy products decrease cholesterol, even in diabetic patients who are refractory to other lipid-lowering regimens, probably reduce the risk of hormone-related cancers, including those of the prostate, breast, and colon, and (more problematically) may decrease postmenopausal bone loss.[29]

TABLE 10.5 *Comparison of soy products for isoflavone and protein contents*

SOY PRODUCT	ISOFLAVONES (MILLIGRAMS)	PROTEIN (GRAMS)
mature soybeans, ½ cup	176	34
soy nuts (roasted soybeans), ½ cup	167	30
green soybeans, ½ cup	70	21
tempeh, 4 oz.	61	19
tofu, 4 oz.	38	18
soy milk, whole, 8 fl. oz.	20	10

A fairly recent addition to the American diet but long a mainstay in Asian cooking, tofu is a good replacement for meat and dairy products, thanks to a somewhat lower percentage of fat (40 percent calories from fat), mostly unsaturated (15 percent saturated, 52 percent polyunsaturated). Soybean curd, which is tofu, is low in calories (72 calories for a three-and-one-half-ounce serving). It goes well in recipes calling for cheese—as examples: in sauces, pasta, or pizza. It will absorb the flavor of anything you cook with it. Scrambled and with salsa added, it can substitute for scrambled eggs, and it contains no cholesterol. Its protein quality approaches or equals that of meat, although slightly low in methionine.

Tofu comes packed in water. The package should bear a date of production. Use the tofu within about two weeks of that date. Once the package has been opened, drain off the liquid, add fresh water, and change the water every one or two days. To see if you like the taste of tofu relatively plain, try the following: place a block of soft tofu on a plate, top with diced shallots fried in a minimal amount of olive oil, and add soy sauce or Worcestershire sauce and fresh chopped cilantro. Serve this as an appetizer.

Evidence suggests that the proteins and isoflavones of tofu may help prevent heart disease. Other soy products may contain relatively more or less of these substances. (See Table 10.5.) The evidence is now good enough that the FDA allows soy foods to be labeled with such a health claim. Experts disagree whether it's the protein or isoflavone that has this effect. Phytoestrogens may also be partly responsible for the cholesterol-lowering effect. Phytoestrogens can inhibit the oxidation of LDLs. Population studies suggest soy can help reduce the incidence of hormone-related cancers, including those of the prostate and breast, and possibly colorectal polyps. Soy contains the isoflavone genistein.[30] But recent evidence suggests that a more effective anticancer substance in soy products may not be the isoflavones but saponins (cholesterol-related plant compounds).[31] In any case, an increase in soy products in the diet has been considered a good move.

All well and good, but you should review the warning note about tofu found in Chapter 7. It is hard to know what to make of this, except to keep one's ears open for confirmation or denial by further work. Meantime, however, I have not abandoned a moderate soy products intake.

Sprouts: These have the nutritive value of greens, rather than that of the seeds they emerged from. For example, soybean sprouts are nutritionally more like broccoli than like soybeans. A sprout from a grain would be nutritionally similar to lettuce. Sprouts are delicious and good for you, but don't use them to replace grains, seeds, or beans in your diet. Broccoli sprouts are noteworthy as they contain 20 to 25 times as much per gram weight as the mature broccoli plant of the potent anticancer phytochemical sulphoraphane.[32] Alfalfa sprouts, on the other hand, contain canavanine, a natural toxin.

Vinegar: Buy only the top quality. Even the most expensive vinegar is comparatively cheap, and top quality will pay handsomely in the excellence of your salads and other dishes. (See Readings and Resources.)

Water: Bottled waters have increased remarkably in popularity in the United States in the past several decades. A great deal of this is due to advertising, which has popularized and internalized the most famous myth in gerontology, the Fountain of Youth. There is also a growing fear of contamination of city water. Whole sections of cities have suddenly discovered that industrial pollutants have crept into their local aquifer. The underground march of the infamous Stringfellow acid pits in eastern Los Angeles is one gruesome example. Bottled water from carefully controlled springs or other sources should be free of this danger, or so it is hoped.

In fact, only a fourth of the bottled water sold in the United States is truly spring water. Again, labels can be deceiving. If a label carries the word *spring* merely in the company's name, rather than on the product, it's not spring water. If the label says "spring-type," "spring-fresh," or "spring-pure," it is not spring water. Look for a product that is designated specifically as "spring water" or "natural spring water." Anything labeled "natural mineral water" usually comes from a spring. "Mineral water" generally refers more to the total dissolved solids than to the source. In California, whatever is labeled as "mineral water" must contain 500 parts per million or more of total dissolved solids.

Certain areas of the United States are characterized by greater average longevities and lower death rates than other areas. In general, the southeastern United States (Georgia, the Carolinas, and parts of Alabama, but not Florida) shows *decreased* longevity in the population. The uppermiddle portion of the United States (Nebraska, Colorado, South Dakota, Minnesota, and neighboring states to some extent) plus Alaska generally shows *increased* longevity. The rest of the country follows a hodgepodge pattern, with longevity varying from county to county. Trace elements in the soil or differences in the quality of the drinking water may be of paramount importance in accounting for these differences.

There is a relation between the extent of heart disease in a population and the hardness of water in the area, although it's not easy to pin down just what chemical or chemicals are involved.[33] In the areas of greater longevity the water supplies are characterized by a high density of dissolved solids (over 300 milligrams per liter), very hard water (over 200 milligrams of inorganic matter per liter), high calcium content (over 50 milligrams per liter), high magnesium content (over 30 milligrams per liter), a variable but often high sodium content (10 to

1,000 milligrams per liter), and a low level of dissolved organic compounds.[34] A high chromium and manganese content might also be important.[35] You can find out about your own water by writing to the Department of Water and Power in your county. Table 10.6 lists some of the characteristics of a number of popular bottled waters and, for comparison, tap waters of Los Angeles and New York City. To my knowledge, these all come from good sources. The term *bottled waters* refers to quart-sized or one-half gallon bottles. So-called "jug water," which comes in the five-gallon home or office plastic jug, doesn't necessarily come from a pristine source, such as a mountain spring.[36]

These data are assembled from various sources, not all of which are in complete agreement, but should be approximately correct. Make your own judgment among the waters. Vichy and Calso are simply too high in sodium to be good choices. Vittel, Deep Rock, Indian Head, Evian, San Pellegrino, and a few others all look good. Rocky Minerals water comes from the Big Rock Candy Mountain spring in Utah, and might suit those who wish to drink so-called "glacial milk," like the Hunza peoples of India.

We were born in water and we go to dust. The Fountain of Youth is the enduring legend. Take a good drink of water, therefore, and thank your stars you were not born too early in human history to participate in the life-extension revolution.

TABLE 10.7 *Characteristics of selected bottled and tap waters (milligrams/liter)*

WATER SOURCE	DISSOLVED SOLIDS TOTAL	HARDNESS	CALCIUM	MAGNESIUM	SODIUM
Appolinaris	2,250	1,200	180	240	570
Arrowhead	112	96	16	3	9
Badoit	—	1,550	355	198	205
Calistoga	540	240	80	3	120
Calso	2,910	670	230	3	1,325
Deep Rock	547	320	73	25	55
Deer Park	29	15	3	3	4
Evian	330	295	78	25	7
Fiuggi	120	400	118	25	68
Indian Head	654	367	74	32	33
Los Angeles tap	186	61	21	5	31
Mendocino	2080	—	380	120	105
Mountain Valley	205	230	79	11	3
New York tap	127	65	18	6	1
Perrier	545	290	88	13	5
Polanco Spring	125	50	19	7	4
Pamlosa	—	1	0.2	0.1	3
Rocky Minerals	12,120	—	1501	281	112
San Peligrino	1,100	776	212	60	4
Saratoga	400	—	64	6	7
Silver Springs	150	95	31	7	1
Sparkletts	18	12	1	1	4
Vichy	3,400	105	162	12	1,223
Vittel	465	755	181	41	7

APPENDIX A

FOOD COMBINATIONS AND TASTY MENUS FOR THE
HEALTHIEST FOURTEEN DAYS OF YOUR LIFE

===

MENUS

(An asterisk indicates that a recipe is provided.)

DAY ONE

Breakfast

1 Sherm's MegaMuffin*

8 oz. nonfat plain yogurt

6 large strawberries, or 5 oz. frozen, defrosted

Lunch

1 cup succotash (frozen corn and lima beans) with

    2 slices grilled Canadian-style bacon and

    1 cup prepared kale, fresh or frozen

½ cup prepared okra, fresh or frozen

1 slice whole-wheat bread

Dinner

½ turkey breast, deli meat or roasted, no skin

½ baked sweet potato

1 large broccoli spear, steamed

2–3 cups green salad, any combination greens with

    1 tbsp. low-fat salad dressing

3.5 oz. red table wine or concord grape juice

1 orange

% OF RDA'S				NUTRITIONAL INFORMATION	
Vitamin A	938	Iron	106		
Vitamin B6	190	Magnesium	186	Total calories	1182
Vitamin B12	120	Manganese	253	% calories from	
Vitamin C	790	Phosphorus	135	protein	32
Vitamin E	99	Potassium	255	% calories from fat	12
Thiamine	166	Zinc	88	% calories from	
Folacin	352	Selenium	167	carbohydrates	57
Riboflavin	152	Sodium	64	Total protein	94 gm
Niacin	155			Total fat	15 gm
Pantothenic Acid	152			Total	
Calcium	97			carbohydrate	168 gm
Copper	86			Fiber	37 gm
				Cholesterol	140 mg

DAY TWO

Breakfast

Oatmeal and Fruit:

¼ cup cooked oat bran,

1 cup cooked oatmeal, ·

2 oz. (½ cup) blueberries (frozen or fresh),

2 tbsp. raisins,

¼ banana

1 cup skim milk

Lunch

1 serving MegaMeal Fruit Salad 400*

1 slice whole-wheat toast

Dinner

3 oz. pink salmon, broiled, with

6 oz. (¾ cup) Spanish-style tomato sauce

1 medium sweet potato, baked

1 cup peas and onions (frozen, prepared)

1 cup red wine (optional, add 80 calories)

% OF RDA'S				NUTRITIONAL INFORMATION	
Vitamin A	691	Iron	105		
Vitamin B6	170	Magnesium	143	Total calories	1316
Vitamin B12	224	Manganese	181	% calories from protein	22
Vitamin C	399	Phosphorus	122		
Vitamin E	168	Potassium	209	% calories from fat	19
Thiamine	134	Zinc	70	% calories from carbohydrates	59
Folacin	168	Selenium	248		
Riboflavin	152	Sodium	tk	Total protein	66 gm
Niacin	116			Total fat	33 gm
Pantothenic Acid	135			Total carbohydrate	201 gm
Calcium	80			Fiber	26 gm
Copper	79			Cholesterol	79 gm

DAY THREE

Breakfast

1 ¼ cups rolled oats, cooked, with
    ¼ cup wheat bran,
    1 banana, sliced
1 glass skim milk

Lunch

3 oz. grilled halibut
½ cup cabbage (as cole slaw) with
    1 tbsp. low-fat dressing
1 slice whole-wheat bread
1 glass skim milk

Dinner

Oyster cocktail (4 to 8 oysters, depending on size)
Pasta Primavera*
6–8 leaves kale, steamed, with sauce of choice
    (see Sauces in Chapter 10)
1 slice watermelon, equivalent of 2 cups, or other fruit

% OF RDA'S				NUTRITIONAL INFORMATION	
Vitamin A	427	Iron	133		
Vitamin B6	156	Magnesium	203	Total calories	1374
Vitamin B12	832	Manganese	203	% calories from	
Vitamin C	561	Phosphorus	135	protein	14
Vitamin E	111	Potassium	217	% calories from fat	21
Thiamine	146	Zinc	335	% calories from	
Folacin	145	Selenium	380	carbohydrates	64
Riboflavin	145	Sodium	tk	Total protein	78 gm
Niacin	125			Total fat	23 gm
Pantothenic Acid	116			Total	
Calcium	96			carbohydrate	235 gm
Copper	112			Fiber	43 gm
				Cholesterol	75 gm

DAY FOUR

Breakfast

½ cantaloupe

½ cup blueberries

1 poached egg

1 slice whole-wheat bread

Lunch

Chicken Sandwich:

2 slices whole-wheat bread,

3½ oz. chicken, white meat,

3 leaves romaine lettuce,

1 slice tomato,

2 tsp. mustard (optional) or nonfat mayonnaise

Dinner

Saffron SLS Soup* (2 bowls) with

2 tsp. yeast added and garnished with

¼ cup chopped parsley

1–2 cups steamed collard greens (fresh or frozen)

1 slice mixed-grain bread or dinner roll

1 glass skim milk

% OF RDA'S				NUTRITIONAL INFORMATION	
Vitamin A	640	Iron	82		
Vitamin B6	134	Magnesium	106	Total calories	1101
Vitamin B12	120	Manganese	142	% calories from protein	27
Vitamin C	341	Phosphorus	106		
Vitamin E	53	Potassium	255	% calories from fat	15
Thiamine	176	Zinc	67	% calories from carbohydrates	58
Folacin	317	Selenium	192		
Riboflavin	144	Sodium	88	Total protein	77 gm
Niacin	171			Total fat	19 gm
Pantothenic Acid	119			Total carbohydrate	167 gm
Calcium	82			Fiber	24 gm
Copper	66			Cholesterol	302 mg

DAY FIVE

Breakfast

½ cup cooked millet

1 small banana

1 tbsp. sunflower seeds

1 cup skim milk

Lunch

Sardine Sandwich:

2 slices mixed-grain bread,

¼ can sardines, canned in tomato or mustard sauce,

1 slice tomato (optional),

2 leaves romaine lettuce

Dinner

2 bowls Vegetable Salad*

1 dinner roll (optional, will add approximately 100 calories)

Dessert

1 cup nonfat yogurt

5–6 dry apricots

% OF RDA'S				NUTRITIONAL INFORMATION	
Vitamin A	384	Iron	89		
Vitamin B6	134	Magnesium	163	Total calories	1249
Vitamin B12	549	Manganese	173	% calories from protein	21
Vitamin C	382	Phosphorus	153	% calories from fat	17
Vitamin E	147	Potassium	202	% calories from carbohydrates	62
Thiamine	142	Zinc	93		
Folacin	250	Selenium	182	Total protein	70 gm
Riboflavin	158	Sodium	46	Total fat	25 gm
Niacin	100			Total carbohydrate	207 gm
Pantothenic Acid	138			Fiber	25 gm
Calcium	113			Cholesterol	75 mg
Copper	80				

DAY SIX

Breakfast

1 serving Scrambled Tofu*
1 slice mixed-grain bread
½ grapefruit

Lunch

2 bowls Vegetable Salad* (from the night before)
1 slice rye toast
1 cup skim milk or buttermilk (optional, will add 80 calories)

Dinner

½ cup cooked millet (or other grain) with ¼ cup peas, prepared
3 oz. oysters, cooked with
  ¼ cup onions
2 stalks broccoli, steamed
1 cup collard greens, steamed

Snack

½ cup nonfat yogurt with 1 tbsp. nonfat dry milk
  (necessary for calcium)
½ tsp. cinnamon or other spice

% OF RDA'S				NUTRITIONAL INFORMATION	
Vitamin A	556	Iron	160		
Vitamin B6	137	Magnesium	183	Total calories	1245
Vitamin B12	1702	Manganese	271	% calories from protein	24
Vitamin C	1118	Phosphorus	139	% calories from fat	12
Vitamin E	125	Potassium	215	% calories from	
Thiamine	156	Zinc	400	carbohydrates	64
Folacin	350	Selenium	440	Total protein	82 gm
Riboflavin	180	Sodium	48	Total fat	17 gm
Niacin	112			Total	
Pantothenic Acid	180			carbohydrate	214 gm
Calcium	90			Fiber	40 gm
Copper	248			Cholesterol	127 mg

DAY SEVEN

Breakfast

2 Sherm's MegaMuffins*

Lunch

Turkey sandwich:

2 slices whole wheat-bread or 1 pita bread,

3 oz. cooked turkey breast,

lettuce, sliced tomato,

1 tbsp. nonfat mayonnaise,

1 tbsp. tomato paste

Dill pickle (optional)

1 glass skim milk

Dinner

Steamed Vegetables:

1 spear broccoli, 1 carrot,

½ sweet potato,

¼ head cabbage, 4 leaves kale

¼ cup cooked adzuki beans mixed with

¾ cup cooked brown rice and

¼ cup cooked wild rice, with one of the Sauces
(optional, see Sauces in Chapter 10)

1 tbsp. sunflower seeds

Snack

apricots, 1 cup water packed or 4 dried Turkish apricots

% OF RDA'S				NUTRITIONAL INFORMATION	
Vitamin A	925	Iron	104		
Vitamin B6	175	Magnesium	179	Total calories	1130
Vitamin B12	81	Manganese	258	% calories from protein	25
Vitamin C	535	Phosphorus	124		
Vitamin E	170	Potassium	200	% calories from fat	15
Thiamine	126	Zinc	85	% calories from carbohydrates	60
Folacin	243	Selenium	142		
Riboflavin	118	Sodium	32	Total protein	75 gm
Niacin	131			Total fat	20 gm
Pantothenic Acid	128			Total carbohydrate	178 gm
Calcium	71			Fiber	33 mg
Copper	91			Cholesterol	104 mg

DAY EIGHT

Breakfast

1 poached egg
1 slice whole-wheat bread
½ grapefruit

Lunch

2 oz. chicken, light meat
Chilled Leafy Potage* (1 bowl) with
     1 tsp. brewer's yeast
1 slice whole-wheat bread

Dinner

Stuffed Bell Peppers in Beer Sauce*
4 Brussels sprouts
1 cup skim milk

% OF RDA'S				NUTRITIONAL INFORMATION	
Vitamin A	819	Iron	147		
Vitamin B6	194	Magnesium	173	Total calories	1216
Vitamin B12	145	Manganese	173	% calories from protein	28
Vitamin C	1100	Phosphorus	131	% calories from fat	19
Vitamin E	166	Potassium	251	% calories from carbohydrates	54
Thiamine	183	Zinc	80		
Folacin	467	Selenium	145	Total protein	88 gm
Riboflavin	177	Sodium	65	Total fat	27 gm
Niacin	161			Total carbohydrate	171 gm
Pantothenic Acid	121				
Calcium	98			Fiber	38 gm
Copper	118			Cholesterol	270 mg

DAY NINE

Breakfast

1 poached egg

1 slice whole-wheat bread

½ papaya

Lunch

Falafel Sandwich:

1 whole-wheat pita bread with

2 tbsp. Hummus,*

1 large Falafel patty,*

1 slice tomato,

1 slice onion (optional),

1 tbsp. tomato paste,

spinach leaves, lettuce, or sprouts

Coleslaw:

1 cup shredded cabbage with

1 carrot, grated,

½ stalk celery, ⅓ red pepper,

1 tbsp. nonfat salad dressing or mayonnaise,

½ cup nonfat yogurt

Dinner

3 oz. pink salmon, broiled with lemon

1 small yam, baked, with

½ cup nonfat yogurt

1 ½ cups kale

1 stalk broccoli

1 serving Roasted Vegetables*

% OF RDA'S				NUTRITIONAL INFORMATION	
Vitamin A	1000	Iron	116		
Vitamin B6	213	Magnesium	194	Total calories	1257
Vitamin B12	238	Manganese	187	% calories from protein	23
Vitamin C	1128	Phosphorus	130		
Vitamin E	186	Potassium	349	% calories from fat	18
Thiamine	174	Zinc	76	% calories from carbohydrates	59
Folacin	436	Selenium	200		
Riboflavin	155	Sodium	59	Total protein	79 gm
Niacin	138			Total fat	26 gm
Pantothenic Acid	160			Total carbohydrate	227 gm
Calcium	114			Fiber	51 gm
Copper	94			Cholesterol	93 mg

DAY TEN

Breakfast

1 packet instant oatmeal (plain), or regular oatmeal, 1 cup, with
  1 tbsp. wheat germ,
  5 fresh or frozen strawberries
1 cup nonfat milk

Lunch

1 serving California Corn Salad*

Dinner

Tempeh Burger:
  1 tempeh burger,
  1 mixed-grain hamburger bun,
  1 tbsp. tomato paste,
  1 tsp. mustard, 1 slice onion, romaine lettuce leaves
Banana Milkshake:
  1 cup nonfat milk whipped with
    1 banana

% OF RDA'S				NUTRITIONAL INFORMATION	
Vitamin A	351	Iron	120		
Vitamin B6	216	Magnesium	160	Total calories	1044
Vitamin B12	197	Manganese	231	% calories from protein	27
Vitamin C	1048	Phosphorus	130		
Vitamin E	66	Potassium	216	% calories from fat	15
Thiamine	199	Zinc	83	% calories from carbohydrates	58
Folacin	374	Selenium	143	Total protein	76 gm
Riboflavin	164	Sodium	182	Total fat	18 gm
Niacin	136			Total carbohydrate	161 gm
Pantothenic Acid	107				
Calcium	100			Fiber	33 gm
Copper	94			Cholesterol	37 mg

DAY ELEVEN

Breakfast

> 1 CRONshake,* with
>> 1 tbsp. wheat germ
>
> 1 slice mixed-grain bread

Lunch

> 3 cups+ Green Grain Salad with
>> Mustard Dressing*
>
> 1 small baked sweet potato

Dinner

> 2 bowls Eternal Youth Chili*
>
> 1 corn tortilla
>
> 1 cup skim milk or beer (optional, add 80 calories)

% OF RDA'S				NUTRITIONAL INFORMATION	
Vitamin A	1089	Iron	116	Total calories	1089
Vitamin B6	179	Magnesium	160	% calories from	
Vitamin B12	133	Manganese	201	protein	126
Vitamin C	829	Phosphorus	107	% calories from fat	39
Vitamin E	82	Potassium	215	% calories from	
Thiamine	148	Zinc	92	carbohydrates	69
Folacin	361	Selenium	122	Total protein	25 gm
Riboflavin	136	Sodium	75	Total fat	150 gm
Niacin	111			Total	
Pantothenic Acid	99			carbohydrate	150 gm
Calcium	100			Fiber	23 gm
Copper	91			Cholesterol	77 mg

DAY TWELVE

Breakfast

½ cup millet with
    2 tbsp. wheat germ
1 medium peach or other seasonal fresh fruit
1 glass skim milk

Lunch

Salmon Sandwich:
    3 ½ oz. canned salmon,
    2 slices whole-wheat bread,
    2 leaves romaine lettuce,
    1 slice onion (optional),
    ¼ tomato

Dinner

Green Grain Salad with Mustard Dressing*
½ pound (1 large stalk) broccoli
1 glass skim milk

% OF RDA'S				NUTRITIONAL INFORMATION	
Vitamin A	168	Iron	88		
Vitamin B6	12495	Magnesium	143	Total calories	1059
Vitamin B12	282	Manganese	202	% calories from protein	25
Vitamin C	505	Phosphorus	136		
Vitamin E	123	Potassium	162	% calories from fat	15
Thiamine	140	Zinc	81	% calories from carbohydrates	60
Folacin	273	Selenium	177		
Riboflavin	147	Sodium	tk	Total protein	70 gm
Niacin	127			Total fat	18 gm
Pantothenic Acid	134			Total carbohydrate	168 gm
Calcium	91			Fiber	32 gm
Copper	76			Cholesterol	48 mg

DAY THIRTEEN

Breakfast

½ cantaloupe

⅓ cup blueberries, frozen or fresh

1 slice mixed-grain bread

1 poached egg

1 cup skim milk

Lunch

1 large bowl Cape Cod Chowder*

1 whole-grain roll

Dinner

Steamed Vegetables:

⅓ cup cauliflower, 3–4 florets,

½ cup broccoli,

1 ½ carrots,

¾ cup (¼ lb.) kale,

½ medium sweet potato,

½ cup snap green beans,

1 small leek, bulb and lower leaf portion,

⅓ cup Almond Sauce* with

½ cup plain nonfat yogurt

½ cup cooked millet

% OF RDA'S				NUTRITIONAL INFORMATION	
Vitamin A	1189	Iron	70		
Vitamin B6	155	Magnesium	75	Total calories	1257
Vitamin B12	190	Manganese	136	% calories from	
Vitamin C	432	Phosphorus	152	protein	27
Vitamin E	66	Potassium	114	% calories from fat	13
Thiamine	122	Zinc	202	% calories from	
Folacin	200	Selenium	68	carbohydrates	60
Riboflavin	147	Sodium	204	Total protein	86 gm
Niacin	107			Total fat	19 gm
Pantothenic Acid	111			Total	
Calcium	87			carbohydrate	194 gm
Copper	70			Fiber	318 gm
				Cholesterol	29 mg

DAY FOURTEEN

Breakfast

Omelet:

2 egg whites and 1 whole egg

1 slice tomato

1 slice mixed-grain bread

1 cup nonfat milk

Lunch

1 serving MegaMeal Fruit Salad 400*

2 crackers (optional, whole-wheat,
low-fat, will add 50–100 calories)

Dinner

Vegetables and Salmon:

1 lb. mixed frozen vegetables, cooked

¼ lb. (1 ¼ cups) mushrooms, sliced and cooked,

⅓ can pink salmon, water-packed, drained,

½ cup pasta sauce

% OF RDA'S				NUTRITIONAL INFORMATION	
Vitamin A	603	Iron	78		
Vitamin B6	134	Magnesium	136	Total calories	1190
Vitamin B12	280	Manganese	137	% calories from protein	24
Vitamin C	396	Phosphorus	131		
Vitamin E	120	Potassium	211	% calories from fat	21
Thiamine	129	Zinc	78	% calories from carbohydrates	55
Folacin	207	Chromium	132		
Riboflavin	215	Selenium	309	Total protein	77 gm
Niacin	141	Sodium	tk	Total fat	28 gm
Pantothenic Acid	158			Total carbohydrate	172 gm
Calcium	93			Fiber	250 gm
Copper	93			Cholesterol	35 mg

RECIPES

BREAKFASTS

CRONshake (1 serving)

⅔ cup frozen or fresh strawberries
1 cup low-fat milk
1½ oz. tofu (roughly ¼ block)
½ banana
Cinnamon
Stevia powder

Blend strawberries, milk, tofu, and banana. Add cinnamon and/or stevia powder to taste.

% OF RDA'S PER SWERVING				NUTRITIONAL INFORMATION	
Vitamin A	13	Manganese	24	Total calories	222
Vitamin B6	25	Phosphorus	28	% calories from protein	27
Vitamin B12	47	Potassium	37	% calories from fat	24
Vitamin C	54	Selenium	25	% calories from carbohydrates	50
Vitamin E	13	Sodium	6		
Thiamine	18	Zinc	15	Total protein	16 gm
Folacin	24			Total fat	6 gm
Riboflavin	41			Saturated fat	2 gm
Niacin	6			Monounsaturated fat	2 gm
Pantothenic Acid	21			Polyunsaturated fat	2 gm
Calcium	50			Carbohydrate	29 gm
Copper	13			Fiber	3 gm
Iron	33			Cholesterol	9 mg
Magnesium	28				

Scrambled Tofu (1 serving)

2 fresh shiitake mushrooms
⅓ red onion
½ small red pepper, cored and seeded
1 clove garlic, minced
Canola or olive-oil based spray
4 oz. firm tofu
½ tsp. turmeric
½ tsp. ground thyme
Barbecue sauce

Finely chop the mushrooms, onion, and red pepper. Spray a nonstick skillet with oil. Saute the garlic, mushrooms, onions, and red peppers. Add the tofu and mash until it is scrambled and all the ingredients are blended. Season with turmeric and thyme. Garnish with barbecue sauce, to taste.

% OF RDA'S PER SERVING				NUTRITIONAL INFORMATION	
Vitamin A	97	Phosphorus	20	Total calories	141
Vitamin B6	24	Potassium	8	% calories from protein	27
Vitamin B12	0	Selenium	20		
Vitamin C	268	Sodium	8	% calories from fat	23
Vitamin E	13	Zinc	12	% calories from carbohydrates	56
Thiamine	18				
Folacin	38			Total protein	9.5 gm
Riboflavin	11			Total fat	3.6 gm
Niacin	10			Saturated fat	0.6 gm
Pantothenic Acid	32			Monounsaturated fat	0.8 gm
Calcium	21			Polyunsaturated fat	1.8 gm
Copper	19				
Iron	45			Carbohydrate	19.8 gm
Magnesium	12			Fiber	4 gm
Manganese	26			Cholesterol	0 mg

Sherm's Megamuffins (18 muffins)

We are grateful to Sherman of the Internet CR society for providing this well-balanced, nutrient-dense recipe for delicious muffins.

Canola- or olive-oil based spray
4 cups frozen strawberries
2 gm. calcium supplement
30 mg. zinc supplement
1 tbsp. potassium based baking powder
   (no sodium)
1 tbsp. cinnamon
1 tsp. ginger
1 tsp. nutmeg
1 tsp. powdered pure stevia extract (sweetener)
1 cup rice bran
1 cup soy protein isolate powder
¾ cup flax meal

5 tbsp. brewer's yeast

¾ cup psyllium husk

½ cup wheat bran

¼ cup raw wheat germ

3 tbsp. raw sunflower seeds (whole or ground)

⅓ cup nonfat dry milk

¾ cup nonfat plain yogurt

½ cup water

3 oz. frozen orange juice concentrate

3 large egg whites

1 large egg

1 medium carrot

¼ medium avocado

2 cups dehydrated unsweetened blueberries

3 tbsp. raisins (or cherries)

Preheat oven to 325. Spray muffin trays (18 medium-size muffin forms, preferably nonstick) lightly with canola or olive oil-based spray like Pam. Use a paper towel to spread the oil evenly and absorb excess. Defrost the strawberries in the microwave for 3 minutes on full power (to avoid destroying your blender). If the supplements are not already in powdered form, crush them to a fine powder. Thoroughly mix supplements with baking powder, cinnamon, ginger, nutmeg, and stevia extract in a small bowl. Set aside.

Mix together the rice bran, soy protein, flax meal, brewer's yeast, psyllium husk, wheat bran, raw wheat germ, raw sunflower seeds, and nonfat dry milk in a large bowl. Mix thoroughly and break up any lumps (the soy protein is particularly prone to form lumps). Add the set aside dry ingredients to the rice bran mixture and mix thoroughly until ingredients are uniformly distributed. Set aside.

In a blender, mix the strawberries, yogurt, water, orange juice concentrate, egg whites and eggs, carrot, and avocado. Run blender on high to create a smooth texture. Pour the blender mix into the dry ingredients. Mix thoroughly for about five minutes by hand until uniform. Make sure there are no dry spots left. Finally, add in the dehydrated blueberries and raisins (or cherries) and mix until well distributed. This must be done last because otherwise bits of dry powder will hide inside the crevasses of the dried fruit. Quickly distribute the now-rising dough evenly into 18 medium-size muffin forms. Make sure that every muffin ends up with some of the dried fruit in it. Bake at 325 degrees for 40 minutes. Remove from oven and let stand until cool enough to touch (2 to 3 minutes). Then take muffins out of muffin tins and place on a cooling rack for at least 10 minutes. Pack in ziploc freezer bags to retain moisture. Keep refrigerated or frozen. To eat, microwave frozen muffins 60 seconds on high. (We found that they taste better after freezing and microwaving than they do when eaten hot out of the oven.)

% OF RDA'S PER SERVING				NUTRITIONAL INFORMATION	
Vitamin A	26	Phosphorus	15	Total calories	150
Vitamin B6	23	Potassium	26	% calories from protein	21
Vitamin B12	20	Selenium	27	% calories from fat	30
Vitamin C	33	Sodium	3	% calories from carbohydrates	28
Vitamin E	22	Zinc	24		
Thiamine	31			Total protein	11.2 gm
Folacin	28			Total fat	5 gm
Riboflavin	27			Saturated fat	0.7 gm
Niacin	24			Monounsaturated fat	1.2 gm
Pantothenic Acid	19			Polyunsaturated fat	2.8 gm
Calcium	20				
Copper	15			Carbohydrate	21 gm
Iron	15			Fiber	8 gm
Magnesium	21			Cholesterol	12 mg
Manganese	36				

SAUCES AND SPREADS

Almond Sauce (4+ Servings [⅓ cup per serving])
  ½ cup almonds
  ½ large red pepper, cored and seeded
  ½ medium onion, diced
* 1 tbsp. olive oil
  2 cloves garlic, minced
  3 tbsp. chili powder
  Juice of 1 lime
  ⅓ cup white wine
  1 cup spicy tomato sauce
  2 cups vegetable broth
  1 tbsp. almond butter
  1 tbsp. cornstarch
  1 29-oz. can tomato puree

Grind the almonds in a blender. (There are half as many calories and fat in ground almonds as in almond butter.) Saute the peppers and onion in the olive oil until golden. Add the garlic, chili powder, and ground almonds and saute an additional 2 minutes. Add the lime juice and wine and boil until the mixture is almost dry. Add the tomato sauce and broth, reserving 2 tbsp. of the broth, and simmer for 15 minutes. Stir in the almond butter. Mix the cornstarch in the reserved broth and add it to the almond sauce. Cook until the mix is slightly thickened. Serve hot over vegetables of your choice.

% OF RDA'S PER SERVING				NUTRITIONAL INFORMATION	
Vitamin A	4,522	Phosphorus	19	Total calories	289
Vitamin B6	30	Potassium	60	% calories from protein	13
Vitamin B12	0	Selenium	7		
Vitamin C	111	Sodium	33	% calories from fat	50
Vitamin E	138	Zinc	11	% calories from carbohydrates	45
Thiamine	21				
Folacin	26			Total protein	10 gm
Riboflavin	24			Total fat	16 gm
Niacin	32			Saturated fat	2 gm
Pantothenic Acid	21			Monounsaturated fat	10 gm
Calcium	10				
Copper	30			Polyunsaturated fat	32 gm
Iron	28			Carbohydrate	32 gm
Magnesium	46			Fiber	8 gm
Manganese	42			Cholesterol	0 mg

Hummus (5 Servings)

1 cup dry chick peas

1 carrot

3 scallions

2 tbsp. parsley

⅓ cup (or more) water

¼ cup lemon juice

2 tbsp. tamari

1 tbsp. Vegit seasoning

½ clove garlic, mashed (optional)

Dash of cayenne pepper (optional)

Soak the chick peas overnight. Discard soak water. Put the beans in 2 ½ cups of fresh water in a saucepan. Bring to a boil. Reduce heat and simmer, partially covered, for 1 hour or until the beans are tender. Shred the carrot and set aside. (It is a good idea to use a food processor, if you have one, from here on.) Finely chop the scallions and parsley. Add the cooked and cooled chick peas and grind them, with some water to help mash the beans. Also add the lemon juice, tamari, and Vegit, and mix. (Add more water if necessary to achieve the texture you desire.) By hand, mix in the shredded carrot. For added flavor, add garlic and cayenne. Use this as a spread for sandwiches or as a dip for steamed vegetables.

% OF RDA'S PER SERVING				NUTRITIONAL INFORMATION	
Vitamin A	184	Phosphorus	60	Total calories	855
Vitamin B6	63	Potassium	113	% calories from protein	22
Vitamin B12	0	Selenium	29		
Vitamin C	117	Sodium	32	% calories from fat	12
Vitamin E	12	Zinc	37	% calories from carbohydrates	66
Thiamine	52				
Folacin	113			Total protein	45 gm
Riboflavin	22			Total fat	11 gm
Niacin	26			Saturated fat	2 gm
Pantothenic Acid	77			Monounsaturated fat	3 gm
Calcium	31			Polyunsaturated fat	6 gm
Copper	79				
Iron	86			Carbohydrate	142 gm
Magnesium	85			Fiber	142 gm
Manganese	101			Cholesterol	0 mg

SALADS

Asparagus and Red Bell Pepper Salad (4 servings)

Grated peel from ½ large orange

1 medium red bell pepper

1 lb. asparagus with 2–3 inches of
   stalks discarded

2 tbsp. red wine vinegar

1 tsp. Dijon mustard

½ tbsp. olive oil or safflower oil

1 tbsp. water

Place orange gratings in boiling water for 3 to 5 minutes, drain, and set aside. Broil pepper until skin is black all around. Rub off the blackened skin, cut pepper into strips, and set aside. Steam asparagus spears until tender. Allow to cool, then cut into 1-inch lengths. Mix vinegar, mustard, oil, and water in a bowl. Mix all ingredients thoroughly by hand.

% OF RDA'S PER SERVING				NUTRITIONAL INFORMATION	
Vitamin A	59	Phosphorus	5	Total calories	46
Vitamin B6	7	Potassium	12	% calories from protein	24
Vitamin B12	0	Selenium	5	% calories from fat	32
Vitamin C	161	Sodium	0	% calories from carbohydrates	61
Vitamin E	17	Zinc	4		
Thiamine	7			Total protein	27 gm
Folacin	60			Total fat	1.6 gm
Riboflavin	7			Saturated fat	0.2 gm
Niacin	7			Monounsaturated fat	0.9 gm
Pantothenic Acid	3			Polyunsaturated fat	0.3 gm
Calcium	2				
Copper	8			Carbohydrate	7 gm
Iron	5			Fiber	2 gm
Magnesium	6			Cholesterol	0 mg
Manganese	7				

California Corn Salad (2 Servings)

1 ½ large red peppers, cored and seeded

1 ½ large green peppers, cored and seeded

2 zucchini

2 summer squash

1 cup eggplant

1 ½ ears corn

1 cup lettuce

1 cup nonfat cottage cheese

1 large stalk celery, chopped

½ tbsp. black walnuts, chopped

This recipe can be prepared with raw or cooked vegetables.

To serve raw, chop the peppers, zucchini, and squash (omit the eggplant) into corn kernel size pieces. Remove the kernels from the corn cob. Mix the vegetables together.

To serve cooked, cut the peppers into strips and drop into boiling water for 1 minute. Remove with a slotted spoon and drop into cold water. Dice the zucchini, squash, and eggplant, and remove the kernels from the corn cob. Add to boiling water. Parboil for 2 minutes. Set aside.

Tear the lettuce leaves into pieces and mix with the raw or cooked vegetables and the cottage cheese. Garnish with chopped celery and walnuts.

% OF RDA'S PER SERVING				NUTRITIONAL INFORMATION	
Vitamin A	189	Phosphorus	32	Total calories	301
Vitamin B6	71	Potassium	87	% calories from protein	39
Vitamin B12	47	Selenium	27	% calories from fat	11
Vitamin C	622	Sodium	3	% calories from carbohydrates	61
Vitamin E	30	Zinc	18	Total protein	30 gm
Thiamine	57			Total fat	3.5 gm
Folacin	132			Saturated fat	0.7 gm
Riboflavin	34			Monounsaturated fat	0.6 gm
Niacin	31			Polyunsaturated fat	1.5 gm
Pantothenic Acid	26			Carbohydrate	45 gm
Calcium	13			Fiber	14 gm
Copper	28			Cholesterol	7.5 mg
Iron	26				
Magnesium	53				
Manganese	42				

Creamed Cole Slaw (8 Servings)

1 small head cabbage

4 medium carrots

⅓ cup raw sunflower or pumpkin seeds

⅓ cup raisins

½ cup buttermilk

1 tbsp. apple cider vinegar

1 sprig fresh or 1 tbsp. dry dill

Grate or thinly slice the cabbage and grate the carrots. Mix the cabbage, carrots, sunflower seeds, and raisins. In a shaker jar, mix the buttermilk, vinegar, and dill. Shake well. Use the dressing to moisten only, you will have more than you need. Use the extra dressing as a dip or all purpose salad dressing. Let the slaw marinate in the refrigerator for several hours or overnight.

% OF RDA'S PER SERVING				NUTRITIONAL INFORMATION	
Vitamin A	174	Phosphorus	7	Total Calories	89
Vitamin B6	12	Potassium	21	% calories from protein	16
Vitamin B12	2	Selenium	9	% calories from fat	32
Vitamin C	54	Sodium	2	% calories from carbohydrates	63
Vitamin E	37	Zinc	5	Total protein	3.5 gm
Thiamine	19			Total fat	3 gm
Folacin	31			Saturated fat	.4 gm
Riboflavin	8			Monounsaturated fat	.5 gm
Niacin	6			Polyunsatured fat	2 gm
Pantothenic Acid	12			Carbohydrate	14 gm
Calcium	6			Fiber	4 gm
Copper	7			Cholesterol	0.5 mg
Iron	8				
Magnesium	15				
Manganese	10				

Green Grain Salad with Mustard Dressing (2 Servings)

¼ cup dried lentils

¼ cup brown rice

¼ cup dry bulgur

5 mushrooms, chopped

1 medium red pepper, cored, seeded, and chopped
4 tbsp. minced parsley
1 large scallion, chopped
2 stalks celery, minced
1 can water chestnuts (8–12 nuts)
1 tbsp. oat bran
1 tsp. sunflower seeds
⅓ cup apple cider vinegar
2 tbsp. Dijon mustard
1 tsp. cumin seed
1 tsp. ground oregano

Cook the lentils in 1 ½ cups of water for 45 minutes or until soft. Drain and cool. Cook the brown rice in ½ cup water for 30 minutes. Let cool. Soak the bulgur in water until soft, about 20 minutes, then drain. Mix the mushrooms, peppers, parsley, scallions, celery, and water chestnuts (reserving a few for garnish). Add the lentils, rice, bulgur, and oat bran. In a food processor or blender, combine the sunflower seeds, vinegar, mustard, cumin seed, and oregano. Pour the mustard dressing over the grains and vegetables and let marinate for 30 minutes.

% OF RDA'S PER SERVING				NUTRITIONAL INFORMATION	
Vitamin A	82	Phosphorus	34	Total calories	345
Vitamin B6	43	Potassium	53	% calories from protein	19
Vitamin B12	0	Selenium	28		
Vitamin C	230	Sodium	3	% calories from fat	14
Vitamin E	55	Zinc	25	% calories from carbohydrates	77
Thiamine	55				
Folacin	108			Total protein	16 gm
Riboflavin	31			Total fat	0.7 gm
Niacin	37			Saturated fat	0.7 gm
Pantothenic Acid	55			Monounsaturated fat	1 gm
Calcium	10			Polyunsaturated fat	3 gm
Copper	41				
Iron	46			Carbohydrate	66 gm
Magnesium	58			Fiber	17 gm
Manganese	88			Cholesterol	0 mg

SOUPS

Borscht with Greens (2 Servings)

3 medium beets, grated

½ sweet potato, grated

1 vegetable bouillon cube

2 tbsp. tamari

3 cups water

1 cup chopped beet greens

1 tsp. chopped fresh dill

1 scallion, chopped

1 ½ cups nonfat plain yogurt

Combine beets, sweet potato, vegetable bouillon cube, and tamari in water in a soup pot. Bring to a boil, cover, and simmer for 10 minutes. Add the beet greens, dill, and scallion, and simmer another 5 minutes. Remove from heat and let cool to room temperature. Chill in refrigerator. Stir in yogurt just before serving.

% OF RDA'S PER SERVING				NUTRITIONAL INFORMATION	
Vitamin A	204	Phosphorus	29	Total calories	197
Vitamin B6	21	Potassium	72	% calories from protein	29
Vitamin B12	53	Selenium	20		
Vitamin C	52	Sodium	38	% calories from fat	4
Vitamin E	11	Zinc	20	% calories from carbohydrates	72
Thiamine	20			Total protein	14 gm
Folacin	58			Total fat	0.8 gm
Riboflavin	55			Saturated fat	0.3 gm
Niacin	9			Monounsaturated fat	0.2 gm
Pantothenic Acid	34				
Calcium	38			Polyunsaturated fat	0.2 gm
Copper	17				
Iron	18			Carbohydrate	35 gm
Magnesium	38			Fiber	5 gm
Manganese	27			Cholesterol	3 mg

Cape Cod Chowder (6 Servings)

    3 tbsp. or 1 strip wakame or kombu seaweed

    3 medium potatoes

    ½ cup millet

    3 cups boiling water

    Canola- or olive-oil based spray

    4 medium leeks, bulb and lower leaf

    1 stalk celery, chopped

    ½ red pepper, cored, seeded, and chopped

    4 carrots, chopped

    1 bay leaf

    1 tsp. ground basil

    1 tsp. paprika

    ½ tsp. nutmeg

    1 lb. 3 oz. Atlantic cod

    1 tbsp. wheat germ

    2 cups skim milk

Soak seaweed in warm water for 10 minutes and cut into bite-size pieces. Add potatoes and millet to boiling water and boil for 15 minutes. Spray nonstick skillet with oil and saute leeks, celery, and peppers for 2 to 3 minutes. Add the contents of the skillet to the soup. Drain the seaweed. Add seaweed, carrots, bay leaf, basil, paprika, and nutmeg to the soup and simmer for 10 minutes. Cut cod into bite-size pieces. Add wheat germ and cod and simmer for 20 minutes. Remove bay leaf and gradually stir in milk.

% OF RDA'S PER SERVING				NUTRITIONAL INFORMATION	
Vitamin A	136	Phosphorus	28	Total calories	296
Vitamin B6	46	Potassium	41	% calories from protein	41
Vitamin B12	68	Selenium	77	% calories from fat	9
Vitamin C	32	Sodium	8	% calories from carbohydrates	50
Vitamin E	8	Zinc	15	Total protein	30 gm
Thiamine	30			Total fat	3 gm
Folacin	33			Saturated fat	0.9 gm
Riboflavin	24			Monounsaturated fat	0.5 gm
Niacin	33			Polyunsaturated fat	0.9 gm
Pantothenic Acid	23				
Calcium	12			Carbohydrate	37 gm
Copper	19			Fiber	4.5 gm
Iron	14			Cholesterol	58 mg
Magnesium	37				
Manganese	35				

Chilled Leafy Pottage (Serves 2)

1 bunch fresh spinach, cleaned, or 1 10-oz. package frozen

1 medium summer squash, cubed

1 medium cucumber, peeled and cut in quarters

3 cups lettuce

2 cups low-fat buttermilk

2 tbsp. chopped parsley

¼ small onion, minced

Steam spinach in 1 cup of water for 5 minutes. Add the squash and steam for 5 minutes. Reserve the cooking water. Combine the spinach, squash, cooking water, and cucumber in a blender. If your blender is large enough, add the lettuce and 1 cup of the buttermilk. Otherwise, blend separately. Combine all ingredients with remaining buttermilk, parsley, and onion in a large bowl. Chill.

% OF RDA'S PER SERVING				NUTRITIONAL INFORMATION	
Vitamin A	185	Phosphorus	30	Total calories	170
Vitamin B6	32	Potassium	77	% calories from protein	33
Vitamin B12	27	Selenium	11	% calories from fat	16
Vitamin C	121	Sodium	14	% calories from carbohydrates	60
Vitamin E	33	Zinc	18	Total protein	14 gm
Thiamine	30			Total fat	3 gm
Folacin	200			Saturated fat	1.5 gm
Riboflavin	54			Monounsaturated fat	0.6 gm
Niacin	13				
Pantothenic Acid	26			Polyunsaturated fat	0.4 gm
Calcium	38			Carbohydrate	25 gm
Copper	15				
Iron	30			Fiber	7 gm
Magnesium	53			Cholesterol	8.5 mg
Manganese	55				

Saffron SLS Soup (4 Servings)

¼ cup (approximately 1 oz.) dry kelp, kombu, or wakame
  seaweed

2 cups chopped leeks (approximately 8 leeks), bulb and
  lower leaf

1 ½ medium onions, chopped

2 cloves garlic, minced

1 tbsp. grated ginger root

4 cups chicken or vegetable broth

1 medium sweet potato

1 ½ cups skinned, seeded, and chopped winter squash
  (1 acorn, butternut, or small kaboshi)

½ tsp. pepper

½ tsp. cinnamon

1 tsp. saffron

1 cup nonfat yogurt

Preheat oven to 400. Soak the seaweed in warm water for 10 minutes. In a large nonstick skillet stir-fry the leeks, onion, garlic, and ginger in a little broth until the leeks are soft and the onion is translucent. Add the rest of the broth and the sweet potato, squash, pepper, and cinnamon.

Add the seaweed. Heat the saffron in the oven for 2 minutes, then add to soup. Cook 20 to 25 minutes until all is tender. Transfer the soup to a blender and puree. Add the yogurt and blend again. Return the soup to the pot and reheat if desired.

% OF RDA'S PER SERVING				NUTRITIONAL INFORMATION	
Vitamin A	183	Phosphorus	12	Total calories	144
Vitamin B6	19	Potassium	34	% calories from protein	17
Vitamin B12	18	Selenium	7	% calories from fat	8
Vitamin C	33	Sodium	23	% calories from carbohydrates	82
Vitamin E	5	Zinc	9		
Thiamine	14			Total protein	6 gm
Folacin	35			Total fat	1.2 gm
Riboflavin	19			Saturated fat	0.3 gm
Niacin	7			Monounsaturated fat	0.2 gm
Pantothenic Acid	19				
Calcium	14			Polyunsaturated fat	0.4 gm
Copper	11			Carbohydrate	30 gm
Iron	10			Fiber	4 gm
Magnesium	15			Cholesterol	1 mg
Manganese	20				

MAIN DISHES

Beef and Green Bean Stir-Fry (1 Serving)
¾ lb. snap beans, ends trimmed
4 carrots
1 large red pepper
Canola- or olive-oil based spray
2 cloves garlic
4 tbsp. water
1 medium onion
8 oz. beef, top round, fat trimmed
½ tsp. ground oregano
½ tsp. ground basil
1 tsp. red pepper flakes (or more, to taste)
½ cup mirin (Japanese rice wine)
3 tsp. soy sauce

Slice the beans into 2-inch pieces. Scrub and slice the carrots into ¼-inch rounds. Julienne the red pepper. Steam the green beans and carrots for 6 to 8 minutes. Spray a medium skillet with oil. Heat the skillet over a medium flame.

Mince or press the garlic and put it in a tablespoon of water. Slice the onion into thin slivers and place onion and garlic into the hot pan and fry for 3 to 4 minutes. Cut the round steak into ½-inch slices. Add the meat to the skillet, stirring constantly for 2 minutes to sear in flavors. Add the steamed vegetables along with the red pepper, oregano, basil, and red pepper flakes. Add a few tablespoons of water and cover. Reduce heat to low and cook for 3 minutes. Add the mirin and soy sauce and simmer for a final 3 minutes.

% OF RDA'S PER SERVING				NUTRITIONAL INFORMATION	
Vitamin A	405	Phosphorus	19	Total calories	225
Vitamin B6	39	Potassium	40	% calories from protein	39
Vitamin B12	68	Selenium	22	% calories from fat	24
Vitamin C	171	Sodium	13	% calories from carbohydrates	38
Vitamin E	14	Zinc	29		
Thiamine	23			Total protein	21 gm
Folacin	38			Total fat	6 gm
Riboflavin	25			Saturated fat	2 gm
Niacin	34			Monounsaturated fat	2 gm
Pantothenic Acid	11				
Calcium	6			Polyunsaturated fat	0.4 gm
Copper	11			Carbohydrate	20 gm
Iron	23			Fiber	7 gm
Magnesium	22			Cholesterol	47 mg
Manganese	16				

Eternal Youth Chili (10 Servings)

1 cup dried pinto beans

5 cups chicken or vegetable broth

2 cups beer

tk oregano

6 red chili peppers

8 medium tomatoes, quartered

5 stalks celery, chopped

Canola- or olive-oil based spray

3 large green peppers, chopped

3 medium onions, chopped

10 cloves garlic, minced

½ cup chopped parsley

½ lb. extra lean ground beef, cut into small cubes

1 lb. eye of round steak, fat trimmed, cut into small cubes

1 lb. lean pork, cut into small cubes

⅓ cup chili powder

¼ cup ground cumin

2 tbsp. coriander seeds

1 6-oz. can tomato paste

1 8-oz. can tomato sauce

6 to 8 oz. prepared salsa
1 tbsp. yellow cornmeal or masa harina flour
1 square unsweetened baking chocolate
¼ cup chili salsa with chopped onions (optional garnish)
2 tbsp. chopped fresh cilantro (optional garnish)
Lime wedges (optional garnish)

Soak pinto beans overnight and discard water. In a large stock pot, bring broth and beer to boil. Add oregano and beans and simmer for 1 hour. Remove the stems and seeds from the red chilis and boil them for 30 minutes. (When handling chilis, you may want to wear gloves. Do not rub your eyes at any time, as the oil in chilis is hot.)   Remove and discard the skins. Blend the pulp in a blender.

Blend the tomatoes in a blender or food processor and add them to the pot along with the celery. Spray a nonstick skillet with olive oil and saute the green peppers and chopped onions until tender, stir frequently. Add the garlic and parsley. Mix and remove from the stove. Spray a nonstick skillet with olive oil and sear all meat, stirring constantly until browned. Add the meat to the stock pot.

Dissolve the chili powder, cumin, and coriander in a small amount stock to remove lumps. Add this mixture to the pot as well as the tomato paste, sauce, and salsa. Dissolve the cornmeal or masa harina flour in enough water to make a paste and add it to the pot. Add the chocolate and simmer for 45 minutes. Garnish with salsa and onions, cilantro, or lime wedges.

% OF RDA'S PER SERVING				NUTRITIONAL INFORMATION	
Vitamin A	210	Manganese	41	Total Calories	472
Vitamin B6	77	Phosphorus	40	% calories from protein	33
Vitamin B12	84	Potassium	90	% calories from fat	31
Vitamin C	441	Selenium	42	% calories from carbohydrate	38
Vitamin E	39	Sodium	54	Total protein	38 gm
Thiamine	64	Zinc	47	Total fat	16 gm
Folacin	100			Saturated fat	6 gm
Riboflavin	43			Monounsaturated fat	6.7 gm
Niacin	65			Polyunsatured fat	2 gm
Pantothenic Acid	26			Carbohydrate	44 gm
Calcium	12			Fiber	13 gm
Copper	46			Cholesterol	67 mg
Iron	55				
Magnesium	51				

Falafels (8 Servings)

⅔ cup dried chickpeas (soaked in 5 cups water with ¼ cup kelp
   for 24 hours) or 24 oz. canned

¼ cup dried soybeans (cooked in 1½ cups water for 1 hour)
   or ⅔ cup canned

1 medium sweet potato, grated

1 tsp. baking soda

¼ medium onion, minced

½ cup parsley, minced

4 cloves garlic, peeled, pressed or minced

1 lemon, juiced

4 oz. tomato paste

2 tsp. ground cumin

2 tsp. ground coriander

1 tsp. cayenne pepper

½ cup wheat germ

Black pepper, to taste

Canola- or olive-oil based spray

Preheat the oven to 350. Drain the beans and kelp and combine with
the cooked soybeans in a food processor. Add the sweet potato and
baking soda. Use the pulse mode on the food processor and mix until
you have a texture like coarse bread crumbs. Do not puree.

In a large bowl, combine the processed beans, onion, parsley, garlic,
lemon juice, tomato paste, cumin, coriander, cayenne, wheat germ,
and black pepper to taste. Mix gently with a fork. Spray a large cookie
sheet with oil. Use your hands to shape falafels into 16 meatball-
shaped patties. Bake for 15 minutes, until moist on the inside and
crisp on the outside.

% OF RDA'S PER SERVING				NUTRITIONAL INFORMATION	
Vitamin A	75	Phosphorus	15	Total calories	141
Vitamin B6	19	Potassium	24	% calories from protein	21
Vitamin B12	0	Selenium	16	% calories from fat	19
Vitamin C	28	Sodium	7	% calories from carbohydrates	60
Vitamin E	9	Zinc	16	Total protein	8 gm
Thiamine	27			Total fat	3 gm
Folacin	79			Saturated fat	0.4 gm
Riboflavin	13			Monounsaturated fat	0.7 gm
Niacin	9			Polyunsaturated fat	1.6 gm
Pantothenic Acid	13			Carbohydrate	23 gm
Calcium	5			Fiber	6 gm
Copper	19			Cholesterol	0 mg
Iron	22				
Magnesium	23				
Manganese	54				

Fast Fish-n-Veggies (1 Serving)

Practical and versatile, you may use frozen vegetables in this dish for convenience, or prepare the vegie mix in bulk and store it in the refrigerator. If you do use frozen, choose a mix with a variety of colorful vegetables. This indicates a good phytonutrient mix. You can also use salsa and olive oil instead of the pasta sauce for a spicier dish.
We thank Sherm for this fabulous contribution.

1 small spear broccoli
¼ head cauliflower
1 ½ medium zucchinis
1 medium yellow summer squash
1 cup peppers (use one or an assortment of red, green, or yellow)
1 medium carrot
1 medium stalk celery
1 spear asparagus (or other vegetable of choice)
1 ¼ cup sliced mushrooms
⅓ cup canned pink salmon
½ cup pasta sauce (store-bought or homemade)

Coarsely chop the vegetables. Put vegetables into a large (1.5 quarts or larger) microwaveable bowl. Cover and steam in microwave on high for 5 minutes. Mix in the salmon and pasta sauce and steam for 1 minute more. Stir the mixture at least once during heating to avoid possible hot spots from microwaving

% OF RDA'S PER SERVING				NUTRITIONAL INFORMATION	
Vitamin A	421	Phosphorus	38	Total calories	300
Vitamin B6	73	Potassium	106	% calories from protein	29
Vitamin B12	150	Selenium	73	% calories from fat	25
Vitamin C	439	Sodium	32	% calories from carbohydrates	46
Vitamin E	73	Zinc	19		
Thiamine	47			Total protein	24 gm
Folacin	113			Total fat	8.5 gm
Riboflavin	70			Saturated fat	2 gm
Niacin	89			Monounsaturated fat	2 gm
Pantothenic Acid	83			Polyunsaturated fat	3 gm
Calcium	29			Carbohydrate	39 gm
Copper	53			Fiber	11.5 gm
Iron	34			Cholesterol	44 mg
Magnesium	44				
Manganese	35				

MegaMeal Fruit Salad 400 (1 Serving)

Another contribution by Sherm, this nutrient-packed recipe has a good omega-6/omega-3 ratio. The topping can be mixed and matched with many other recipe.

Fruit salad:
    1 ⅓ cups chopped strawberries
    ¾ cup cubed cantaloupe
    ⅓ cup sliced mango (or any sweet fruit)
    1 small kiwi, chopped
Nut topping mix:
    8 raw almonds
    1 brazil nut
    4 tsp. raw wheat germ
    2 tsp. flax meal (ground flax seed)

2 tsp. brewer's yeast

¼ tsp. nutmeg (or use cinnamon, ginger, or allspice)

⅔ cup plain nonfat yogurt

⅓ cup water

Mix the fruit in a large bowl. You may substitute any sweet fruit for the mango and kiwi (e.g., apple, pear, pineapple, banana, peach, grapes—even better, add some blueberries). Don't, however, use substitutions for the strawberries or cantaloupe.

Chop or grind the nuts in a food processor. Mix nuts with wheat germ, flax meal, brewer's yeast, and nutmeg. Set aside. Mix together yogurt, topping mix, and water in a small bowl and pour over the fruit.

% OF RDA'S PER SERVING				NUTRITIONAL INFORMATION	
Vitamin A	125	Phosphorus	40	Total calories	400
Vitamin B6	40	Potassium	60	% calories from protein	16
Vitamin B12	60	Selenium	150	% calories from fat	30
Vitamin C	350	Sodium	13	% calories from carbohydrates	59
Vitamin E	75	Zinc	30		
Thiamine	40			Total protein	19 gm
Folacin	60			Total fat	12.5 gm
Riboflavin	60			Saturated fat	1.5 gm
Niacin	30			Monounsaturated fat	5 gm
Pantothenic Acid	46			Polyunsaturated fat	4.5 gm
Calcium	30				
Copper	30			Carbohydrate	60 gm
Iron	20			Fiber	12.5 gm
Magnesium	60			Cholesterol	2.5 mg
Manganese	60				

Roasted Vegetables (4 Servings)

1 tbsp. olive oil

1 cup vegetable bouillon, prepared with ¼ cup water

3 medium onions

24 cloves garlic

1 tsp. sweet potato

1 tsp. large parsnips

1 tsp. carrots

2 small eggplants

2 green peppers

4 celery stalks

3 tbsp. balsamic vinegar

1 tsp. rosemary

1 tsp. thyme

1 tsp. pepper

Preheat oven to 400 degrees. Mix olive oil with vegetable broth. Set aside. Peel and slice the onions into ¼-inch rounds. Peel and separate the garlic cloves. Slice the sweet potato into ½-inch rounds. Slice the parsnips and carrots into ¼-inch rounds. Cube the eggplant. Seed and quarter the peppers. Slice the celery into 1 inch pieces.

Mix the onions, the garlic, sweet potato, parsnip, carrots, and eggplant together in a large baking pan. Add the olive oil and broth and mix thoroughly. Bake for 20 minutes. Add the green peppers and celery and cook another 10 minutes. All vegetables should be slightly browned. Remove from the oven and drizzle with balsamic vinegar and toss with rosemary, thyme, and pepper. Serve hot or at room temperature.

% OF RDA'S PER SERVING				NUTRITIONAL INFORMATION	
Vitamin A	487	Phosphorus	18	Total calories	271
Vitamin B6	59	Potassium	76	% calories from protein	11
Vitamin B12	0	Selenium	12	% calories from fat	10
Vitamin C	161	Sodium	5	% calories from carbohydrates	88
Vitamin E	18	Zinc	12	Total protein	7.5 gm
Thiamine	36			Total fat	3 gm
Folacin	82			Saturated fat	0.4 gm
Riboflavin	21			Monounsaturated fat	1 gm
Niacin	23			Polyunsaturated fat	0.6 gm
Pantothenic Acid	33			Carbohydrate	60 gm
Calcium	12			Fiber	16 gm
Copper	23			Cholesterol	0 mg
Iron	17				
Magnesium	33				
Manganese	48				

Stuffed Bell Peppers in Beer Sauce (2 Servings)

Stuffed peppers:

　　½ cup dry soybeans or 1 8-oz. can prepared soybeans

　　2 medium green peppers

　　2 medium red peppers

　　½ oz., 2 strips, wakame, kombu, or kelp seaweed

　　½ cup millet

　　1 cup diced tempeh

　　½ cup chopped onions

　　1 medium carrot, grated

　　¼ cup chopped parsley

　　⅓ cup, 2 oz.+, tomato paste

　　1 tsp. ground allspice

Sauce:

　　½ cup minced onions

　　Canola- or olive-oil based spray

　　⅔ cup ketchup or ½ cup tomato paste

　　2 tsp. Worcestershire sauce

　　⅓ cup beer

　　Black pepper to taste

If using dry soybeans, soak overnight and simmer in a medium pot with 2 cups of water for 1 hour. Drain and set aside. Preheat the oven to 350 degrees. Cut the tops off the peppers and reserve the tops. Clean out the seeds inside the pepper. Soak the seaweed in warm water for 10 minutes. Drain and cut it into bite size pieces.

Cook the millet in 1 ½ cups of water for 30 minutes, until all the water is absorbed. Add the seaweed and tempeh for the last 15 minutes. In a large bowl combine the canned (or fresh prepared) soybeans, the millet mixture, chopped onion, carrot, parsley, tomato paste, and allspice. Stuff each pepper until it bulges. Top with reserved caps and bake for 40 minutes.

For the sauce, stir fry the onion in a nonstick skillet sprayed with olive oil. Add the ketchup or tomato paste and the Worcestershire sauce. If the sauce is too thick, add beer for desired thickness and black pepper to taste. Simmer for a few minutes, then pour over the stuffed peppers and serve.

% OF RDA'S PER SERVING					NUTRITIONAL INFORMATION	
Vitamin A	610	Phosphorus	46		Total Calories	550
Vitamin B6	105	Potassium	110		% calories from protein	24
Vitamin B12	42	Selenium	27		% calories from fat	21
Vitamin C	789	Sodium	25		% calories from carbohydrate	61
Vitamin E	101	Zinc	32		Total protein	33 gm
Thiamine	65				Total fat	13 gm
Folacin	128				Saturated fat	1.8 gm
Riboflavin	45				Monounsatured fat	2.6 gm
Niacin	68				Polyunsaturated fat	7 gm
Pantothenic Acid	34				Carbohydrate	84 gm
Calcium	20				Fiber	23 gm
Copper	79				Cholesterol	0 mg
Iron	81					
Magnesium	79					
Manganese	98					

Vegetable Salad (4 Servings)

⅓ cup dry chickpeas
⅓ cup dry black-eyed peas
⅓ cup brown rice
¼ cup wild rice
1 carrot
1 spear broccoli
1 small sweet potato
6 medium mushrooms
8 cherry tomatoes or 1 large tomato
6 large leaves romaine lettuce
1 medium green or red bell pepper
1 zucchini or other summer squash
¼ small head red cabbage
½ cup chopped parsley
1 small red onion, chopped
1 hard boiled egg
¾ cup plain nonfat yogurt
½ cup buttermilk
⅓ cup balsamic vinegar
Assorted herbs

Soak the chickpeas and black-eyed peas in water overnight. Discard the water, and, in a large pot, add water to cover. Bring to a boil. Reduce the heat, cover, and simmer for 15 minutes. Add the brown and wild rice to the beans and cook for an additional hour.

Meanwhile, slice the carrot into ¼-inch rounds and separate the broccoli florets from the stalk. Peel the outer layer of broccoli stalk skin off and chop the spear into bite size pieces. Slice the sweet potato into ½-inch circles. Steam the broccoli spears and carrots for 4 minutes, add the sweet potato and broccoli florets and continue steaming for another 7 to 10 minutes. Drain and cool the vegetables. Place in a large mixing bowl.

Slice the mushrooms, tomato, lettuce, bell pepper, squash, and cabbage. Add to the steamed vegetables along with the parsley and onions. Drain the cooled rice and beans and add it to the vegetables. Chop the hard boiled egg and add to salad. Blend the yogurt, buttermilk, and vinegar and add to the salad. Add any herbs you might favor and mix thoroughly.

% OF RDA'S PER SERVING				NUTRITIONAL INFORMATION	
Vitamin A	285	Phosphorus	46	Total Calories	378
Vitamin B6	0.8	Potassium	76	% calories from protein	20
Vitamin B12	15	Selenium	34		
Vitamin C	344	Sodium	4	% calories from fat	9
Vitamin E	28	Zinc	34	% calories from carbohydrate	86
Thiamine	60				
Folacin	134			Total protein	19 gm
Riboflavin	38			Total fat	4 gm
Niacin	31			Saturated fat	.7 gm
Pantothenic Acid	45			Monounsaturated fat	.9 gm
Calcium	23				
Copper	27			Polyunsaturated fat	1.5 gm
Iron	33			Carbohydrate	81 gm
Magnesium	72			Fiber	16 gm
Manganese	106			Cholesterol	9 mg

GRAINS, LEGUMES, AND PASTA

Kasha Tabouli (8 Servings)

2 cups kasha (roasted buckwheat)
1 32-oz. can chicken or vegetable broth
3 large tomatoes, seeded, cored, and chopped into ¼-inch pieces
½ medium onion, minced
1 clove garlic, minced
1 cup fresh parsley, chopped
Juice of one lemon
1 tbsp. olive oil
1 tsp. fresh or dried mint or spearmint, minced
½ tsp. black pepper, or to taste
Dash of salt (optional)
½ cup romaine lettuce, shredded

To cook the kasha, heat a large skillet over medium heat. Add the kasha and roast the grains until they smell nutty, stirring constantly. Heat the chicken or vegetable broth in a medium sized saucepan. Add the kasha and simmer for 20 minutes. Remove from heat when all liquid has been absorbed.

Fluff with a fork and cool for 15 minutes. Drain the kasha in a fine-mesh colander, pressing firmly with a large spoon to remove as much liquid as possible. In a large bowl, combine kasha, tomatoes, onions, garlic, parsley, lemon juice, olive oil, mint, black pepper, and salt. Mix thoroughly but gently, so as not to smash the tomatoes. Serve over lettuce leaves.

% OF RDA'S PER SERVING				NUTRITIONAL INFORMATION	
Vitamin A	24	Phosphorus	16	Total calories	198
Vitamin B6	14	Potassium	23	% calories from protein	16
Vitamin B12	6	Selenium	7	% calories from fat	16
Vitamin C	57	Sodium	20	% calories from carbohydrates	68
Vitamin E	14	Zinc	11	Total protein	8 gm
Thiamine	14			Total fat	4 gm
Folacin	32			Saturated fat	0.7 gm
Riboflavin	15			Monounsaturated fat	2 gm
Niacin	29			Polyunsaturated fat	11 gm
Pantothenic Acid	15			Carbohydrate	36 gm
Calcium	3			Fiber	5.5 gm
Copper	19			Cholesterol	0 mg
Iron	17				
Magnesium	38				
Manganese	31				

Pasta Primavera (2 Servings)

    5 oz. Japanese soba noodles, dry

    ½ onion, chopped

    ½ large red pepper, chopped

    4 shiitake mushrooms, sliced

    4 cloves garlic, minced

    ½ tbsp. olive oil

    2 medium tomatoes, chopped

    ¼ cup chopped parsley

    2 tbsp. dill

    ⅔ cup spaghetti or marinara sauce

    3 tbsp. prepared salsa

    1 tbsp. parmesan or soy parmesan cheese (optional, add
       22 calories)

Place noodles in boiling water for 7 minutes. While the noodles cook, fry the onion, pepper, mushrooms, and garlic in olive oil in a nonstick skillet until the onion is translucent. Add the tomato, parsley, and dill. Stir completely. Add the spaghetti sauce and salsa and simmer an additional 3 to 5 minutes. Serve sauce over noodles. Top with cheese, if desired.

% OF RDA'S PER SERVING				NUTRITIONAL INFORMATION	
Vitamin A	101	Phosphorus	25	Total Calories	384
Vitamin B6	36	Potassium	53	% calories from protein	16
Vitamin B12	0	Selenium	114		
Vitamin C	275	Sodium	43	% calories from fat	14
Vitamin E	33	Zinc	19	% calories from carbohydrates	78
Thiamine	48				
Folacin	78			Total protein	15 gm
Riboflavin	29			Total fat	6 gm
Niacin	38			Saturated fat	0.8 gm
Pantothenic Acid	41			Monounsaturated fat	3.3 gm
Calcium	11			Polyunsaturated fat	1 gm
Copper	29				
Iron	40			Carbohydrate	75 gm
Magnesium	42			Fiber	14 gm
Manganese	47			Cholesterol	0 mg

Pasta Fagioli (4 Servings)

¼ cup dry white beans

1 bay leaf

2 cups cold water plus 1 tbsp.

Canola- or olive-oil based spray

6 cloves garlic, minced

¼ onion, finely chopped

1 sweet red pepper, finely chopped

1 bunch fresh spinach, washed and chopped

4 oz. whole-wheat or quinoa elbows, macaroni, or spaghetti, dry

Juice of one lemon

Salt, to taste

Pepper, to taste

Rinse the beans and soak overnight in water to cover. Drain the beans, and place, along with a bay leaf, in a large saucepan with 2 cups cold water. Bring to boil over high heat. Reduce heat and simmer until tender, about 45 minutes. Remove from heat.

Spray a small skillet with olive oil and add the garlic and onions. Over a medium flame, cook for 3 minutes. Stir frequently, scraping the drippings from the bottom of the pan as the onions cook. Add a little water if the onions dry and stick. Add the peppers along with 1 tbsp. water and cover. Simmer for 3 minutes. Add the spinach. Cover, and cook over a low heat for 2 minutes, or until the spinach wilts.

Cook the pasta according to the package directions. Drain the beans and add the spinach mixture to the beans along with the lemon juice and salt or pepper to taste. Combine the pasta with the beans and heat thoroughly.

% OF RDA'S PER SERVING				NUTRITIONAL INFORMATION	
Vitamin A	101	Phosphorus	25	Total Calories	384
Vitamin B6	36	Potassium	53	% calories from protein	16
Vitamin B12	0	Selenium	114		
Vitamin C	275	Sodium	43	% calories from fat	14
Vitamin E	33	Zinc	19	% calories from carbohydrates	78
Thiamine	48				
Folacin	78			Total protein	15 gm
Riboflavin	29			Total fat	6 gm
Niacin	38			Saturated fat	0.8 gm
Pantothenic Acid	41			Monounsaturated fat	3.3 gm
Calcium	11			Polyunsaturated fat	1 gm
Copper	29			Carbohydrate	75 gm
Iron	40			Fiber	14 gm
Magnesium	42			Cholesterol	0 mg
Manganese	47				

APPENDIX B

NUTRITIVE VALUES OF THE BEST FOODS

Food   *Weight of Normal Portion*   *Nutritive Values of Foods (Values per 100 gm)*

CATEGORY & SUBSTANCE	NORMAL PORTION	AMT. GRAMS	CALORIES	PROTEIN (GM)	FAT	CARBOHYDRATE	FIBER	% SATD. FAT	CHOLESTEROL (MG)
VEGETABLES									
Artichoke—boiled	base & ends—leaves	100	26	3	0.2	10	2.5	0	0
Asparagus	4 large spears	100	26	2.5	0.2	5	0.7	0	0
Beets (greens)	cooked 1 cup	150	24	2.2	0.3	5	1.3	0	0
Beets—Red Raw	1 cup diced	140	43	1.6	0.1	10	0.8	0	0
Broccoli	1 med. stalk	180	32	3.6	0.3	6	1.5	0	0
Brussels sprouts	2 large	140	45	5	0.4	8	1.6	0	0
Cabbage	1 cup finely shredded	90	24	1.3	0.2	5	0.1	0	0
Cabbage—Chinese	cup 1 inch pcs.	75	14	1.2	0.1	3	0.6	0	0
Cabbage—Red	1 cup shredded	100	31	2	0.2	7	1	0	0
Carrots	1 carrot 7.5 × 1.125	80	42	1.1	0.2	10	1	0	0
Cauliflower	1 cup whole flowerettes	100	27	2.7	0.2	5	1	0	0
Celeriac	¼ of 1 large	100	40	2	0.3	8.5	1.3	0	0
Celery	1 cup chopped	120	17	.9	0.1	4	0.6	0	0
Chard	¼ lb.	115	25	2.4	0.3	4.5	0.8	0	0
Corn	1 cob 5 × 1.75 (kernels)	140	96	3.5	1	22	0.7	0	0
Cucumber	1 small 6.5 × 1.5	180	15	.9	0.1	3.4	0.6	0	0
Eggplant	1 cup diced	200	25	1.2	0.2	6	0.9	0	0

Garlic	1 clove (1.3 × .5 × .3)	3	137	6.2	0.2	31	1.5	0	0
Kale	¼ lb.	115	38	4.2	0.8	6	1.3	0	0
Leeks	3–4 (5 inches)	100	52	2.2	0.3	11.2	1.3	0	0
Lettuce—Iceberg	wedge .125 of head	90	13	.9	0.1	3	0.5	0	0
Lettuce—Romaine	1 cup chopped	55	18	1.3	0.3	3.5	0.7	0	0
Mushrooms	1 cup sliced or diced	70	28	2.7	0.3	4.4	0.8	0	0
Mushrooms—Shiitake	2 oz.	55	275	12.5	1.6	65	5.5	0	0
Onions	1 cup chopped	160	38	1.5	0.1	9	0.6	0	0
Parsley	1 t. chopped	4	44	3.6	0.6	9	1.5	0	0
Peppers—Green	1 cup strips	100	22	1.2	0.2	5	1.4	0	0
Peppers (red—sweet)	1 large or 1 cup strips	100	31	1.4	0.3	7.1	1.7	0	0
Potato—White	2.75 × 4.25	250	77	2	0.1	17	0.5	0	0
Potato—Sweet	5 × 2	180	114	1.7	0.4	27	0.7	0	0
Radishes (red)	10 small (1 in. diam.)	100	17	1	0.1	3.6	0.7	0	0
Spinach	1 cup chopped	55	26	3.2	0.3	4	0.6	0	0
Squash (summer)	1 cup—cubed	130	19	1.1	0.1	4.2	0.6	0	0
Squash (winter)	1 cup baked	205	50	1.4	0.3	12.4	1.4	0	0
Tomato	2.5 inch diam.	100	22	1.1	0.2	5	0.5	0	0
Turnip Greens	¼ lb.	115	28	3	0.3	5	0.8	0	0
Waterchestnut	4 chestnuts	25	80	1.4	0.2	19	0.8	0	0
Yams	¼ lb.	115	100	2.1	0.2	23.2	0.9	0	0

Food   Weight of Normal Portion   Nutritive Values of Foods (Values per 100 gm)

CATEGORY & SUBSTANCE	NORMAL PORTION	AMT. GRAMS	CALORIES	PROTEIN (GM)	FAT	CARBOHYDRATE	FIBER	% SATD. FAT	CHOLESTEROL (MG)
LEGUMES									
Beans—Garbanzos	¼ cup	50	360	21	5	61	5	9	0
Beans—Green	1 cup	100	32	1.9	0.2	7	1	0	0
Beans—Lima	½ cup	100	345	20.4	1.6	64	4.3	0	0
Beans—Pinto	½ cup	100	349	23	1.2	63.7	4.3	0	0
Cowpeas	½ cup	70	343	23	1.5	62	4.4	0	0
Lentils—Brown	½ cup	100	340	25	1.1	60	4	0	0
Peas	1 cup	140	84	6	0.4	14	2	0	0
Soybeans (mature)	¼ cup	50	403	34	18	34	5	15	0
Soybean Curd (tofu)	1 piece 2.5 × 1 × 2.75	120	72	8	4.2	2.4	0.1	0	0
Split Peas	½ cup	100	345	24.7	0.9	61.8	1.7	0	0
SEAWEED									
Hijiki	¼ cup	8	256	7.5	0.5	46	0	0	0
Kombu	¼ cup	8	219	6	1.2	42	6.7	0	0
Nori	¼ cup	8	235	27	0.8	40	4.7	0	0
Wakami	¼ cup	8	227	12.4	0.3	47.4	3.6	0	0
FISH & SHELLFISH									
Bass—Black Sea	3.5 oz.	100	93	19	1	0	0	0	55

Food	Measure								
Bass—White Sea	3.5 oz.	100	98	18	2	0	0	50	55
Catfish	3.5 oz.	100	103	18	3	0	0	33	55
Clams	4 cherrystone	70	76	13	1.6	2	0	0	50
Cod	3.5 oz.	100	78	18	0.3	0	0	0	50
Crab (steamed)	3.5 oz.	100	93	17	2	0.5	0	0	100
Haddock	3.5 oz.	100	79	18	0.1	0	0	0	60
Halibut	3.5 oz.	100	100	21	1.2	0	0	0	50
Herring (Pacific)	1 herring	50	98	17.5	2.6	0	0	0	85
Lobster	1 cup cubed	145	91	19	1.5	0.5	0	0	77
Mackarel (Atlantic)	3.5 oz.	100	191	19	12	0	0	33	95
Ocean Perch	3.5 oz.	100	88	18	1.2	0	0	0	55
Oysters	med.—2 selects	25	66	8.4	1.8	3.4	0.1	0	50
Perch—White	3.5 oz.	100	118	19	4	0	0	25	55
Red Snapper	3.5 oz.	100	93	20	1	0	0	0	55
Salmon (Atlantic)	3.5 oz.	100	217	23	13	0	0	31	39
Salmon (Atlantic can)	1 can 6.5 oz.	185	203	22	12	0	0	25	37
Sardines (Pacific)	3.5 oz.	100	157	19	9	0	0	22	112
Sardines (Atlantic can)	3.5 oz.	100	203	24	11	0	0	0	130
Scallops—Raw	1 large	25	80	15	0.2	3	0	0	35
Shark	3.5 oz.	100	103	24	0.1	0	0	0	33

Food *Weight of Normal Portion* *Nutritive Values of Foods (Values per 100 gm)*

CATEGORY & SUBSTANCE	NORMAL PORTION	AMT. GRAMS	CALORIES	PROTEIN (GM)	FAT	CARBOHYDRATE	FIBER	% SATD. FAT	CHOLESTEROL (MG)
Shrimp—Raw	3.5 oz.	100	91	18	0.8	1.5	0	0	150
Sole	3.5 oz.	100	79	17	0.8	0	0	0	50
Squid	3.5 oz.	100	84	16.5	1	0	0	0	56
Swordfish	3.5 oz.	100	118	19	4	0	0	25	55
Tuna (canned)	0.5 cup	115	127	28	0.8	0	0	0	63
MEAT & POULTRY									
Beef—Loin/Sirloin	3.5 oz.	100	143	22	6	0	0	46	65
Beef—Round	3.5 oz.	100	135	22	5	0	0	45	65
Calves Liver	3.5 oz.	100	140	19	5	4	0	20	300
Chicken (dark meat)	3.5 oz.	100	130	20	4.3	0	0	25	80
Chicken (light meat)	3.5 oz.	100	117	23	2	0	0	25	58
Ham (canned)	3.5 oz.	100	193	18	12	0.9	0	37	89
Hamburger	3.5 oz.	100	179	21	10	0	0	50	68
Lamb (choice)	3.5 oz.	100	263	17	21	0	0	57	71
Lamb—Loin	3.5 oz.	100	138	20	6	0	0	55	70
Pork (thin)	3.5 oz.	100	165	20	9.1	0	0	36	60
Rabbit (domestic)	3.5 oz.	100	162	21	8	0	0	38	0
Turkey (light meat)	3.5 oz.	100	114	23.4	2	0	0	32	60

Turkey (dark meat)	3.5 oz.	100	123	20	4	0	0	33	75
Veal	3.5 oz.	100	156	20	8	0	0	48	71
Veal—Loin	3.5 oz.	100	156	19.7	8	0	0	48	71
FRUIT									
Apples	1 med. 2.75 in. diam.	150	59	.2	0.4	15	0.8	0	0
Applesauce—Unsweetened	½ cup	100	40	.2	5	11	0.5	0	0
Apricots	1 med.	40	51	1.4	0.4	11	0.6	0	0
Avocado	1 cup	150	167	2	17	7	2.1	0	0
Banana	1 med.	150	85	1	0.5	23	0.5	0	0
Blueberries	1 cup	140	56	.7	0.5	15	1.5	0	0
Cantaloupe	0.5 med.	400	30	.9	0.3	8	0.4	0	0
Cranberries	1 cup	100	49	.4	0.2	13	1.2	0	0
Dates—Nat'l & Dried	5 w/o pits	40	274	2.2	0.5	73	2.3	0	0
Figs—Raw	2 large/3 small	100	74	.8	0.3	19	1.2	20	0
Grapefruit	sections 1 cup	190	41	.7	0.1	8.4	0.2	0	0
Grapes	1 cup	150	67	.6	0.4	17	0.8	0	0
Lemon (peeled)	1 med.	100	29	1.1	0.3	9.3	0.4	0	0
Lime	1 med.	100	30	.7	0.2	10.5	.5	0	0
Nectarine	2 med.	100	49	.9	0.5	12	0.4	0	0
Orange	1 med.	180	47	.9	0.1	12	0.4	0	0

Food　　　Weight of Normal Portion　　　Nutritive Values of Foods (Values per 100 gm)

CATEGORY & SUBSTANCE	NORMAL PORTION	AMT. GRAMS	CALORIES	PROTEIN (GM)	FAT	CARBOHYDRATE	FIBER	% SATD. FAT	CHOLESTEROL (MG)
Papaya	⅓ med.	100	39	.6	0.1	10	0.8	0	0
Peaches	1 med.	100	38	.7	0.1	11	0.6	0	0
Pears	1 small	75	61	.4	0.4	15	1.4	0	0
Persimmon—Native	1 med.	100	127	.8	0.4	33.5	1.5	0	0
Pineapple	1 cup diced	140	52	.4	0.4	12	0.5	0	0
Plums	2 med.	100	55	.79	0.6	13	0.6	0	0
Raisins	2 T.	18	289	3.2	0.5	79	1.3	0	0
Raspberries—Red	¾ cup	100	50	.9	0.6	12	3	0	0
Strawberries	1 cup whole	150	37	.6	0.4	7	0.5	0	0
Watermelon	1 cup diced	160	26	.6	0.4	7	0.3	0	0
Orange Juice	1 cup	248	45	.7	0.2	10.4	0.1	0	0
CEREAL									
Buckwheat	1 cup	100	335	11.7	2.4	73	10	0	0
Grape Nuts	1 cup	224	357	11.7	0.4	82	4.8	0	0
Cereals—Rolled Oats	1 cup	80	391	14	7	68	1.2	29	0
Cereals—Rye	1 cup	80	355	12	1.7	73	2	0	0
Shredded Wheat	1 biscuit	25	360	11	2.2	80	9.3	0	0
Wheat Flakes	1 cup	30	355	10	1.6	81	1.6	0	0

Whole Wheat Hot	1 cup	125	342	11.2	2	75	2	0	0
GRAIN									
Grains—Barley	¼ cup	50	349	8	1	79	0.5	0	0
Bulgur Wheat	½ cup	100	361	11	1.5	76	1.7	0	0
Corn Meal	¼ cup	30	355	9.2	3.9	74	1.6	11	0
Gluten Flour	1 cup	140	378	41.4	1.9	47	0.4	0	0
Millet	¼ cup	25	327	10	2.9	73	3.2	34	0
Popcorn (plain—popd)	3 cups	42	386	12.7	5	77	2.2	20	0
Rice (brown—raw)	short grain—¼ cup	50	356	7.5	2	77	0.9	0	0
Rye Flour	1 cup—sifted	88	357	9.4	1	78	0.4	0	0
Wheat Bran	1 T.	6	213	16	4.6	62	9	21	0
Wheat Flour (enr)	½ cup sifted	55	364	10.5	1	76.1	0.3	0	0
Wheat Flour (wh)	½ cub sifted	55	333	13.3	2	71	2.3	0	0
Wheat Germ	1 T.	6	395	27	11	47	2.5	18	0
Wild Rice	¼ cup	40	353	14.1	0.7	75.3	1	0	0
DAIRY									
Butter Milk	1 cup	244	41	3.3	0.9	4.8	0	67	4
Lowfat Milk (2%)	1 cup	244	50	3.3	1.9	4.8	0	63	8
Skim Milk	1 cup	244	35	3.4	0.2	4.9	0	55	2
Whole Milk	1 cup	244	62	3.3	3.3	4.7	0	61	14

Food   Weight of Normal Portion   Nutritive Values of Foods (Values per 100 gm)

CATEGORY & SUBSTANCE	NORMAL PORTION	AMT. GRAMS	CALORIES	PROTEIN (GM)	FAT	CARBOHYDRATE	FIBER	%SATD. FAT	CHOLESTEROL (MG)
Yogurt (low fat)	1 cup	244	64	5.3	1.6	7	0	63	6
CHEESE									
Cheese—American	1 slice 2.25 × 2.25 × .25	25	375	22	31	1.6	0	64	94
Cheese—Cheddar	1 inch cubed	30	402	25	33	1.3	0	64	105
Cheese (cottage)—Dry Curd	1 cup	200	85	17	0.4	1.9	0	64	7
Cheese—Cottage (1% fat)	¼ cup	60	72	12	1	2.7	0	64	4
Cheese (feta)	1 inch cube	17	264	14	21	4	0	71	89
Cheese—Monterey Jack	1 inch cube	30	373	24	30	0.7	0	62	112
Mozzarella (part skim)	1 inch cube	30	252	24	16	3	0	63	58
Ricotta (part skim)	½ cup	124	140	11	8	5	0	62	31
Cheese—Swiss	1 inch cube	30	369	28	27	3.4	0	66	92
BREAD									
Pumpernickel	1 slice	32	247	9.1	1.3	53	1.3	0	0
Bread—Rye—Amer	1 slice	25	243	9	1.1	52	0.4	0	1
Bread—Wheat	1 slice	25	241	9	2.6	49	1.5	20	3

EGGS

Food	Measure								
Eggs—White	1 med.	15	49	10	0	1.2	0	0	0
Eggs—Whole	1 whole med. refuse 12%	50	158	13	12	1.2	0	28	548
Eggs—Yolk	1 med.	29	369	16	33	0.2	0	30	1602

NUTS & SEEDS

Food	Measure								
Almonds	1 T.	8	598	19	54	20	2.6	8	0
Cashew	14 large	28	561	17	46	29	1.4	17	0
Chestnuts (fresh)	2 lrge or 3 smll	15	194	3	1.5	42	1	0	0
Peanuts (roasted)	1 T. chpd or 15 whl	9	582	26	49	21	2.7	22	0
Pecans	10 large	9	687	9.2	71	14.6	2.3	7	0
Pumpkin Seeds	⅛ cup	17	553	29	47	15	1.9	18	0
Sunflower Seeds	⅛ cup	18	560	24	47	20	4	12	0

OILS

Food	Measure								
Butter—Salted	1 T.	14	717	.9	81	0.1	0	62	219
Corn Oil	1 T.	14	900	0	100	0	0	12.7	0
Olive Oil	1 T.	14	900	0	100	0	0	13.5	0
Safflower Oil	1 T.	14	900	0	100	0	0	9.1	0
Sesame Oil	1 T.	14	884	.8	100	0	0	14.2	0
Soy Oil	1 T.	14	900	0	100	0	0	14.4	0

MISCELLANEOUS

Food	Measure								
Melba Toast	1 slice	4	475	16.7	15	67.5	0	0	0
Yeast	1 oz.	28	283	39	1	38	1.7	0	0

Food   Weight of Normal Portion   Nutritive Values of Foods (Values per 100 gm)
Essential Amino Acids (Mg)

CATEGORY & SUBSTANCE	NORMAL PORTION	AMT. GRAMS	TRYPTOPHAN	THREONINE	ISOLEUCINE	LEUCINE	LYSINE	PHENYLALAN	TYROSINE	VALINE	METHIONINE/ CYSTEINE
VEGETABLES											
Artichoke—boiled	base & ends—leaves	100	0	0	0	0	0	0	0	0	0
Asparagus	4 large spears	100	30	75	90	110	120	78	45	120	55
Beets (greens)	cooked 1 cup	150	26	84	90	140	120	128	0	110	70
Beets—Red Raw	1 cup diced	140	14	34	52	55	86	27	86	49	48
Broccoli	1 med. stalk	180	45	133	137	177	160	175	0	185	90
Brussels sprouts	2 large	140	50	170	206	216	219	162	100	215	137
Cabbage	1 cup finely shredded	90	10	36	50	53	61	27	30	40	38
Cabbage—Chinese	cup 1 inch pcs.	75	10	34	35	49	57	25	25	37	35
Cabbage—Red	1 cup shredded	100	16	56	78	80	94	42	0	60	59
Carrots	1 carrot 7.5 × 1.125	80	8	33	33	50	45	30	25	50	36
Cauliflower	1 cup whole flowerettes	100	40	120	135	200	160	100	34	155	68
Celeriac	¼ of 1 large	100	0	0	0	0	0	0	0	0	0
Celery	1 cup chopped	120	14	40	45	75	27	50	16	55	25
Chard	¼ lb.	115	25	100	100	130	95	80	0	95	7
Corn	1 cob 5 × 1.75 (kernels)	140	21	144	130	390	130	200	170	220	110

Cucumber	1 small 6.5 × 1.5	180	6	21	25	35	35	20	0	28	8
Eggplant	1 cup diced	200	12	45	50	70	32	50	45	60	20
Garlic	1 clove (1.3 × .5 × .3)	3	0	0	0	0	0	0	0	0	0
Kale	¼ lb.	115	50	150	150	280	130	170	0	200	70
Leeks	3-4 (5 inches)	100	0	0	0	0	0	0	0	0	0
Lettuce—Iceberg	wedge .125 of head	90	10	54	50	83	50	67	102	71	29
Lettuce—Romaine	1 cup chopped	55	13	54	50	83	75	67	35	71	42
Mushrooms	1 cup sliced or diced	70	8	100	600	320	0	0	0	425	190
Mushrooms—Shiitake	2 oz.	55	0	0	0	0	0	0	0	0	0
Onions	1 cup chopped	160	20	20	20	35	60	40	46	30	26
Parsley	1 T. chopped	4	75	0	0	0	530	0	0	0	18
Peppers—Green	1 cup strips	100	8	50	46	46	50	55	55	32	35
Peppers (red—sweet)	1 lrg or 1 cup strips	100	10	58	53	53	60	70	60	38	40
Potato—White	2.75 × 4.25	250	21	86	72	105	111	92	43	111	25
Potato—Sweet	5 × 2	180	30	80	82	97	80	90	80	127	58
Radishes (red)	10 small (1 in. diam.)	100	4	49	54	75	28	48	0	25	2
Spinach	1 cup chopped	55	51	141	150	245	200	130	110	176	120
Squash (summer)	1 cup—cubed	130	9	35	35	50	42	30	0	41	14
Squash (winter)	1 cup baked	205	0	0	0	0	0	0	0	0	0
Tomato	2.5 inch diam.	100	9	36	32	45	46	28	14	31	13

Food Weight of Normal Portion Nutritive Values of Foods (Values per 100 gm) Essential Amino Acids (Mg)

CATEGORY & SUBSTANCE	NORMAL PORTION	AMT. GRAMS	TRYPTO-PHAN	THREONINE	ISOLEUCINE	LEUCINE	LYSINE	PHENY-LALAN	TYROSINE	VALINE	METHIO-NINE/CYSTEINE
Turnip Greens	¼ lb.	115	47	127	106	210	133	142	86	154	54
Waterchestnut	4 chestnuts	25	0	0	0	0	0	0	0	0	0
Yams	¼ lb.	115	27	76	79	136	86	84	84	98	58
LEGUMES											
Beans—Garbanzos	¼ cup	50	165	750	1200	1500	1415	1000	700	1000	560
Beans—Green	1 cup	100	26	70	90	110	100	100	80	91	47
Beans—Lima	½ cup	100	184	960	1180	1700	1370	1200	535	1290	630
Beans—Pinto	½ cup	100	210	1000	1310	1980	1710	1270	890	1400	460
Cowpeas	½ cup	70	250	850	1094	1710	1480	1200	600	1530	645
Lentils—Brown	½ cup	100	220	900	1320	1760	1530	1100	670	1360	384
Peas	1 cup	140	65	250	275	455	480	290	200	300	157
Soybeans (mature)	¼ cup	50	525	1470	2010	2900	2350	2050	1300	2000	1065
Soybean Curd (tofu)	1 piece 2.5 × 1 2.75	120	132	233	359	616	458	440	330	363	215
Split Peas	½ cup	100	220	860	1310	1750	1510	1140	660	1330	604
SEAWEED											
Hijiki	¼ cup	8	40	180	350	405	160	320	170	570	180
Kombu	¼ cup	8	130	615	205	230	160	0	0	780	0

Nori	¼ cup	8	280	1030	870	1510	800	0	0	1950	0
Wakami	¼ cup	8	120	550	290	860	375	0	0	700	0
FISH & SHELLFISH											
Bass—Black Sea	3.5 oz.	100	190	830	980	1460	1690	710	620	1020	712
Bass—White Sea	3.5 oz.	100	180	770	920	1370	1580	670	574	950	668
Catfish	3.5 oz.	100	180	790	830	1440	1600	650	600	1160	670
Clams	4 cherrystone	70	170	610	610	1000	1040	540	540	810	545
Cod	3.5 oz.	100	197	900	800	1450	1700	850	650	900	800
Crab (steamed)	3.5 oz.	100	200	730	745	1400	1250	650	600	750	720
Haddock	3.5 oz.	100	180	790	920	1370	1600	680	490	970	775
Halibut	3.5 oz.	100	200	890	1078	1500	1760	750	540	1070	860
Herring (Pacific)	1 herring	50	180	870	1000	1500	1530	740	190	1040	760
Lobster	1 cup cubed	145	220	870	890	1650	1500	770	700	910	780
Mackarel (Atlantic)	3.5 oz.	100	186	810	950	1410	1640	690	500	1000	670
Ocean Perch	3.5 oz.	100	200	700	800	1200	1600	650	625	1100	740
Oysters	med.—2 selects	25	110	390	400	650	670	350	350	530	360
Perch—White	3.5 oz.	100	225	750	840	1290	1630	640	680	1250	780
Red Snapper	3.5 oz.	100	200	850	1010	1490	1740	730	0	1050	570
Salmon (Atlantic)	3.5 oz.	100	225	970	1125	1690	1960	832	700	1200	815
Salmon (Atlantic can)	1 can 6.5 oz.	185	200	875	1025	1500	1800	750	550	1100	785
Sardines (Pacific)	3.5 oz.	100	190	820	960	1430	1660	700	510	1010	750

Food   Weight of Normal Portion   *Nutritive Values of Foods (Values per 100 gm)*
Essential Amino Acids (Mg)

CATEGORY & SUBSTANCE	NORMAL PORTION	AMT. GRAMS	TRYPTOPHAN	THREONINE	ISOLEUCINE	LEUCINE	LYSINE	PHENYLALAN	TYROSINE	VALINE	METHIONINE/CYSTEINE
Sardines (Atlantic can)	3.5 oz.	100	240	1040	1220	1820	2110	890	650	1280	898
Scallops—Raw	1 large	25	190	680	680	1120	1160	600	600	910	673
Shark	3.5 oz.	100	220	820	1390	1710	1930	830	740	1100	570
Shrimp—Raw	3.5 oz.	100	200	800	820	1530	1390	740	640	840	920
Sole	3.5 oz.	100	220	800	800	1350	1650	650	625	900	550
Squid	3.5 oz.	100	347	1368	2096	2900	3280	1500	1500	2665	4293
Swordfish	3.5 oz.	100	220	770	840	1300	1610	630	700	1260	676
Tuna (canned)	0.5 cup	115	320	1100	1200	1850	2300	900	1000	1800	985
MEAT & POULTRY											
Beef—Loin/Sirloin	3.5 oz.	100	260	970	1150	1800	1920	900	750	1220	800
Beef—Round	3.5 oz.	100	260	970	1150	1800	1930	910	750	1220	810
Calves Liver	3.5 oz.	100	300	900	1000	1750	1450	950	700	1200	700
Chicken (dark meat)	3.5 oz.	100	235	850	1060	1500	1700	800	680	1000	1815
Chicken (light meat)	3.5 oz.	100	285	992	1235	1740	2055	920	780	1150	940
Ham (canned)	3.5 oz.	100	200	700	910	1325	1477	710	640	930	740
Hamburger	3.5 oz.	100	242	914	1083	1700	1810	860	710	1150	775
Lamb (choice)	3.5 oz.	100	200	750	800	1200	1275	625	500	800	610

Food	Measure										
Lamb—Loin	3.5 oz.	100	220	780	890	1320	1380	700	600	840	740
Pork (thin)	3.5 oz.	100	250	900	1000	1435	1600	790	700	1014	710
Rabbit (domestic)	3.5 oz.	100	0	1020	1080	1640	1820	790	0	1020	540
Turkey (light meat)	3.5 oz.	100	270	1040	1220	1870	2210	930	930	1240	1020
Turkey (dark meat)	3.5 oz.	100	250	890	1040	1600	1890	800	790	1070	866
Veal	3.5 oz.	100	250	850	1030	1400	1600	800	700	1000	685
Veal—Loin	3.5 oz.	100	260	850	1040	1440	1645	790	720	1020	685
FRUIT											
Apples	1 med. 2.75 in. diam.	150	2	7	8	12	12	5	4	9	5
Applesauce— Unsweetened	½ cup	100	2	6	6	10	10	5	3	8	4
Apricots	1 med.	40	15	47	44	77	97	52	29	47	9
Avocado	1 cup	150	22	70	75	131	100	72	52	103	61
Banana	1 med.	150	12	34	33	71	48	38	24	47	28
Blueberries	1 cup	140	3	18	21	40	12	24	8	28	18
Cantaloupe	0.5 med.	400	6	1	25	34	20	30	20	28	12
Cranberries	1 cup	100	0	0	0	0	0	0	0	0	0
Dates—Nat'l & Dried	5 w/o pits	40	50	52	47	88	60	56	30	66	67
Figs—Raw	2 large/3 small	100	6	25	23	33	30	18	32	28	18
Grapefruit	sections 1 cup	190	2	0	0	0	18	0	0	0	2
Grapes	1 cup	150	3	17	5	13	14	13	11	17	31

Food　　　　Weight of Normal Portion　　　　Nutritive Values of Foods (Values per 100 gm)
Essential Amino Acids (Mg)

CATEGORY & SUBSTANCE	NORMAL PORTION	AMT. GRAMS	TRYPTO-PHAN	THREONINE	ISOLEUCINE	LEUCINE	LYSINE	PHENY-LALAN	TYROSINE	VALINE	METHIONINE / CYSTEINE
Lemon (peeled)	1 med.	100	0	0	0	0	0	0	0	0	0
Lime	1 med.	100	3	0	0	0	14	0	0	0	2
Nectarine	2 med.	100	0	0	0	0	0	0	0	0	0
Orange	1 med.	180	9	15	25	23	47	31	16	40	30
Papaya	⅓ med.	100	8	11	8	16	25	9	5	10	2
Peaches	1 med.	100	2	27	20	40	23	22	18	38	23
Pears	1 small	75	6	10	11	20	14	10	3	14	9
Persimmon—Native	1 med.	100	14	41	35	58	45	36	23	42	25
Pineapple	1 cup diced	140	5	12	13	19	25	12	12	16	13
Plums	2 med.	100	0	16	16	21	17	17	6	19	10
Raisins	2 T.	18	0	0	0	0	0	0	0	0	0
Raspberries—Red	¾ cup	100	0	0	0	0	0	0	0	0	0
Strawberries	1 cup whole	150	7	19	14	31	25	18	21	18	6
Watermelon	1 cup diced	160	7	27	19	18	62	15	12	16	8
Orange Juice	1 cup	248	2	8	8	13	9	9	4	11	8
CEREAL											
Buckwheat	1 cup	100	146	420	400	690	450	450	280	780	430

Grape Nuts	1 cup	224	210	370	480	830	860	590	360	590	306
Cereals—Rolled Oats	1 cup	80	175	460	500	1000	500	700	450	700	520
Cereals—Rye	1 cup	80	137	400	400	700	400	500	225	560	400
Shredded Wheat	1 biscuit	25	210	370	430	760	340	530	320	540	284
Wheat Flakes	1 cup	30	115	330	470	840	340	450	290	540	318
Whole Wheat Hot	1 cup	125	130	303	457	706	289	457	457	488	392
GRAIN											
Grains—Barley	¼ cup	50	103	279	343	570	280	429	247	411	323
Bulgur Wheat	½ cup	100	127	340	390	750	300	480	350	450	392
Corn Meal	¼ cup	30	60	370	430	1190	270	420	560	470	170
Gluten Flour	1 cup	140	440	1100	1900	3100	790	2250	1340	1960	1612
Millet	¼ cup	25	220	400	560	1540	340	450	900	600	480
Popcorn (plain—popd)	3 cups	42	80	510	590	1670	370	580	0	660	400
Rice (brown—raw)	short grain—¼ cup	50	34	300	300	650	300	400	275	400	250
Rye Flour	1 cup—sifted	88	110	350	400	630	380	440	300	490	310
Wheat Bran	1 T.	6	256	500	650	900	600	550	425	680	560
Wheat Flour (enr)	½ cup sifted	55	130	305	485	810	240	580	360	450	320
Wheat Flour (wh)	½ cub sifted	55	160	380	580	890	370	660	500	620	460
Wheat Germ	1 T.	6	260	1430	1270	1700	1600	1000	800	1460	740
Wild Rice	¼ cup	40	240	550	633	1140	660	400	400	930	390

Food   Weight of Normal Portion   Nutritive Values of Foods (Values per 100 gm)
Essential Amino Acids (Mg)

CATEGORY & SUBSTANCE	NORMAL PORTION	AMT. GRAMS	TRYPTO-PHAN	THREONINE	ISOLEUCINE	LEUCINE	LYSINE	PHENY-LALAN	TYROSINE	VALINE	METHIO-NINE/CYSTEINE
DAIRY											
Butter Milk	1 cup	244	35	160	200	330	280	175	140	250	110
Lowfat Milk (2%)	1 cup	244	47	150	200	320	260	160	160	220	120
Skim Milk	1 cup	244	50	150	200	330	270	165	165	230	120
Whole Milk	1 cup	244	45	150	200	300	250	160	160	220	115
Yogurt (low fat)	1 cup	244	30	210	300	500	475	300	275	400	150
CHEESE											
Cheese—American	1 slice 2.25 × 2.25 × .25	25	325	700	1025	2000	2100	1100	1200	1300	715
Cheese—Cheddar	1 inch cubed	30	320	900	1550	2400	2100	1300	1200	1700	780
Cheese (cottage)—Dry Curd	1 cup	200	190	770	1015	1770	1400	930	920	1070	680
Cheese—Cottage (1% fat)	¼ cup	60	140	550	700	1300	1000	670	660	770	490
Cheese (feta)	1 inch cube	17	0	0	0	0	0	0	0	0	0
Cheese—Monterey Jack	1 inch cube	30	300	875	1500	2350	2036	1300	1200	1600	765
Mozzarella (part skim)	1 inch cube	30	310	900	1200	2400	2500	1300	1400	1500	820
Ricotta (part skim)	½ cup	124	145	520	600	1240	1350	560	600	700	385

Food	Measure	g									
Cheese—Swiss	1 inch cube	30	400	1000	1500	3000	2600	1700	1700	2100	1025
BREAD											
Pumpernickel	1 slice	32	100	330	390	610	370	425	350	470	390
Bread—Rye—Amer	1 slice	25	100	400	400	600	290	500	225	475	360
Bread—Wheat	1 slice	25	130	310	475	720	325	550	380	490	385
EGGS											
Eggs—White	1 med.	15	155	450	620	880	625	650	400	760	650
Eggs—Whole	1 whole med. refuse 12%	50	195	600	760	1070	820	700	500	875	680
Eggs—Yolk	1 med.	29	240	890	940	1400	1110	700	700	1000	600
NUTS & SEEDS											
Almonds	1 T.	8	175	500	700	1300	450	1000	600	1100	635
Cashew	14 large	28	375	650	1100	1400	730	870	650	1460	690
Chestnuts (fresh)	2 lrge or 3 smll	15	40	100	110	170	180	60	60	150	30
Peanuts (roasted)	1 T. chpd or 15 whl	9	340	800	1300	1900	1100	1600	1100	1500	625
Pecans	10 large	9	140	390	550	770	440	560	320	530	300
Pumpkin Seeds	⅛ cup	17	530	880	1630	2290	1330	1640	0	1580	780
Sunflower Seeds	⅛ cup	18	360	940	1320	1820	910	1270	380	1410	950
OILS											
Butter—Salted	1 T.	14	12	40	50	80	70	40	40	60	30
Corn Oil	1 T.	14	0	0	0	0	0	0	0	0	0
Olive Oil	1 T.	14	0	0	0	0	0	0	0	0	0

Food   Weight of Normal Portion   Nutritive Values of Foods (Values per 100 gm)
Essential Amino Acids (Mg)

CATEGORY & SUBSTANCE	NORMAL PORTION	AMT. GRAMS	TRYPTO-PHAN	THREONINE	ISOLEUCINE	LEUCINE	LYSINE	PHENY-LALAN	TYROSINE	VALINE	METHIO-NINE / CYSTEINE
Safflower Oil	1 T.	14	0	0	0	0	0	0	0	0	0
Sesame Oil	1 T.	14	0	0	0	0	0	0	0	0	0
Soy Oil	1 T.	14	0	0	0	0	0	0	0	0	0
MISCELLANEOUS											
Melba Toast	1 slice	4	190	440	700	1170	350	700	650	660	505
Yeast	1 oz.	28	700	2300	2400	3200	3300	1900	1900	2700	1380

Food Weight of Normal Portion Nutritive Values of Foods (Values per 100 gm)
Vitamins

CATEGORY & SUBSTANCE	NORMAL PORTION	AMT. GRAMS	A (I.U.)	C (MG)	D (I.U.)	E (I.U.)	K (MCG)	THIAMINE (MG)	RIBOFLAVIN (MG)	NIACIN (MG)	B-6 (MCG)	FOLACIN (MCG)	B-12 (MCG)	PANTOTHENIC (MG)	BIOTIN (MCG)
VEGETABLES															
Artichoke—Boiled	base & ends—leaves	100	150	8	0	0.28	0	0.07	0.04	0.700	0.100	0	0	0.300	4.100
Asparagus	4 large spears	100	900	33	0	3	60	0.18	0.20	1.500	0.150	64	0	0.600	1.700
Beets (greens)	cooked 1 cup	150	6100	30	0	2.20	0	0.10	0.22	0.400	0.100	110	0	0.250	2.700
Beets—Red Raw	1 cup diced	140	20	10	0	0.04	0	0.03	0.05	0.400	0.055	90	0	0.150	2
Broccoli	1 med. stalk	180	2500	110	0	0.69	200	0.10	0.23	0.900	0.200	70	0	1.200	0.500
Brussels sprouts	2 large	140	550	100	0	1.30	570	0.10	0.16	0.900	0.230	78	0	0.700	0.400
Cabbage	1 cup finely shredded	90	130	50	0	2.50	125	0.05	0.05	0.300	0.160	66	0	0.200	2.400
Cabbage—Chinese	cup 1 inch pcs.	75	150	25	0	0	0	0.05	0.04	0.600	0.780	83	0	0	0
Cabbage—Red	1 cup shredded	100	40	60	0	0.20	0	0.09	0.06	0.400	0.200	34	0	0.320	0.100
Carrots	1 carrot 7.5 × 1.125	80	11000	8	0	0.70	80	0.06	0.05	0.600	0.150	32	0	0.280	2.500
Cauliflower	1 cup whole flowerettes	100	60	80	0	0.04	300	0.11	0.10	0.700	0.210	55	0	1	17
Celeriac	¼ of 1 large	100	0	8	0	4	100	0.05	0.06	0.700	0.170	7	0	0	0
Celery	1 cup chopped	120	240	9	0	0.54	0	0	0.03	0.300	0.060	12	0	0.430	0.100
Chard	¼ lb.	115	6500	32	0	0	0	0.06	0.17	0.500	0	0.700	0	0.170	0
Corn	1 cob 5 × 1.75 (kernels)	140	400	12	0	0.73	2	0.15	0.12	1.700	0.160	33	0	0.540	6

Food — Weight of Normal Portion — Nutritive Values of Foods (Values per 100 gm)

Vitamins

CATEGORY & SUBSTANCE	NORMAL PORTION	AMT. GRAMS	A (I.U.)	C (MG)	D (I.U.)	E (I.U.)	K (MCG)	THIA-MINE (MG)	RIBO-FLAVIN (MG)	NIACIN (MG)	B-6 (MCG)	FOLACIN (MCG)	B-12 (MCG)	PANTO-THENIC (MG)	BIOTIN (MCG)
Cucumber	1 small 6.5 × 1.5	180	250	11	0	0.22	5	0.03	0.04	0.200	0.040	15	0	0.250	0.400
Eggplant	1 cup diced	200	10	5	0	0.04	0	0.05	0.05	0.600	0.080	30	0	0.220	0
Garlic	1 clove (1.3 × .5 × .3)	3	0	15	0	0.02	0	0.25	0.08	0.500	0	0	0	0	0
Kale	¼ lb.	115	8900	125	0	8	0	0	0.26	2.100	0.300	60	0	1	0.500
Leeks	3–4 (5 inches)	100	40	17	0	1.40	0	0.11	0.06	0.500	0.200	36	0	0.120	1.400
Lettuce—Iceberg	wedge .125 of head	90	330	6	0	0.80	129	0.06	0.06	0.300	0.055	37	0	0.200	3
Lettuce—Romaine	1 cup chopped	55	1900	18	0	0.50	103	0.05	0.08	0.400	0.055	179	0	0.200	0.700
Mushrooms	1 cup sliced or diced	70	0	3	78	0.10	17	0.10	0.46	4.200	0.130	23	0	2.200	16
Mushrooms—Shiitake	2 oz.	55	0	0	0	0	0	0.32	0.74	10 0	0	0	0	0	4
Onions	1 cup chopped	160	40	10	0	0.18	0	0.03	0.04	0.200	0.130	25	0	0.130	3.5
Parsley	1 T. chopped	4	8500	172	0	2.60	0	0.12	0.26	1.200	0.160	120	0	0.300	0.400
Peppers—Green	1 cup strips	100	420	128	0	1	0	0.08	0.08	0.500	0.260	19	0	0.230	0
Peppers (red—sweet)	1 large or 1 cup strips	100	4450	204	0	0	0	0.08	0.08	0.500	0	0	0	0.270	0
Potato—White	2.75 × 4.25	250	0	20	0	0.09	3	0.10	0.04	1.500	0.250	19	0	0.380	0.400
Potato—Sweet	5 × 2	180	8800	21	0	6.80	0	0.10	0.06	0.600	0.220	50	0	0.820	4.300
Radishes (red)	10 small (1 in. diam.)	100	10	26	0	0	0	0.03	0.03	0.300	0.075	24	0	0.180	0

Food	Measure														
Spinach	1 cup chopped	55	8100	51	0	2.80	89	0.10	0.20	0.600	0.280	193	0	0.300	7
Squash (summer)	1 cup—cubed	130	410	22	0	0.18	0	0.05	0.09	1	0.080	31	0	0.360	0
Squash (winter)	1 cup baked	205	3700	13	0	0	0	0.05	0.11	0.600	0.150	34	0	0.400	0
Tomato	2.5 inch diam.	100	900	23	0	0.51	630	0.06	0.04	0.700	0.100	39	0	0.330	4
Turnip Greens	¼ lb.	115	7600	139	0	3.30	650	0.20	0.40	0.800	0.260	95	0	0.380	0.400
Waterchestnut	4 chestnuts	25	0	4	0	0	0	0.14	0.20	1	0	0	0	0	0
Yams	¼ lb.	115	0	9	0	0	0	0.10	0.04	0.500	0	50	0	0.390	0
LEGUMES															
Beans—Garbanzos	¼ cup	50	50	0	0	0	0	0.31	0.15	2	0.500	200	0	1.300	10
Beans—Green	1 cup	100	600	20	0	0.03	14	0.08	0.11	0.500	0.080	44	0	0.200	0.400
Beans—Lima	½ cup	100	0	0	0	0.66	0	0.48	0.17	1.900	0.600	110	0	1	9.800
Beans—Pinto	½ cup	100	0	0	0	0	0	0.84	0.21	2.200	0.531	26	0	0	0
Cowpeas	½ cup	70	30	6	0	0	0	1	0.20	2.200	0.560	70	0	1	21
Lentils—Brown	½ cup	100	60	0	0	1.90	0	0.37	0.22	2	0.600	36	0	1.400	0
Peas	1 cup	140	640	27	0	0.22	0	0.35	0.14	3	0.160	50	0	0.750	9
Soybeans (mature)	¼ cup	50	80	0	0	23	190	1.10	0.30	2.200	0.800	170	0	1.700	60
Soybean Curd (tofu)	1 piece 2.5 × 1 2.75	120	0	0	0	0	0	0.06	0.03	0.100	0	0	0	0	0
Split Peas	½ cup	100	60	0	0	0	0	0.37	.22	2	0	0	0	0	0
SEAWEED															
Hijiki	¼ cup	8	0	0	0	0	0	0	0	0	0	45	80	0.630	0
Kombu	¼ cup	8	190	13	5400	0	0	0.07	0.26	2.100	10	45	45	0.630	0

Food   Weight of Normal Portion   Nutritive Values of Foods (Values per 100 gm)
                                                                    Vitamins

CATEGORY & SUBSTANCE	NORMAL PORTION	AMT. GRAMS	(I.U.) A	(MG) C	(I.U.) D	(I.U.) E	(MCG) K	(MG) THIA-MINE	(MG) RIBO-FLAVIN	(MG) NIACIN	(MCG) B-6	(MCG) FOLACIN	(MCG) B-12	(MG) PANTO-THENIC	(MCG) BIOTIN
Nori	¼ cup	8	6474	14	5400	0	0	0.28	1.20	5.500	70	45	80	0.630	0
Wakami	¼ cup	8	255	15	5400	0	0	0.11	0.14	10	0	45	80	0.630	0
FISH & SHELLFISH															
Bass—Black Sea	3.5 oz.	100	0	0	0	0	0	0.10	0.80	1.900	0	9	0	0	0
Bass—White Sea	3.5 oz.	100	0	0	0	0	0	0.10	0.03	2.100	0	9	0	0	0
Catfish	3.5 oz.	100	217	0	0	0	0	0.04	0.03	1.500	0.290	20	2.200	0.470	0
Clams	4 cherrystone	70	100	10	0	0	0	0.10	0.18	1.300	0.080	0	19.100	0.300	0
Cod	3.5 oz.	100	33	2	52	0.33	0	0.06	0.07	2.200	0.230	18	0.800	0.140	3
Crab (steamed)	3.5 oz.	100	220	2	0	0	0	0.16	0.08	2.800	0.300	15	10	0.600	0
Haddock	3.5 oz.	100	0	0	0	0.58	0	0.04	0.07	3	0.180	10	1.30	0.130	5
Halibut	3.5 oz.	100	440	0	44	1.27	0	0.07	0.07	8.300	0.430	15	1	0.280	8
Herring (Pacific)	1 herring	50	100	3	315	1.60	0	0.02	0.16	3.500	0.370	11	2	1	4.500
Lobster	1 cup cubed	145	0	0	0	2.20	0	0.10	0.05	1.500	0	17	0.500	1.500	5
Mackarel (Atlantic)	3.5 oz.	100	450	3	1100	2.26	0	0.15	0.33	8.200	0.500	9	9	0.240	13
Ocean Perch	3.5 oz.	100	40	0.80	3	1.86	0	0.10	0.08	1.900	0.230	9	1	0.360	0
Oysters	med.—2 selects	25	300	30	320	1.30	0	0.14	0.18	2.500	0.050	10	18	0.250	9

Food	Serving													
Perch—White	3.5 oz.	100	170	1	0	0	0	0.01	0.04	1.500	0	0	0	0	0
Red Snapper	3.5 oz.	100	0	0	0	0	0	0.17	0.02	3.500	0	0	0	0	0
Salmon (Atlantic)	3.5 oz.	100	310	9	154	2	0	0.18	0.08	7	0.700	26	4	1.300	0.900
Salmon (Atlantic can)	1 can 6.5 oz.	185	230	0	220	1.50	0	0.03	0.16	7.400	0.300	20	7	0.550	15
Sardines (Pacific)	3.5 oz.	100	110	3	1150	0	0	0.02	0.15	3.600	0.240	16	17	1	24
Sardines (Atlantic can)	3.5 oz.	100	220	0	0	2.50	0	0.03	0.20	5.400	0.180	16	10	0.850	5
Scallops—Raw	1 large	25	100	0	0	0	0	0.10	0.06	1.300	0	16	1.200	0.130	0
Shark	3.5 oz.	100	2417	0	0	0	0	0.02	0.03	6.600	0.250	11	0.900	0	0
Shrimp—Raw	3.5 oz.	100	0	1.90	150	6	0	0.02	0.03	3.200	0.100	11	0.900	0.280	1
Sole	3.5 oz.	100	0	0	0	0	0	0.05	0.05	1.7000	0	11	0.800	0.300	0
Squid	3.5 oz.	100	616	0	0	1.8	0	0.02	0.12	3.200	0.060	10	1	0	0
Swordfish	3.5 oz.	100	1600	0	0	0	0	0.05	0.05	8	0	8	1	0.190	0
Tuna (canned)	0.5 cup	115	90	0	250	0	0	0.04	0.10	13	0.430	15	2.200	0.300	3
MEAT & POULTRY															
Beef—Loin/Sirloin	3.5 oz.	100	10	0	0	0.20	0	0.09	0.19	5.200	0.230	7	1	0.500	0
Beef—Round	3.5 oz.	100	10	0	0	0	0	0.09	0.19	5.200	0.400	6	1.850	0.660	5
Calves Liver	3.5 oz.	100	22500	36	15	2	90	0.20	2.70	11	0.700	220	60	8	100
Chicken (dark meat)	3.5 oz.	100	70	3	0	0.40	0	0.08	0.20	6.200	0.330	10	0.360	1.200	10
Chicken (light meat)	3.5 oz.	100	28	1.20	0	0.43	0	0.07	0.09	11	0.540	4	0.380	0.800	11
Ham (canned)	3.5 oz.	100	0	0	0	1	15	0.50	0.20	4	0.400	8	0.600	0.680	5
Hamburger	3.5 oz.	100	20	0	0	0.90	7	0.09	0.18	5	0.400	7	1.800	0.600	0

Food Weight of Normal Portion Nutritive Values of Foods (Values per 100 gm)
Vitamins

CATEGORY & SUBSTANCE	NORMAL PORTION	AMT. GRAMS	(I.U.) A	(MG) C	(I.U.) D	(I.U.) E	(MCG) K	(MG) THIAMINE	(MG) RIBOFLAVIN	(MG) NIACIN	(MCG) B-6	(MCG) FOLACIN	(MCG) B-12	(MG) PANTOTHENIC	(MCG) BIOTIN
Lamb (choice)	3.5 oz.	100	0	0	0	0.90	0	0.15	0.20	5	0.280	4	2	0.550	6
Lamb—Loin	3.5 oz.	100	0	0	0	0	0	0.18	0.25	5.800	0.280	4	2.200	0.280	0
Pork (thin)	3.5 oz.	100	0	0	0	0.90	11	0.95	0.20	5.100	0.450	8	0.700	0.800	5
Rabbit (domestic)	3.5 oz.	100	0	0	0	0.60	0	0.08	0.06	12.800	0.440	0	0	.780	0
Turkey (light meat)	3.5 oz.	100	40	0	0	0.13	0	0.07	0.11	6	0.550	8	0.450	0.680	0
Turkey (dark meat)	3.5 oz.	100	140	0	0	0.95	0	0.09	0.22	3.300	0.360	11	0.400	1.200	0
Veal	3.5 oz.	100	0	0	152	0	0	0.14	0.25	6	0.340	5	1.600	0.900	2
Veal—Loin	3.5 oz.	100	0	0	0	0	0	0.14	0.26	6.600	0.0.340	5	1.750	0.900	0
FRUIT															
Apples	1 med. 2.75 in. diam.	150	52	6	0	0.90	0	0.02	0.01	0.077	0.048	2.800	0	0.061	0.900
Applesauce— Unsweetened	½ cup	100	30	1	0	0.20	2	0.01	0.03	0.200	0.026	0.600	0	0.100	0.300
Apricots	1 med.	40	2612	10	0	0.75	0	0.03	0.04	0.600	0.054	8.600	0	0.240	0
Avocado	1 cup	150	612	8	0	2	8	0.11	0.12	1.900	0.280	62	0	1	5.500
Banana	1 med.	150	81	9	0	0.40	2	0.05	0.10	0.500	0.580	19	9	0.260	4.400
Blueberries	1 cup	140	100	13	6.40	0	0	0.05	0.05	0.400	0.036	6.400	0	0.090	0
Cantaloupe	0.5 med.	400	3220	42	0	0.20	0	0.04	0.02	0.600	0.120	17	0	0.130	3

Food	Measure														
Cranberries	1 cup	100	46	14	0	0	0	0.03	0.02	0.100	0.065	1.700	0	0.220	0
Dates—Nat'l & Dried	5 w/o pits	40	50	3	0	0	0	0.09	0.10	2.200	0.190	12.600	0	0.780	0
Figs—Raw	2 large/3 small	100	142	2	0	0	0	0.06	0.05	0.400	0.110	6.700	0	0.300	0.300
Grapefruit	sections 1 cup	190	10	33	0	0.37	0	0.04	0.02	0.200	0.043	10	0	0.280	3
Grapes	1 cup	150	100	4	0	0	0	0.09	0.06	0.300	0.110	4	0	0.024	1.600
Lemon (peeled)	1 med.	100	30	53	0	1.20	0	0.04	0.02	0.100	0.080	10.600	0	0.190	0
Lime	1 med.	100	10	29	0	0	0	0.03	0.02	0.200	0	8.200	0	0.220	0
Nectarine	2 med.	100	736	5.40	0	0	0	0.02	0.04	1	0.025	13.700	0	0.160	0
Orange	1 med.	180	200	53	0	0.36	1	0.09	0.04	0.300	0.060	30	0	0.250	1.900
Papaya	⅓ med.	100	2010	62	0	0	0	0.03	0.03	0.400	0.019	0	0	0.220	0
Peaches	1 med.	100	535	7	0	0.90	8	0.02	0.04	1	0.018	3.400	0	0.170	1.700
Pears	1 small	75	20	4	0	0.80	0	0.02	0.04	0.100	0.018	7.300	0	0.070	0.100
Persimmon—Native	1 med.	100	0	66	0	0	0	0.02	0.03	0.200	0	0	0	0	0
Pineapple	1 cup diced	140	25	15	0	0.15	0	0.09	0.04	0.400	0.080	11	0	0.160	0
Plums	2 med.	100	320	9.50	0	0.70	0	0.04	0.10	0.500	0.080	2.200	0	0.180	0.100
Raisins	2 T.	18	8	3	0	1	6	0.16	0.09	0.800	0.250	3.300	0	0.045	4.500
Raspberries—Red	¾ cup	100	130	25	0	0.45	0	0.03	0.09	0.900	0.057	0	0	0.240	1.900
Strawberries	1 cup whole	150	27	57	0	0.18	13	0.02	0.07	0.200	0.054	17.700	0	0.340	4
Watermelon	1 cup diced	160	370	9.60	0	0	0	0.08	0.02	0.200	0.140	2.200	0	0.200	3.600
Orange Juice	1 cup	248	200	50	0	0.06	0	0.09	0.03	0.400	0.040	55	0	0.190	0.800

Food   *Weight of Normal Portion*   *Nutritive Values of Foods (Values per 100 gm)*

Vitamins

CATEGORY & SUBSTANCE	NORMAL PORTION	AMT. GRAMS	(I.U.) A	(MG) C	(I.U.) D	(I.U.) E	(MCG) K	(MG) THIA-MINE	(MG) RIBO-FLAVIN	(MG) NIACIN	(MCG) B-6	(MCG) FOLACIN	(MCG) B-12	(MG) PANTO-THENIC	(MCG) BIOTIN
CEREAL															
Buckwheat	1 cup	100	0	0	0	5.50	0	0.60	0.15	4.400	0.300	0	0	1.500	0
Grape Nuts	1 cup	224	4409	0	143	1.60	0	1.30	1.50	17.600	1.800	353	5.300	0.950	0
Cereals—Rolled Oats	1 cup	80	0	0	0	1.60	20	0.60	0.14	1	0.140	52	0	1.090	24
Cereals—Rye	1 cup	80	0	0	0	1.80	0	0.40	0.22	1.600	0.350	78	0	1	6
Shredded Wheat	1 biscuit	25	0	0	0	0.54	0	0.26	0.28	5.300	0.250	50	0	0.830	0
Wheat Flakes	1 cup	30	0	0	0	0.63	0	0.64	0.14	4.900	0.300	0	0	0.470	0
Whole Wheat Hot	1 cup	125	0	0	0	1.6	17	0.40	0.30	4.900	0.019	78	0	0.920	0
GRAIN															
Grains—Barley	¼ cup	50	0	0	0	0.85	0	0.12	0.05	3	0.220	20	0	0.500	31
Bulgur Wheat	½ cup	100	0	0	0	0,09	0	0.30	0.15	4	0.200	46	0	0.700	0
Corn Meal	¼ cup	30	510	0	0	0.22	0	0.38	0.11	2	0.250	24	0	0.580	6.600
Gluten Flour	1 cup	140	0	0	0	0	0	0.03	0.03	0.500	0	25	0	0	0
Millet	¼ cup	25	0	0	0	0.07	0	0.73	0.38	2.300	0.750	0	0	0	0
Popcorn (plain—popd)	3 cups	42	0	0	0	0	0	0.37	0.12	2.200	0.200	0	0	0	0

Food	Measure														
Rice (brown—raw)	short grain—¼ cup	50	0	0	0	2	0	0.34	0.05	5	0.550	16	0	.100	12
Rye Flour	1 cup—sifted	88	0	0	0	0.64	0	0.15	0.07	0.600	0.090	12	0	0.720	6
Wheat Bran	1 T.	6	0	0	0	2.20	80	0.70	0.35	20	0.800	260	0	3	14
Wheat Flour (enr)	½ cup sifted	55	0	0	0	0.04	0	0.44	0.26	3.500	0.060	21	0	0.470	1
Wheat Flour (wh)	½ cub sifted	55	0	0	0	0.37	4	0.55	0.12	4.300	0.340	54	0	1.100	9
Wheat Germ	1 T.	6	0	0	0	90	350	2	0.70	4	1.200	330	0	1.200	17
Wild Rice	¼ cup	40	0	0	0	0	0	0.45	0.63	6.200	0	0	0	1.020	0
DAIRY															
Butter Milk	1 cup	244	33	1	0	0.07	0	0.03	0.15	0.100	0.034	5	0.220	0.280	1.500
Lowfat Milk (2%)	1 cup	244	210	1	42	0	2	0.04	0.17	0.100	0.040	5	0.360	0.320	0
Skim Milk	1 cup	244	210	1	42	0.01	0	0.04	0.14	0.100	0.040	5	0.380	0.330	1.500
Whole Milk	1 cup	244	210	0.90	42	0.09	3	0.04	0.16	0.100	0.040	5	0.360	0.310	5
Yogurt (low fat)	1 cup	244	70	0.80	1.12	0.06	0	0.04	0.20	0.200	0.050	11	0.600	0.600	3.300
CHEESE															
Cheese—American	1 slice 2.25 × 2.25 ×.25	25	1200	0	12	1	35	0.03	0.35	0.100	0.070	8	0.700	0.500	0
Cheese—Cheddar	1 inch cubed	30	110	0	12	1	35	0.03	0.38	0.100	0.070	18	0.800	0.400	3.600
Cheese (cottage)—Dry Curd	1 cup	200	30	0	12	1	35	0.03	0.14	0.200	0.080	15	0.830	0.160	0
Cheese—Cottage (1% fat)	¼ cup	60	37	0	12	1	35	0.02	0.17	0.130	0.070	12	0.630	0.200	0
Cheese (feta)	1 inch cube	17	0	0	12	1	35	0	0	0	0	0	0	0	0

Food   Weight of Normal Portion   Nutritive Values of Foods (Values per 100 gm)
Vitamins

CATEGORY & SUBSTANCE	NORMAL PORTION	AMT. GRAMS	A (I.U.)	C (MG)	D (I.U.)	E (I.U.)	K (MCG)	THIAMINE (MG)	RIBOFLAVIN (MG)	NIACIN (MG)	B-6 (MCG)	FOLACIN (MCG)	B-12 (MCG)	PANTOTHENIC (MG)	BIOTIN (MCG)
Cheese—Monterey Jack	1 inch cube	30	950	0	12	1	35	0	0.40	0	0	0	0	0	0
Mozzarella (part skim)	1 inch cube	30	600	0	12	1	35	0.02	0.30	0.100	0.070	9	0.800	0.080	0
Ricotta (part skim)	½ cup	124	430	0	12	1	35	0.02	0.19	0.080	0.020	0	0.290	0	0
Cheese—Swiss	1 inch cube	30	800	0	12	1	35	0.02	0.37	-.090	0.080	6	1.700	0.400	0
BREAD															
Pumpernickel	1 slice	32	0	0	0	0	4	0.22	0.13	1.250	0.160	0	0	0.500	0
Bread—Rye—Amer	1 slice	25	0	0	0	0	4	0.18	0.07	1.400	0.100	23	0	0.450	0
Bread—Wheat	1 slice	25	0	0	0	0.15	4	0.30	0.10	2.800	0.180	58	0	0.800	2
EGGS															
Eggs—White	1 med.	15	0	0.30	0	0	0	1	0.29	0.100	0.003	16	0.070	0.240	7
Eggs—Whole	1 whole med. refuse 12%	50	520	0	56	1	11	0.09	0.30	0.062	0.120	65	1.500	1.700	23
Eggs—Yolk	1 med.	29	1839	0	100	3.10	0	0.25	0.44	0.070	0.300	152	3.800	4.400	52
NUTS & SEEDS															
Almonds	1 T.	8	0	0	0	36	0	0.24	0.90	3.500	0.100	100	0	0.500	18
Cashew	14 large	28	100	0	0	0.28	0	0.43	0.25	1.800	0	70	0	1.300	0
Chestnuts (fresh)	2 lrge or 3 smll	15	0	27	0	0.70	0	0.22	0.22	0.600	0.330	0	0	0.470	1.500

						C									
Peanuts (roasted)	1 T. chpd or 15 whl	9	0	0	0	10	0	0	0.13	17	0.300	100	0	2	35
Pecans	10 large	9	130	2	0	1.80	0	0.86	0.13	0.900	0.180	24	0	1.710	27
Pumpkin Seeds	⅛ cup	17	70	0	0	0	0	0.24	0.19	2.400	0.090	0	0	0	0
Sunflower Seeds	⅓ cup	18	50	0	0	74	0	2	0.23	5.400	1.300	234	0	1.400	0
OILS															
Butter—Salted	1 T.	14	3000	0.20	35	2.40	30	0.01	0.03	0.042	0.003	3	0	0.050	0
Corn Oil	1 T.	14	0	0	0	21	0	0	0	0	0	0	0	0	0
Olive Oil	1 T.	14	0	0	0	17.80	0	0	0	0	0	0	0	0	0
Olive Oil	1 T.	14	0	0	0	50	0	0	0	0	0	0	0	0	0
Sesame Oil	1 T.	14	0	0	0	1.40	0	0	0	0	0	0	0	0	0
Soy Oil	1 T.	14	0	0	0	16	0	0	0	0	0	0	0	0	0
MISCELLANEOUS															
Melba Toast	1 slice	4	0	0	0	0	0	0.16	0.16	0	0	0	0	0	0
Yeast	1 oz.	28	0	0	0	0	0	16	4	40	2.500	3900	0	12	110

Food   Weight of Normal Portion   Nutritive Values of Foods (Values per 100 gm)

Minerals

CATEGORY & SUBSTANCE	NORMAL PORTION	AMT. GRAMS	(MG) Ca	(MG) P	(MG) Mg	(MG) K	(MG) Na	(MG) Fe	(MG) Cu	(MG) Mn	(MG) Zn	(MG) Se	(MG) Cr
VEGETABLES													
Artichoke—boiled	base & ends—leaves	100	50	70	12	300	30	1.100	0.310	0.360	0.350	0	0
Asparagus	4 large spears	100	22	60	20	280	2	1	0.210	0.180	0.800	0	4
Beets (greens)	cooked 1 cup	150	120	40	106	570	130	3.300	0.090	0.900	0	0	4
Beets—Red Raw	1 cup diced	140	16	33	29.500	335	60	0.700	0.130	1.260	1.090	0	5
Broccoli	1 med. stalk	180	100	80	24	380	15	1.100	0.011	0.056	0.270	0	11
Brussels sprouts	2 large	140	36	80	30	390	14	1.500	0.011	0.110	0.370	18	10
Cabbage	1 cup finely shredded	90	50	30	13	230	20	0.560	0.060	0.060	0.140	2.300	8
Cabbage—Chinese	cup 1 inch pcs.	75	43	40	14	253	23	0.600	0	0	0.270	0	5
Cabbage—Red	1 cup shredded	100	40	35	13	270	25	0.800	0.090	0	0.460	0	5
Carrots	1 carrot 7.5 × 1.125	80	37	36	23	340	47	0.510	0.011	0.020	0.120	2.200	5
Cauliflower	1 cup whl flowerettes	100	25	56	24	300	13	0.580	0.011	0.160	0.460	0.700	3
Celeriac	¼ of 1 large	100	43	115	0	300	100	0.600	0.020	0.150	0.310	10	4
Celery	1 cup chopped	120	40	28	22	340	130	0.480	0.010	0.020	0.070	0.600	8
Chard	¼ lb.	115	90	40	65	550	145	3.200	0.110	0.800	0	0	0
Corn	1 cob 5 × 1.75 (kernels)	140	3	110	50	280	0.300	0.700	0.011	0.020	0.400	0.400	9
Cucumber	1 small 6.5 × 1.5	180	25	27	11	160	6	1.100	0.010	0.060	0.100	0	1

Food	Serving												
Eggplant	1 cup diced	200	12	26	16	200	2	0.700	0.090	0.190	0.280	0	2
Garlic	1 clove (1.3 × .5 × .3)	3	30	200	27	530	19	1.500	0.170	0.330	1.330	27.600	4
Kale	¼ lb	115	180	70	37	380	75	2.200	0.090	0.550	0	2.300	4
Leeks	3-4 (5 inches)	100	50	50	23	350	5	1.100	0.100	0	0.100	0	8
Lettuce—Iceberg	wedge .125 of head	90	20	22	11	175	9	0.500	0.037	0.070	0.250	0.800	4
Lettuce—Romaine	1 cup chopped	55	68	26	11	264	9	1.100	0.040	0.310	0.360	0	7
Mushrooms	1 cup sliced or diced	70	6	120	13	400	15	1.700	0.260	0.030	1.100	13	14
Mushrooms—Shiitake	2 oz.	55	16	240	0	2590	100	3.900	0	0	0	0	14
Onions	1 cup chopped	160	27	36	12	160	10	0.500	0.100	0.080	0.110	1.500	11
Parsley	1 T. chopped	4	200	60	40	700	45	6.200	0.520	0.940	0.900	0	4
Peppers—Green	1 cup strips	100	9	22	18	210	13	0.700	0.070	0.150	0.100	0.600	10
Pepper (red—sweet)	1 large or 1 cup strips	100	13	30	9.460	213	0	0.600	0.040	0.150	0.210	0	10
Potato—White	2.75 × 4.25	250	7	50	35	400	3	0.760	0.050	0.040	0.200	0.500	21
Potato—Sweet	5 × 2	180	30	50	30	240	10	0.700	0.060	0.620	0.160	0.700	20
Radishes (red)	10 small (1 in. diam)	100	30	30	15	320	18	0	0.130	0.040	0.180	4	3
Spinach	1 cup chopped	55	90	50	90	470	70	3	0.080	0.600	0.400	18	10
Squash (summer)	1 cup—cubed	130	28	29	16	200	1	0.400	0.140	0.100	0.300	0	1
Squash (winter)	1 cup baked	205	22	38	17	370	1	0.600	0.100	0.220	0.440	0	3
Tomato	2.5 inch diam.	100	13	27	14	240	3	0.500	0.010	0.020	0.046	0.500	9
Turnip Greens	¼ lb.	115	250	60	60	470	71	1.800	0.090	1.420	0	0	5
Waterchestnut	4 chstnts	25	4	65	0	500	20	0.600	0	0	0	0	4

Food | Weight of Normal Portion | Nutritive Values of Foods (Values per 100 gm) Minerals

CATEGORY & SUBSTANCE	NORMAL PORTION	AMT. GRAMS	(MG) Ca	(MG) P	(MG) Mg	(MG) K	(MG) Na	(MG) Fe	(MG) Cu	(MG) Mn	(MG) Zn	(MG) Se	(MG) Cr
Yams	¼ lb.	115	20	70	40	600	10	0.600	0.160	0	0.400	0	20
LEGUMES													
Beans—Garbanzos	¼ cup	50	150	330	144	800	26	7	0.740	1.220	2.700	0	10
Beans—Green	1 cup	100	56	44	30	240	7	0.800	0.040	0.270	0.300	0.600	4
Beans—Lima	½ cup	100	72	385	180	1530	4	7.800	0.180	0.540	2.800	0	10
Beans—Pinto	½ cup	100	135	457	0	984	10	6.400	0	0	4.400	0	17
Cowpeas	½ cup	70	75	430	230	1000	35	5.800	0	0	2.800	0	10
Lentils—Brown	½ cup	100	80	377	80	790	30	6.800	0.660	0	3.100	11	1
Peas	1 cup	140	26	120	35	300	2	2	0.130	0.110	1.300	0.300	4
Soybeans (mature)	¼ cup	50	230	550	265	1700	5	8	0.110	2.800	3.600	60	10
Soybean Curd(tofu)	1 piece 2.5 x 1 x 2.75	120	130	130	110	40	7	2	0	0	0	0	0
Split Peas	½ cup	100	0	260	80	670	36	7.600	0.580	0	3.100	0	18
SEAWEED													
Hijiki	¼ cup	8	0	0	0	0	0	60	0	0	0	0	0
Kombu	¼ cup	8	950	360	1670	10600	2500	7	0	0	0	3.500	0
Nori	¼ cup	8	350	510	2040	3300	1290	74	0	4	0	1.300	0
Wakami	¼ cup	8	1162	195	3050	4200	2500	43	0	0	0	5.900	0

FISH AND SHELLFISH

Bass—Black Sea	3.5 oz.	100	20	207	0	255	70	1	0	0	0.700	0	0
Bass—White Sea	3.5 oz.	100	20	212	0	256	68	1	0	0	0.700	0	0
Catfish	3.5 oz.	100	37	187	19.060	330	60	0.400	0.100	0.060	0.700	0	0
Clams	4 cherrystone	70	70	160	0	180	120	6	0	0	1.500	0	40
Cod	3.5 oz.	100	10	200	28	400	70	0.400	0.230	0.010	14.600	43	7
Crab (steamed)	3.5 oz.	100	43	175	34	180	210	0.800	0.270	0.020	3.600	0	0
Haddock	3.5 oz.	100	25	200	24	300	60	0.700	0.011	0.020	0.320	20	5
Halibut	3.5 oz.	100	13	211	23	449	54	0.700	0.230	0.010	0.700	0	1
Herring (Pacific)	½ herring	50	45	225	0	420	74	1.300	0	0	0.700	143	0
Lobster	1 cup cubed	145	29	200	22	180	210	0.600	0.730	0.040	1.800	63	2
Mackerel (Atlantic)	3.5 oz.	100	5	230	28	420	100	1	0.160	0.020	0.500	120	4
Ocean Perch	3.5 oz.	100	20	200	32	270	80	1	0	0	0.700	196	0
Oysters	med—2 selects	25	90	140	32	120	70	5.500	3.070	0.210	40	65	13
Perch—White	3.5 oz.	100	50	192	0	286	50	0.900	0	0	0.700	0	0
Red Snapper	3.5 oz.	100	16	214	28	323	67	0.800	0	0	0.700	0	0
Salmon (Atlantic)	3.5 oz.	100	80	190	29	420	74	0.900	0.200	0	0.930	0	1
Salmon (Atlantic can)	1 can 6.5 oz.	185	154	300	30	400	74	0.900	0.080	0.020	1.100	0	0
Sardines (Pacific)	3.5 oz.	100	33	215	24	420	74	1.800	0.170	0	2.300	85	20
Sardines (Atlantic can)	3.5 oz.	100	437	500	52	590	823	2.900	0.040	0	3	0	20
Scallops—Raw	1 large	25	26	210	38	396	255	1.800	0	0	0.850	0	11

Food   Weight of Normal Portion   Nutritive Values of Foods (Values per 100 gm)
Minerals

CATEGORY & SUBSTANCE	NORMAL PORTION	AMT. GRAMS	(MG) Ca	(MG) P	(MG) Mg	(MG) K	(MG) Na	(MG) Fe	(MG) Cu	(MG) Mn	(MG) Zn	(MG) Se	(MG) Cr
Shark	3.5 oz.	100	14	204	27.300	549	79	1.100	0.030	0.020	0.310	0	0
Shrimp—Raw	3.5 oz.	100	60	170	50	220	140	1.600	0.240	0.030	1.500	60	12
Sole	3.5 oz.	100	12	200	73	340	80	0.800	0.010	0.020	0.300	0	16
Squid	3.5 oz.	100	12	120	20.460	223	158	0.500	1.670	0.050	1.560	0	0
Swordfish	3.5 oz.	100	19	200	0	449	54	0.900	0	0	0.700	0	0
Tuna (canned)	½ cup	115	16	200	23	280	40	1.600	0.010	0.020	0.400	130	5
MEAT AND POULTRY													
Beef—Loin/Sirloin	3.5 oz.	100	112	200	22	355	65	3.200	0.040	0.020	4.200	0	7
Beef—Round	3.5 oz.	100	13	220	16	355	65	3.20	0.050	0.020	3	36	44
Calves Liver	3.5 oz.	100	8	330	16	280	70	9	5	0.170	4	43	40
Chicken (dark meat)	1 w	12	160	23	220	85	1	0.063	0.021	2	12	13
Chicken (light meat)	3.5 oz.	100	12	187	27	240	68	0.730	0.040	0.020	0.970	11	12
Ham (canned)	3.5 oz.	100	11	160	19	340	1100	2.700	0.340	0.020	1.700	0	26
Hamburger	3.5 oz.	100	12	200	21	350	65	3	0.060;	0.020	3.400	20	6
Lamb (choice)	3.5 oz.	100	10	150	15	295	75	1.200	0.060	0.020	3	18	8
Lamb—Loin	3.5 oz.	100	6.800	185	16	300	75	1.300	0.045	0.020	2.400	0	9
Pork (thin)	3.5 oz.	100	11	226	22	285	70	2.900	0.011	0.020	1.400	24	10

Rabbit (domestic)	3.5 oz.	100	20	350	25	385	43	1.300	0.540	0	1.400	0	0
Turkey (light meat)	3.5 oz.	100	12	210	27	314	67	1	0.060	0.020	1.700	0	11
Turkey (dark meat)	3.5 oz.	100	17	185	21	290	80	1.600	0.140	0.020	3.400	0	11
Veal	3.5 oz.	100	11	200	15	320	90	3	0.050	0.020	3	0	7
Veal—Loin	3.5 oz;	100	11	200	16	320	90	0.670	0	0	2.160	0	7
FRUIT													
Apples	1 med 2.75 in. diam.	150	7	7	5	115	1	0.200	0.040	0.045	0.040	0.300	2
Applesauce—Unsweetened	1 cup	100	3	7	3	75	2	0.120	0.030	0.080	0.030	0.200	8
Apricots	1 med.	40	14	19	12	296	1	0.500	0.040	0.080	0.260	0	0
Avocado	1 cup	150	11	42	39	634	10	1.020	0.270	0.230	0.420	0	0
Banana	1 med.	150	6	20	29	400	1	0.300	0.100	0.150	0.160	1	9
Blueberries	1 cup	140	6	10	5	90	6	0.200	0.060	0.300	0.110	0	5
Cantaloupe	½ med.	400	11	17	11	310	9	0.200	0.042	0.047	0.160	0	2
Cranberries	1 cup	100	7	10	5	70	1	0.200	0.060	0.160	0.130	0	0
Dates—Nat'l & Dried	5 w/o pits	40	32	40	35	650	3	1.200	0.290	0.300	0.300	0	19
Figs—Raw	2 large/3 small	100	35	14	17	230	1	0.370	0.070	0.130	0.200	0	0
Grapefruit sections	1 cup	190	12	8	9	148	1	0.060	0.050	0.010	0.070	0	0.500
Grapes	1 cup	150	14	10	5	190	2	0.300	0.040	0.718	0.040	0	3
Lemon (peeled)	1 med.	100	26	16	28	140	2	0.600	0.040	0	0.060	12	1
Lime	1 med.	100	33	18	0	100	2	0.600	0.070	0	0.110	0	1

Food   Weight of Normal Portion   Nutritive Values of Foods (Values per 100 gm)

Minerals

CATEGORY & SUBSTANCE	NORMAL PORTION	AMT. GRAMS	(MG) Ca	(MG) P	(MG) Mg	(MG) K	(MG) Na	(MG) Fe	(MG) Cu	(MG) Mn	(MG) Zn	(MG) Se	(MG) Cr
Nectarine	2 med.	100	4	16	8	212	0	0.150	0.070	0.044	0.090	0	0
Orange	1 med.	180	40	14	10	180	1	0.100	0.045	0.025	0.070	1.300	3
Papaya	173 med.	100	24	5	10	260	3	0.100	0.016	0.011	0.070	0	0
Peaches	1 med.	100	5	12	7	200	1	0.110	0.070	0.050	0.140	0.400	2
Pears	1 small	75	11	11	6	130	2	0.300	0.110	0.080	0.120	0.600	2
Persimmon—Native	1 med.	100	27	26	0.800	310	1	2.500	0	0	0	0	0
Pineapple	1 cup diced	140	7	7	14	110	1	0.400	0.110	1.700	0.080	0.600	0
Plums	2 med.	100	4	10	7	172	2	0.100	0.043	0.049	0.100	0	2
Raisins	2 T.	18	50	100	33	750	12	2.100	0.310	0.310	0.270	0	6
Raspberries—Red	¾ cup	100	22	12	18	150	0	0.900	0.074	1.010	0.460	0	0
Strawberries	1 cup whole	150	14	19	10	170	1	0.400	0.120	0.290	0.130	0	3
Watermelon	1 cup diced	160	8	9	11	116	2	0.200	0.032	0.037	0.070	0	2
Orange Juice	1 cup	248	11	17	11	200	1	0.200	0.044	0.014	0.050	0	12
CEREAL													
Buckwheat	1 cup	100	114	280	253	450	0	3.100	0.430	2.090	0.870	18	38
Grape Nuts	1 cup	224	38	250	67	334	695	4.300	0.330	0	2.200	0	0
Cereals—Rolled Oats	1 cup	80	50	400	140	350	2	4.500	0.343	3.630	3.400	0	9

Food	Measure												
Cereals—Rye	1 cup	80	40	375	115	470	1	3.700	0.420	0	2.800	0	4
Shredded Wheat	1 biscuit	25	38	353	132	360	10	4.200	0.660	2.390	3.300	0	0
Wheat Flakes	1 cup	30	40	310	111	0	1032	4.400	0.450	1.500	2.300	0	0
Whole Wheat Hot	1 cup	125	40	380	122	390	2	3.400	0.460	3.200	2.700	0	0
GRAIN													
Grains—Barley	¼ cup	50	16	200	37	160	3	2	0.370	1600	2	66	8
Bulgur Wheat	1 cup	100	30	350	0	230	4	3	0	0	0	0	8
Cornmeal	¼ cup	30	20	256	47	284	1	2.400	0.200	0.280	1.840	0	10
Gluten Flour	1 cup	140	40	140	0	60	2	0.400	0	0	1.650	0	8
Millet	¼ cup	25	20	311	162	430	1	6.800	0.850	1.900	1.800	0	8
Popcorn (plain—popd)	3 cups	42	11	281	0	256	3	2.700	0	0	3.900	0	0
Rice (brown—raw) short grain	¼ cup	50	30	220	90	210	91	1.800	0.360	1.700	1.800	39	8
Rye Flour	1 cup—sifted	88	22	185	92	156	1	1.100	0.420	1.940	2.800	0	9
Wheat Bran	6	120	1300	490	1100	9	9	10.800	1.170	9.110	9.800	0	29
Wheat Flour (enr)	½ cup sifted	55	16	87	27	95	2	2.900	0.130	0.400	0.700	19.200	5
Wheat Flour (wh)	½ cup sifted	55	41	372	113	370	3	3.300	0	0	2.400	63	11
Wheat Germ	1 T.	6	70	1100	340	800	3	5.600	0.950	9.300	14.300	111	14
Wild Rice	¼ cup	40	19	339	130	220	7	4.200	0	0	4.650	0	0

Food   Weight of Normal Portion   Nutritive Values of Foods (Values per 100 gm)

Minerals

CATEGORY & SUBSTANCE	NORMAL PORTION	AMT. GRAMS	(MG) Ca	(MG) P	(MG) Mg	(MG) K	(MG) Na	(MG) Fe	(MG) Cu	(MG) Mn	(MG) Zn	(MG) Se	(MG) Cr
DAIRY													
Butter Milk	1 cup	244	116	89	11	150	50	0.050	0.005	0.010	0.400	0	1
Low fat Milk (2%)	1 cup	244	120	95	14	150	50	0.050	0.010	0.003	0.400	0	0
Skim Milk	1 cup	244	120	100	11	166	52	0.040	0.005	0.010	0.400	4.800	1
Whole Milk	1 cup	244	120	90	13	150	50	0.050	0.005	0.010	0.400	1.200	1
Yogurt (low fat)	1 cup	244	180	140	17	230	70	0.080	0.009	0.002	0.900	0	0
CHEESE													
Cheese—American	1 slice 2.25 × 2.25 × .25	25	600	750	22	160	11400	0.400	0.110	0.400	3	9	56
Cheese—Cheddar	1 inch cubed	30	720	500	28	100	620	0.700	0.050	0.110	3	0	29
Cheese (cottage)—Dry Curd	1 cup	200	32	100	4	32	13	0.230	0	0	0.470	0	3
Cheese—Cottage (1 % fat)	¼ cup	60	60	130	5	90	400	0.140	0.020	0	0.400	5.400	0
Cheese (feta)	1 inch cube	17	490	340	19	60	1115	0.650	0	0	2.900	0	36
Cheese—Monterey Jack	1 inch cube	30	750	440	27	80	500	0.700	0	0	3	0	36
Mozzarella(part skim)	1 inch cube	30	650	460	23	84	470	0.200	0	0	3	0	36
Ricotta (part skim)	2 cup	124	270	180	15	125	125	0.440	0	0	1.300	0	0

Cheese—Swiss	1 inch cube	30	960	600	36	110	260	0.170	0.110	0.040	4	11	36
BREAD													
Pumpernickel	1 slice	32	84	230	72	450	570	2.500	0	0	1.100	0	7
Bread—Rye—Amer	1 slice	25	75	150	40	145	560	2.700	0.017	0.500	1.600	0	7
Bread—Wheat	1 slice	25	80	250	80	260	530	3.200	0.170	1.200	1.800	70	8
EGGS													
Eggs—White	1 med.	15	11	11	9	140	150	0.030	0.050	0.010	0.020	5	8
Eggs—Whole	1 whl med. refuse 12%	50	55	200	12	130	140	2.100	0.050	0.020	1.400	10,400	22
Eggs—Yolk	1 med.	29	152	500	16	90	50	6	0.010	0.020	3.400	18	30
NUTS & SEEDS													
Almonds	1 T.	8	230	500	270	775	4	5	1.240	1.900	3.570	2	0
Cashew	14 large	28	40	375	270	460	15	6.400	2.170	0.840	5.120	0	0
Chestnuts (fresh)	2 lrge 3 smll	15	30	90	33	454	6	1.700	0.060	3.670	0	0	0
Peanuts (roasted)	1 T. chpd or 15 whl	9	70	400	175	700	5	2.200	0.400	1.500	3	0	0
Pecans	10 large	9	70	290	110	600	0	2.600	1.100	1.500	4.100	3	0
Pumpkin Seeds	1/8 cup	17	50	1140	0	0	0	10	0	0	0	0	7
Sunflower Seeds	1/8 cup	18	120	800	40	920	30	4.500	5	0.400	11	71	7
OILS													
Butter—Salted	1 T.	14	24	23	2	26	800	0.160	0.030	0.040	0.050	146	17
Corn Oil	1 T.	14	0	0	0	0	0	0	0	0	0.200	0	47
Olive Oil	1 T.	14	0.180	1.200	0.010	0	0.040	0.400	0.070	0	0.060	0	0

	Amount												
Safflower Oil	1 T.	14	0	0	0	0	0	0	0	0	0	0.200	7
Sesame Oil	1 T.	14	0	0	0	0	0	0	0	0	0	0	0
Soy Oil	1 T.	14	0.040	0.250	0.030	0.250	0	0.020	0	0	0	0.200	0
MISCELLANEOUS													
Melba Toast	1 slice	4	84	100	0	225	75	0	1.600	0	0	0	0
Yeast	11 oz.	28	210	1750	230	1900	120	17	5.300	0.400	11	71	1

READINGS AND RESOURCES

Dr. Walford's Interactive Diet Planner

Popularly known as DWIDiP, this software package is the companion to this book. Using the latest U.S. Department of Agriculture database of over 6,000 foods, including whole, name-brand, processed, and fast foods, it is designed to allow you to put together optimal daily or weekly food combinations to achieve highest quality and full RDA values at lowest calorie intake. The unique powerhouse of DWIDiP, not found in any other nutrition software, is the Search feature, which works like this: suppose you are on a 1,600-calorie diet and today's food list comes to 1,200 calories, 25 percent derived from fat, and DWIDiP tells you the RDAs for selenium, vitamin B6, and calcium have not been reached. What single food or two foods can you add, 400 calories of which will make up the difference, and also be low in fat? DWIDiP will tell you this, or any other combination of desires, and no other program will. You can *maximize*, *minimize*, or *optimize* one or many items, and at the same time. Twenty-eight nutrients are covered in the program. The References section lists additional, newly researched nutrients like lycopene, isoflavones, and omega-3 fatty acids, not yet in the USDA database, and foods that contain them, and gives mail order sources for foods hard to find in ordinary markets. A Glossary introduces you to new foods along with simple cooking instructions. A Tutorial and Help program guide you through the interactive capabilities of DWIDiP. Up to 99 users may each have a personal profile based on height, age, frame-size, and desired percentage of fat. A Recipe feature (over 70 nutrient-dense recipes are included, and you can add to or modify these) and Shopping List complete the computer-to-store-to-stove practical application of cooking with a personal computer. Available from the Longbrook Company, Suite 1215, 1015 Gayley Avenue, Los Angeles, CA 90095, at $71.00 postage paid. It can also be ordered online at www.walford.com. Longbrook provides phone and email technical support, as well as updates and upgrades when appropriate. System requirements include: 386 or higher IBM PC or compatible, 4 MB RAM minimum, 8 recommended, 5 MB hard drive space, a VGA monitor, and Microsoft Windows 3.1, 95, 98, or NT. Please specify your operating system when ordering or making inquiries. To view sample screens from DWIDiP or to download a demonstration version, visit the www.walford.com/software.

BOOKS

Maximum Life Span by Roy L. Walford, M.D.

Originally published in 1983 by W.W. Norton (hardcover) and Avon Books (paperback), the book is now out of print but limited copies are available through the Longbrook Company (address above). This is a basic background book on the science of aging research: the colorful history of gerontology, the different theories of aging, the sociopolitical aspects of the long-living society when it is achieved, and anecdotal stories of the author's life as a gerontologist.

The Anti-Aging Plan by Roy L. Walford, M.D., and Lisa Walford
New York: Four Walls Eight Windows, 1996

Sequel to the first edition of *The 120-Year Diet*, this book focuses somewhat less on the scientific literature and more on the practical implementation of low-calorie nutrition, including cooking in bulk and freezing of "megameals." There are over 100 nutrient-dense, freezable recipes.

The Omega Diet by Artemis P. Simopoulos, M.D., and Jo Robinson
New York: Harper Perrenial, 1998

> The best popular book on the Mediterranean diet and the role of the omega-3 and omega-6 fatty acids in health and nutrition. Simopoulos has published fairly extensively in the scientific literature; Robinson is a professional writer.

The Glucose Revolution by J. Brand-Miller et al.
New York: Marlowe & Company, 1999

> Despite the title (The words *revolution* or *miracle* in titles of diet books are always dubious.), this is the best popular book dealing with the glycemic index. The book is well written, and the authors have good scientific credentials.

Fasting and Eating for Health by Joel Fuhrman, M.D.
New York: St. Martin's Griffin, 1995

> Although not updated on the fatty acids and glycemic index, the book is otherwise an excellent and well-referenced book for those interested in short– or relatively long-term fasting. And all diabetics should read Fuhrman's Chapter 7.

MAGAZINES

Nutrition Reviews (published by International Life Sciences Institute, 1126 Sixteenth St., N.W. Washington, D.C. 20035-4810)

> Superb, informative publication, slanted towards the nutritional scientific community but still understandable by an educated lay public, this journal contains concise, very well-balanced reviews of nutritional research at both laboratory and epidemiological levels. I find articles of interest in almost every issue.

Life Extension (published by the Life Extension Foundation, P. O. Box 229120, Hollywood, Florida 33022-9120)

Excellent up-to-date coverage, including good bibliographic referencing, of research in life extension, but overly weighted towards supplements, so that if you follow all their advice, your supplement intake will increase exponentially. So read this magazine, but temper it with the articles from *Nutrition Reviews* and you'll come out okay. I should add that the Life Extension Foundation is, so far as I know, the *only* mail-order or health-food-store supplement company that gives extensively to support university research into life extension, including both basic research and the unbiased testing of their own products (the 45-month-old-mouse test). They are truly interested in *aging*, whereas most such companies are in it for the money.

INTERNET INFORMATION SOURCES

http://infinitefaculty.org/crsociety: This is the prime informational site for the Internet Calorie Restriction Group. A *must* for CRON dieters, it is excellent to browse, but don't post unless you are very seriously into or contemplating a CRON dietary regime.

http://members.aol.com/johnfurber/aging.html: This is a good site for general information about aging, with links to other major instructive sites.

http://www.mendosa.com/gi.htm: This excellent site covers the glycemic index, with extensive listings of GIs of various foods, therefore a good companion to the book *The Glycemic Revolution*, which is listed above.

http://www.nih.gov/health/chip/nia/aging/: Maintained by the National Institute on Aging, and called "In Search of the Secrets of Aging," this site provides excellent, easily understood brief surveys of what's going on in aging research. It includes a section on caloric restriction.

INSTRUMENTATION

For scales for measuring weight, and percentage body fat by imped-ance:

www.bodytrends.com: A variety of Tanita scales are listed, which measure both weight and percent body fat.

For measuring percent body fat based on skin fold thicknesses:

www.bodytrends.com: A variety of skin calipers are listed. Both the Slim-Guide and the Fat Gun models are reasonably satisfactory and inexpensive

SPECIAL FOOD SOURCES

Apples:
Kilcherman's Christmas Cove Farm, 11573 N. Kilcherman Rd., North-port, MI 49670-9722. Telephone: 616-386-5637. Over 200 varieties of apples. Try their Antique Apple Gift Box to realize what agribusiness, which limits itself to six to eight varieties, is doing to biodiveristy.

Beans (legumes):
Zursun, 754 Canyon Park Ave., Twin Falls, ID 83301. Telephone: 800-424-8881. Many unusual heirloom varieties of dried beans, including the very low glycemic index Chana Dal bean (split baby garbonzos).

Garlic:
www.garlicgourmet.com
www.gourmetgarlicgardens.com: There are 20 varieties available from this source.

Grains, cereals, seaweeds:
Gold Mine Natural Food Co., 7805 Arjons Drive, San Diego, CA 92126-4368. Try their "forbidden black rice."

Meat:
www.goodheart.com: A good source of bison, ostrich, boar, and other types of low-fat meats.
www.sayersbrook.com: A good source of bison, emu, elk, and other types of low-fat meat.

Tea:

Upton Tea Imports, 231 South Street, Hopkinton, MA 01748. Phone orders: 800-234-8327. This is a source of a wide variety of green and black teas, at all prices and from many places around the world.

Vinegar (Balsamic) and olive oil of high quality:

www.debruno.com

www.deandeluca.com

Note that by Italian law the top grade balsamic vinegar must bear the stamp "traditional."

REFERENCES AND NOTES

PREFACE

1. Or in my essay, "Children of the Elderberry Bush," *Experimenal Gerontology* 33:189, 1998.

2. C. Canto and O. Faliu, *The History of the Future*. Paris: Flammarion Press, 1993.

CHAPTER 1

1. In the first edition of this book, called at that time *The 120-Year Diet*, I used the term *high/low diet*, to stand for high in quality, low in calories, but the term *CRON diet* has been popularized, largely by the Internet CR-society, and will be adopted in this second edition, as it now represents common use. *CR*, standing for "calorie restriction" has also been used, but could be met simply by eating less of a bad diet. CRON, or caloric restriction with optimal nutrition, seems better.

2. P. Starr, *The Social Transformation of American Medicine*. New York: Basic Books, 1982.

3. Ibid.

4. I am of course aware that very recent actuarial analyses of mortality rates at the extreme ends of life span show a flattening of the curve, even a downturn, which may mean that in fact there is no absolute species-specific maximum life span. For practical purposes at the present time, however, this is irrelevant. (Vaupel et al. , "Biodemographic Trajectories of Longevity," *Science* 280:855–860, 1998.)

5. T.S. Eliot, interview in the *New York Times*, September 21, 1958.

6. C.P. Snow, *The New Physicists*. Boston: Little, Brown, 1981.

7. R.L. Walford, in *Trends in U.S. Life Expectancy*, Hearing before Committee on Finance, U.S. Senate, 98th Congress, July 15, 1983. Washington, D.C.: Senate Hearing 98-359, 1983, p.116–31.

8. Population Reference Bureau, Inc., *Death and Taxes: The Public Policy of Living Longer*. Washington, D.C.: Population Reference Bureau, Inc., September 1984.

9. C. Finch, *Longevity, Senescence, and the Genome*. Chicago: University of Chicago Press, 1994.

10. My comments about *general* processes can be illustrated by reference to nongeneral, that is to say, narrower and more specific processes. These often cannot be translated between species. Humans, guinea pigs, apes, and monkeys, for example, do not manufacture vitamin C in their bodies. They have to get it in their diet. Other mammals, like rats, mice, dogs, and goats, synthesize vitamin C in their own bodies. It would obviously be hazardous to assume that a vitamin C experiment in rats had any direct applicability to humans.

11. Quoted by Claudia Wallis, "Hold the Eggs and Butter," *Time*, March 26, 1984, p. 61.

12. S.B. Eaton and M. Konner, *New England Journal of Medicine* 312:283, 1985.

13. Ibid.

14. D. Ornish, "Can Lifestyle Changes Reverse Coronary Atherosclerosis?" *Hospital Practice*, 15 May 1991, p. 109; D. Ornish et al., "Intensive Lifestyle Changes for Reversal of Coronary Heart Disease," *J. Am. Medical Association* 280:2001, 1998; D. Ornish et al., *Am. J. of Cardiology* 82:72T, 1998.

15. "Healing Broken Hearts," an interview with Dean Ornish, in *Nutrition Action*, June 1999, p. 3.

16. He gives quite a few tables—for example, Table 2.1 of *Enter the Zone*, and Tables 8.2 to 8.5 of *The Anti-Aging Zone*—showing data declared to be highly statistically significant, and indeed they are so, if the given p-values are correct. Well, if the data are in reality that good, they would surely allow for convincing papers in the regular medical literature. Sears knows this, and he also knows how to write such papers, judging from his publications in the '70s. That he has not taken this route—of presenting his diet work before knowledgeable peers—which would greatly strengthen his case, leaves me in the uncomfortable position of a disbeliever. Besides these unsatisfactorily documented tables, most of Sears' "evidence" is testimonial and anecdotal, which is the worst kind of evidence. He also knows this of course, but is in the irritating habit of making statements (for example, on pages 186 and 194 of *Enter the Zone*) that may be paraphrased as "I know testimonial evidence is highly questionable, but . . ." and then he proceeds to lay out testimonial evidence.

17. For an example of an excellent presentation of a theory (in contrast to Sears'), see D. Harman, *Journal of Anti-Aging Med.* 2:15, 1999.

18. B. Rolls et al., *American J. Clinical Nutrition* 69:862, 1999 (editorialized in *Science Daily*, May 24, 1999, as "energy density—not fat—is key to feeling full while managing weight").

19. R. L. Walford et al., *Toxicological Sciences* 52 (suppl.):61,1999.

20. R. L. Walford et al., *Receptor* 5:29–33, 1995.

21. Of course there are plenty of people not at all on a Zone diet who feel fine, are not groggy in the morning, etc. Sears wholly disregards this negative evidence.

CHAPTER 2

1. There are a number of conditions in which part of the body ages faster than the whole. Most of these are genetic in origin and are referred to both as *segmental aging* and as the *progeroid syndromes*. Examples would include progeria, a horrible malady you have probably seen photographs of, where children eight to ten years of age look like scrawny old persons, and Down's syndrome. More mundane examples include maturity-onset diabetes and some of the autoimmune diseases. None of these illnesses show all of the features of accelerated aging, and their lopsidedness illustrates that aging itself is probably multifactorial. The individual who has done the most to categorize these maladies is Dr. George Martin of the University of Seattle. (G.M. Martin. in *Genetic Effects on Aging*, eds. D. Bergsma and D.E. Harrison. Alan R. Liss, Inc., 1978, p. 5.

2. S. Whittingham, J. Irwin, and I. MacKay, *Austrailian J. Medicine* 18:30, 1969.

3. R. Weindruch and R.L. Walford, *The Retardation of Aging and Disease by Dietary Restriction*. Springfield, IL: Charles C. Thomas, 1988.

4. N.W. Shock et al., ed., *Normal Human Aging: The Baltimore Longitudinal Study of Aging*, NIH Publication No. 84-2450, November 1984, is of course a gold mine for the human biomarker area. Other useful books on human biomarkers are R.F. Morgan's *The Adult Growth Examination*. Fresno, CA: International Assn. Applied Psychology, 1986; and particularly W. Dean's *Biological Aging Measurement*. El Toro, CA: The Aging Research Inst., 1986.

5. J. W. Hollingsworth et al., *Yale J. Biol. Med.* 38:11, 1965.

6. R. A. Defronzo, in *Biological Markers of Aging*, ed. M. E. Reff and E. L. Schneider, NIH Publication No. 82-2221, 1982, p. 98.

7. M.A. Lane et al., *J. Clin. Endrocrinol. & Metab.* 82:2093–2096, 1997.

8. Whittingham et al., op.cit.

9. R. Weindruch et al., *Age* 5:111, 1982.

10. There are a number of tests of cognitive function many of which show age-related changes: for example, tests for performance speed and for short-term memory. I have not included these here as they require administration by a specialist in psychometric testing. If you are interested, see H. Liebermeister and K. Schroter, *Internat. J. Obesity* 7:45, 1983.

11. See note 3 above.

12. R. Weindruch, *Toxicol. Pathol.* 24:742–745, 1996; R. Weindruch, *Scientific American* 274:46–52. 1996; H.K. Ortmeyer et al., *J. Basic Clin. Physiol. Pharmacol.* 9:309–323, 1998.

13. R.L. Walford et al., *Proc. National Acad. Sci.* 89:11533–11537, 1992; R.L. Walford et al., *Toxicological Sci.* 52: 61–65, 1999; R. Verdery and R.L. Walford, *Arch. Internal Med.* 158:900–906, 1998; C. Weyer and R.L. Walford et al., *Am. J. Clinical Nutr.* (in press, 2000)

14. G. B. Leyton, *Lancet* 2:73–79, 1946; A. Keys et al., *The Biology of Human Starvation*. Minneapolis: University of Minnesota Press, 1950.

15. R.L. Walford et al., *Aviation, Space and Environmental Med.* 67:609–617, 1996.

16. I only promise you it will work, not that it's easy as pie.

CHAPTER 3

1. C. M. McCay, in *Cowdry's Problems of Aging, Biological and Medical Aspects,* ed. A. I. Lansing. Baltimore: Williams and Wilkins, 1952, p. 130.

2. B. J. Merry and A. M. Holehan, Thirteenth International Congress of Gerontology, New York, July 12–17, 1985.

3. In the 1940s two University of Chicago professors (Carlson and Hoelzel, 1946) introduced the technique of intermittent fasting. Beginning at 42 days of age, and using a high-quality diet, rats were fasted one day in four, one day in three, and every other day. Maximum life span was increased by 20 to 30 percent in all instances, and there was no stunting of growth on any of the regimens. A. H. Carlson and F. Hoelzel, *J. Nutrition* 31:363, 1946.

4. Genes that seem to regulate basic aging are now being found in insects (houseflies, fruit flies), and in particular in the vinegar worm, *C. elegans,* which no doubt have homologues in higher animals, including humans. It will be a long time before this work reaches the stage of direct human applicability, but eventually it will. Meantime, it points in the right direction. For information on the flies, see W. C. Orr and R. S. Sohol, *Science* 263:1128, 1994. For a good popular account of the situation in the vinegar worm, see S. English, *Life Extension* 4:24, February 1998.

5. R. Weindruch and R. L. Walford, *The Retardation of Aging and Disease by Dietary Restriction.* Springfield, IL: Charles C. Thomas, 1988.

6. E. U. Masoro, ed., *Handbook of Physiology,* Section 11: Aging. London: Oxford University Press, 1995.

7. R. Weindruch, *Scientific American* 274: 46, 1996.

8. With caloric restriction beginning at time of weaning, scientists at the University of Texas (Yu et al., 1982; Bertrand et al., 1980) extended average life spans in rats from 32 months out to 47 months. In similar experiments scientists at the National Institute on Aging extended average life spans in rats by more than 83 percent (Goodrick et al., 1982).

    B. P. Yu et al., *J. Gerontology* 37:130, 1982. H. A. Bertrand, *J. Gerontology* 35:827, 1980. C. L. Goodrick et al., *Gerontology* 28:233, 1982.

9. G. Fernandes et al., in *Immunology and Aging,* ed. T. Makinodan and E. J. Yunis. New York: Plenum Press, 1977, p. 111. C. Kubo, B. C. Johnson et al., *J. Nutrition* 114:1884, 1984. R. A. Good, Thirteenth Internat. Congress Gerontol., New York, July 12–17, 1985.

10. E. J. Masoro, *J. Nutrition* 115:842, 1985.

11. Goodrick et al., op. cit.

12. C. Kubo et al., *Proceedings Natl. Acad. Sci.,* USA 81:5831, 1984. C. Kubo, B.C. Johnson et al., op cit.

13. R. Weindruch and R. L. Walford, *Science* 215:1415, 1982.

14. M. H. Ross, *Am. J. Clin. Nutr.* 25:834, 1972.

15. D. E. Harrison et al., *Proceedings Natl. Acad. Sci., U.S.A.* 81:1835, 1984. C. L. Goodrick et al., *AGE* 6:145, 1983.

16. McCay, op. cit.

17. A. Tannenbaum, *Am. J. Cancer* 38:335, 1940.

18. C. H. Barrows, Jr., and G. C. Kokkone, in *Nutritional Approach to Aging Research*, ed. G. B. Moment. Boca Raton, FL: CRC Press, 1982, p. 219.

19. N. H. Sarkar et al., *Proceedings Natl. Acad. Sci., U.S.A.* 79:7758, 1982.

20. Yu, op. cit.

21. K. E. Cheney et al., *J. Gerontology* 38:420, 1983. M. H. Ross and G. J. Bras, *J. Nutrition* 103:944, 1973.

22. Sarkar, op. cit.

23. McCay, op. cit.

24. B. N. Berg and H. S. Simms in *Biological Aspects of Aging*, ed. N. Shock. New York: Columbia University Press, 1962, p. 35.

25. J. B. Young et al., *Metabolism* 27:1711, 1978.

26. A. V. Everitt, *Mechanisms of Ageing and Development* 12:161, 1980.

27. M. T. R. Subbiah and R. G. Siekert, Jr., *J. Nutrition* 41:1, 1979.

28. J. E. Johnson, Jr., and C. H. Barrows, Jr., *Anatomical Record* 196:145, 1980.

    A. V. Everitt, in *Nutritional Approach to Aging Research*, ed. G. B. Moment. Boca Raton, FL: CRC Press, 1982, p. 245. J. R. Wyndham et al., *Archives of Gerontology and Geriatrics* 2:317, 1983.

29. R. L. Walford, *The Immunologic Theory of Aging*. Copenhagen: Munksgaard 1969.

    R. L. Walford, *Maximum Life Span*. New York: W. W. Norton, 1983. S. R. S. Gottesman and R. L. Walford, in *Methods in Aging Research*, ed. R. C. Adelman and G. S. Roth. Boca Raton, FL: CRC Press, 1982, p. 233.

30. An idea that has received much play in gerontology is that of so-called *antagonistic pleiotropy*, which means systems that operate to your benefit in youth become perverted with age, react in ways actually harmful to the body, and in fact are causally related to aging. If you look for concrete examples of antagonistic pleiotropy, however, you will find it unarguably present only in the immune system.

31. Sufai-Kutti et al., *Clinical Immunology and Immunopathology* 15:293, 1980. R. Weinruch et al., *AGE* 5:111, 1982. G. Fernandes et al., *Proceedings Natl. Acad. Sci. U.S.A.* 80:874, 1983. J. A. Levy and W. J. W. Morrow, *Immunology Today* 4:249, 1983.

32. K. Nandy, *Mechanisms of Ageing and Development* 18:97, 1982.

33. Caloric restriction not only will slow the rate of immune system aging, but may even bring about some rejuvenation. One good test measures the response of white blood cells (lymphocytes) to certain plant extracts. At UCLA we have investigated the extracts known as PHA and Con-A. They stimulate lymphocytes to produce fresh DNA (the hereditary double helix material in each cell) and then to divide into two new cells. We have found that the lymphocytes of 16-month-old mice that had been on the CRON diet since 12 months of age respond to PHA and Con-A to the same degree as six- to eight-month-old fully fed mice (Weindruch et al., 1979). Evidently this rejuvenation does not involve all bodily systems, since the maximum life span of this lot of mice was extended by only 20 percent.

Nevertheless, the results—actual rejuvenation of at least one important age-deteriorating function—are highly encouraging. Rejuvenation of one system is even better than retardation, but I would not call it *reversing aging*. That term implies unlinking of cross links, for example, and repair of mitochondrial damage, etc. (R. Weindruch and R. L. Walford, *Federation Proceedings* 38:2007, 1979.)

34. D. N. Kalu et al., *Mechanisms of Ageing and Development* 26:103, 1984. D. N. Kalu et al., *Endocrinology* 115:1239, 1984.

35. Ibid.

36. P. J. Leveille et al., *Science* 224:1247, 1984.

37. S. Chipalkatti et al., *J. Nutrition* 113:944, 1983.

38. D. E. Harrison and J. R. Archer, *Experimental Aging Research* 9:245, 1984.

39. G. M. Reavan and E. P. Reaven, *Metabolism* 30:982, 1981.

40. R. J. McCarter et al., *Am. J. Physiol.* 242: R89, 1982.

41. E. J. Masoro. *J. Am. Geriatric Soc.* 32:296, 1984.

42. Ibid.

43. Two of these features deserve an illustration. We see in the left panel of the figure on the next page that the cholesterol level of a 24-month-old rat on a CRON diet is the same as that of a fully fed rat merely 12 months old; and in the right panel, the response of fat cells to the hormone glucagon falls to zero by 6 months of age in fully fed rats, but on a CRON diet the response is held at a very youthful level until 12 months, and then declines slowly.

44. J. A. Joseph et al., *Neurobiology of Aging* 4:191, 1983.

45. D. K. Ingram et al., *J. Gerontology* 42:78–81, 1987.

46. R. F. Mervis et al., *AGE* 7:144, 1984.

47. R. L. Walford, *Maximum Life Span*. New York: W. W. Norton, 1983.

48. C. L. Goodrick et al., *AGE* 7:1, 1984.

49. D. K. Ingram et al., op. cit.

50. J.W. Kemnitz et al., *Am. J. Physiology* 266 (Endocrinol. Metab. 29): E540, 1994.

51. B. C. Hansen et al., *Diabetes* 42:1809, 1993. N.L. Bodkin et al., *J. Gerontol.* 50A, 3:B142, 1995.

52. M.A. Lane et al., *Proc. Nat. Acad. Science* 93:4159, 1996. M.A. Lane et al., *Age* 20:45, 1997. R. Weindruch et al., *Aging* 4:304, 1997.

53. Merry and Holehan, op. cit.

54. J.F. Nelson et al., *Neurobiology of Aging* 16:837, 1995.

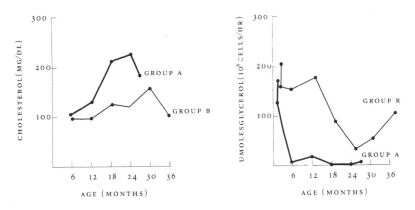

NOTE 43 FIGURE Effect of a CRON diet on blood cholesterol in rats, and on the response of fat cells to the hormone glucagon.

Left Panel, Cholesterol: The age-related rise that occurs in rats on a regular diet is much less in rats on the CRON diet.

Right Panel, Response to the hormone glucagon: In rats fed a regular diet the response falls rapidly after birth, and is negligible by six months; on the CRON diet even 12-month-old animals are responding like weanlings, and 18-month-old animals like three-month-old animals (adapted from E.J. Masoro, *J. Am. Geriatrics Society* 32:296, 1984).

55. Among the major contemporary theories of aging I would include the following:

a. Disposable soma. Evolution favors reproductive performance over maintenance and repair mechanisms, so damage gradually accumulates.

b. Telomeres. A portion of the ends of chromosomes (the telomere) is lost with each cell division. When these are sufficiently diminished or lost, the cell senesces, and so do we.

c. Free radical. Aging is due to accumulating injury from the oxidative stress (free radical generation) secondary to normal metabolism.

d. Glycemic theory. Aging is due to reactions of glucose with other components (proteins and DNA) of the body, with the formation of *Advanced Glycation End Products* (so-called AGE's), which gum up the machinery.

e. Angioplastic pleotropy. Genes whose expression support us during our early years turn against us in later life.

f. Immunologic theory. An example of, or extension of, angioplastic pleotropy. The immune response, which combats infection and cancer in early life, turns against the body itself later in life. Aging thus partakes of an *auto*immune response.

g. System or chaos theory. Aging is an emergent property arising in the nonlinear dynamic system of the body. In this sense, evolution may select "coupling constants" rather than genes. (See note 62 below.)

56. R.S. Sohal and R. Weindruch, *Science* 273:59, 1996; D. Harman, *Journal of Anti-Aging Med.* 2:15–36, 1999.

57. A.T. Lee and A. Cerami, *A. Annual N.Y. Acad. Sci.* 21:663:63–70, 1992.

58. R.L. Walford, *The Immunological Theory of Aging.* Copenhagen: Munksgard, 1969.

59. T. Kirkwood, *Time of Our Lives.* London: Weidenfield and Nicolson, 1999.

60. W.E. Roush, *Science* 277:897, 1997.

61. Sohal and Weindruch, op. cit.

62. A.R. Hibbs and R.L. Walford, *Mech. Aging & Develop.* 50:193, 1989.

63. C. Lee, R.G. Klopp, R. Weindruch, and T.A. Prolla, *Science* 285: 1390, 1999.

CHAPTER 4

1. *Scientific American* interview with Dr. R.L. Leibel, 1996. On-line at www.sciam.com/interview/0896Leibel.html

2. I. Wickelgren, *Science* 280:1364, 1998.

3. Body Mass Index, or BMI, is a measurement giving a relation between weight and height that indirectly reflects how thin or fat you are. A much used parameter, it will be explained at some length in Chapter 5.

4. W.W. Gibbs, *Scientific American*, August 1996.

5. T. Gura, *Science* 280:1369, 1998.

6. Ibid.

7. W. Edmundson, *Ecology Food Nutr.* 8:189, 1979.

8. See note 1 above.

9. R. R. Recker and R. P. Heanen, *Am. J. Clin. Nutr.* 41:254, 1985.

10. *Consumer Reports*, February 1981, p. 68.

11. P. B. Swan, *Annual Review of Nutrition* 3:413, 1983.

12. W. Mertz, *Nutrition Today* 19:22, 1984.

13. M. A. Walker and L. Page, *Journal of the American Dietetic Association* 66:146, 1975.

14. The table given below shows what percentages of the Recommended Daily Allowances for seven essential nutrients are achieved by a number of popular diets and, for comparison, by the CRON diet. There are of course a lot more than merely seven essential nutrients. But even at this level, it seems that the Atkins, Beverly Hills, Scarsdale, and Stillman diets are grossly deficient in multiple nutrients. (The Simmons looks low but would be reasonably good at a higher caloric level.) All except the CRON diet are deficient in one or more nutrients, and would be more so if other nutrients were included in the comparison.

NOTE 14 TABLE. *Values in Percentage of Recommended Daily Allowances*

DIET	THIAMINE	VITAMIN B6	VITAMIN B12	CALCIUM	MAGNESIUM	IRON	ZINC
Atkins	34	37	68	37	25	32	43
Beverly Hills	37	60	0	31	68	60	24
Carbohydrate Cravers	78	58	52	81	73	63	59
California	86	56	36	78	72	62	52
Omega	64	65	354	27	45	45	27
Pritikin	92	85	31	86	97	88	66
Simmons	68	63	123	76	64	65	60
Scarsdale	60	65	37	52	74	56	52
Stillman	46	50	579	35	77	65	90
Zone	303	158	323	40	85	77	48
CRON diet	136	133	306	79	105	85	85

Values for all but the Zone, Omega, and CRON diets are adapted from M.C. Fisher and P.A. Lachance, *Journal of American Dietetic Association* 85:450, 1985.

Values for the Zone and Omega diets are from the respective books. Values for the CRON diet are from the 14 days of food combinations, Appendix A, of this book.

For comparative purposes, all values have been normalized to a 1,000 calorie baseline.

15. J. S. Goodwin et al., *J. Am. Med. Assn.* 249:2917, 1983.

16. J. M. Hsu, *World Rev. Nutr. Dietetics* 33:42, 1979.

17. M. H. Ross and G. J. Bras, *Nature* 250:263, 1974.

18. M. H. Ross, in *Nutrition and Aging*, ed. M. Winick. New York: Wiley & Sons, 1976, p. 43.

19. R. Weindruch and R. L. Walford, *Science* 215:1415, 1982.

20. R.L. Walford et al., *Toxicological Sciences*, 1999 (in press).

21. D. MacKenzie, *New Scientist*, 26 June 1999, p. 19.

22. A. Keys et al., *Biology of Human Starvation*. Minneapolis: University of Minnesota Press, 1950. It is worth noting that the foods eaten, i.e. the menu, in this classic study mimicked those available to semistarved European populations immediately after World War II, and consisted mainly of cabbage and potatoes, not enough to avoid actual malnutrition. The subjects not only lost weight but were sluggish, lethargic, and had peripheral edema. This is quite unlike the situation with the CRON diet of Biosphere 2, for example, under whose influence the crew members were

able to sustain an intense mental and physical work schedule for two straight years,

23. J.O. Hill and J.C. Peters, *Science* 280: 1371, 1998.

24. Ibid.

25. A. Garg et al., *Curr. Opin. Lipidology* 8:23, 1997. G.M. Reaven, *Metabolism* 48:1482, 1994.

26. Metabolic rate is a good example. On short-term calorie reduction, and if measured per lean body mass (fat-free mass), it declines; but on long-term, it returns to normal. R.J. McCarter and J.R. McGee, *Am. J. Physiol.* 257 (Endocrinol. Metab. 20): E175, 1989, although this is now questioned.

27. M.L. Klem et al., *Am. J. Clin. Nutrition* 66: 239, 1997.

28. Gura, op. cit.

29. See note 20 above.

30. T. J. Thomson et al., *Lancet* 2:992, 1966.

31. But in some cases body-protein loss during prolonged dieting has resulted in cardiac-muscle loss and sudden death.

32. H. L. Taylor, *Am. J. Physiol.* 143:148, 1945.

33. S.C. Woods et al., *Science* 280:1378, 1998.

34. A. J. Stunkard, *Nutrition, Longevity, and Aging,* ed. M. Rockstein and M. L. Sussman. New York: Academic Press, 1976, p. 253

35. K.H. Duncan et al., *Am. J. Clin. Nutr.* 37:763, 1983.

36. Ibid.

37. M. Krotkiewski, *Brit. J. Nutr.* 52:97, 1984.

38. A. S. Levine and J. E. Morley, *Nutrition Today,* January/February 1983, p. 6.

39. S. D. Morrison, *Nutrition Reviews* 41:133, 1983.

40. R. Carmena et al., *International J. Obesity* 8:135, 1984; T. A. Hughes et al., *Am. J. Med.* 77:7, 1984; J. Zimmerman et al., *Arteriosclerosis* 4:115, 1984.

41. M. J. Pertshuk et al., *Am. J. Clin. Nutr.* 35:968, 1982.

42. N. A. Ricotti et al., *New Eng. J. Med.* 34:1601, 1984.

43. J. A. Golla et al., *Am. J. Clin. Nutr.* 34:2756, 1981.

44. R. Weindruch et al., *Proceedings Natl. Acad. Sci., U.S.A.* 79:898, 1982.

45. Y. Kagawa, *Preventive Medicine* 7:205, 1978.

46. Y. Kagawa et al., *J. Nutr. Sci. Vitaminol.* 28:441, 1982.

47. Y. Kagawa, *Preventive Medicine,* op. cit.

48. E. A. Vallejo, *Revista Clinica Espanola* 63:25, 1957.

CHAPTER 5

1. J. Constant, *Internal Medicine for the Specialist* 8:95, 1987.

2. *Nutrition Action Newsletter*, April 1999, p. 8.

3. Ibid.

4. G. Taubes, *Science* 280:1369, 1998.

5. R. Andres, in *Aging, Cancer and Cell Membranes*, Vol.7 of *Adv. Pathobiology*, ed. C. Borek, C. M. Fenoglio, and D. W. King. New York: Thieme-Stratton, 1980, p. 238.

6. A. J. Stunkard, *Internatl. J. Obesity* 7:201, 1983.

7. W. P. Catelli (Director of Framingham Heart Study), cited by *Wall Street Journal*, December 1, 1982, p. 32.

8. G. G. Roads and A. Kagan, *Lancet* 1:492, 1983.

9. *Nutrition Reviews* 43:61, 1985.

10. J. Manson et al., *N. Engl. J. Med.* 333:677, 1995

11. I. Wickelgren, *Science* 280: 1365, 1998.

12. A. P. Simopoulos, *Nutrition Reviews* 2:33, 1985; G. Kolata, *Science* 227:1019, 1985.

13. A series of first-rate reviews (pro and con) of the Glycemic Index concept is given in *Nutrition Today* 34 March/April 1999.

14. S.H.A. Holt et al., *Am J. Clin. Nutr.* 66:1264, 1007.

15. T. Parr, *Gerontology* 43:182,1997

16. G.M. Reaven, *Metabolism* 43:1481, 1994.

17. It is worth noting that the GI of the average Greek diet is about 40; the Italian diet, 50; Indian, 60; Chinese, 70; Western, 75; Lebanese, 90 (I. Chew et al, *Am. J. Clin. Nutr.* 47:53, 1988.).

18. See note 2 above.

19. T.J. Horton et al, *Am. J. Clin. Nutr.* 62:19, 1995

20. Constant, op. cit.

21. See note 13 above.

22. Manson, op. cit.

23. D. P. Burkitt in *Nutrition and Killer Diseases*, ed. J. Rose. Park Ridge, NJ: Noyes Publishing, 1982, p. 1.

24. M. J. Gibney and P. G. Burstyn, *Atherosclerosis* 35:339, 1980.

25. W. Dock, *New Eng. J. Med.* 285:58, 1971.

26. *Nutrition Reviews* 9:317, 1984.

27. M. S. Brown and J. L. Goldstein, *Scientific American*, November 1984, p 58.

28. D. J. Namara, *J. Am. Coll. Nutr.* 16:530, 1997

29. B.E. Millen et al., *J. Clin. Epidemiol.* 49:657, 1996

30. Ibid.

31. R. Meleady et al., *Nutrition Reviews* 57:299, 1999. I recommend this article

as an example of a well-balanced review of a controversial subject, contrasting to the jump-to-conclusions reviews one often encounters in the lay, semilay, or advocacy press.

32. A. Keys, *Am. J. Clin. Nutr.* 40:351, 1984.

33. M. Liebman and T. L. Bazzarre, *Amer. J. Clin. Nutr.* 38:612, 1983.

34. R. S. Goor and B. M. Rifkind, in *Nutrition and Killer Diseases*, ed. J. Rose. Park Ridge, NJ: Noyes Publishing, 1982, p. 84.

35. E. Hietanen, ed., *Regulation of Serum Lipids by Physical Exercise.* Boca Raton, FL: CRC Press, 1982.

36. R. Saynor et al., *Atherosclerosis* 50:3, 1984.

37. B. E. Phillipson et al., *New Eng. J. Med.* 312:1210, 1985.

38. D. Kromhout et al., *New Eng. J. Med.* 312:1205, 1985.

39. K. K. Carroll, *Federation Proceedings* 41:2792, 1982.

40. R. A. Anderson and A. S. Kozlovsky, *Am. J. Clin. Nutr.* 41:1177, 1985.

41. M. S. Seelig, in *Intervention in the Aging Process. Part A: Quantitation, Epidemiology and Clinical Research*, ed. W. Regelson and F. M. Sinex. New York: Alan R. Liss, 1983, p. 279.

42. M.A. Eastwood and R. Passmore, *Nutrition Today* 19:6, 1984.

43. *Environmentral Nutrition*, March 1999, p. 7.

44. *Consumer Reports*, February 1980, p. 68.

45. K. M. Behall et al., *Am. J. Clin. Nutr.* 39:209, 1984. A. Aro et al., *Am.J. Clin. Nutr.* 39:911, 1984.

46. H.B. Hubert, *Circulation* 67:986, 1983

47. M.D. Holmes, *J. Am. Med. Assn.* 281:914, 1999.

48. J. L. Marx, *Science* 219:158, 1983; B.B. Beckman and B.N. Ames, *Physiol. Rev.* 78:548, 1998.

49. J. D. Potter, *New Eng. J. Med.* 340:223, 1999.

50. *Nutr. Rev.* 43:170, 1985. C. Garland et al., *Lancet* 1:307, 1985.

51. G. A. Colditz et al., *Am. J. Clinical Nutrition* 41:32, 1985

52. On the other hand, certain procarcinogens such as the chemicals benzo(a)pyrene, AAF, and DMBA are actually *activated* into carcinogens by the mixed-function oxidases. And the Brassicaceae family effect might equally be due to stimulation of the enzyme glutathione transferase. So the beneficial anticancer effect of these vegetables seems real, but the mechanism is not yet clear.

53. D. A. Denton, in *Mechanisms of Hypertension*, ed. M. P. Sambhi, *Excerpta Medica Amsterdam*, 1973, p. 46. H. Blackburn and R. Prineas, *Karger Gazette* 44–45:1, 1983.

54. *Nutr. Action*, March 1985.

55. J. Z. Miller et. al., *Hypertension* 5:790, 1983.

56. G. Berglund, *Acta Medica Scandinavia* (Suppl.) 672: 117, 1983.

57. *Env. Nutr.*, December 1998, p. 1 and 6.

58. J.M. Iacono et al., *Am. J. Clin. Nutr.* 38:860, 1983.

59. P. Puska, *Lancet* 1:1, 1983.

60. K. T. Khaw et al., *Lancet* 2:1127, 1982.

61. G.W. Williams, in *Harrison's Principles of Internal Medicine*, 14th edition. New York: McGraw Hill, 1998.

62. J. M. Belizan et al., *J. Am. Med. Assn.* 249:1161, 1983.

63. C.D. Berdanier, *Nutrition Today* 34:89, 1999

64. S. Goldstein, *Pathologie Biologie* (Paris) 32:99, 1984.

65. S. Pongor et al., *Proceedings Natl. Acad. Sci. U.S.A.* 81:2684, 1984.

66. Glucose-induced activation of a form of protein kinase (PKC) in vascular tissue is a key step in the cascade of events that damage blood vessels and peripheral nerves, leading to higher risk of heart attack, stroke, blindness, and kidney failure. PKC activation may lead to long-term hyperfusion of the retina and kidney, with eventual hypoxia and down-closure of the vessels. The aldose-reductase pathway may also be involved in glucose toxicity. Thus one may postulate three separate pathways to the complications of diabetes: protein glycosylation (the AGEs), the PKC system, and the aldose reductase system. D. Porte and M.W. Schwartz, *Science* 272:699, 1996.

67. E. Reaven et al., *Diabetes* 32:175, 1983.

68. See note 13 above.

69. J. W. Anderson, in *Dietary Fiber in Health and Disease*, ed. G. V. Vahouny and D. Kritchevsky. New York: Plenum Press, 1982, p. 151; G. Ricardi et al., *Diabetologia* 26:116, 1984.

70. J. F. Potter, *Metabolism* 34:199, 1985.

71. T. A. Hughes et al., *Am. J. Med.* 77:7, 1984.

72. Ibid.

73. E. L. Radin and L. E. Lanyon, in *Lectures on Gerontology*, Vol. 1, Part B, ed. A. Viidik. New York: Academic Press, 1982, p. 379.

74. R. R. Recker and R. P. Heaner, *Am. J. Clin. Nutr.* 41:254, 1985.

75. Kruger et al., *Aging* 10:385, 1998

76. D. Kalu et al., *AGE* 6:141, 1983.

77. M.A. Lane et al., *J. Nutr.* 125:1600, 1995.

78. J.C. Matthews and A.C. Scallet, *NeuroToxicology* 12:547,1991.

79. A.J. Bruce-Keller et al., *Ann . Neurol.* 45:8, 1999.

80. R. Mayeux et al., *Neurology* 52 (Suppl. 2): A296, 1999.

81. *Environmental Nutrition* 22 (July): 1, 1999.

82. R.L. Walford et al., *Proc. Nat. Acad. Sci, USA* 89:11533, 1992.

83. R. Verdery and R. L. Walford, *Archives Int. Med.* 158:900, 1998

84. R.L. Walford et al., *J. Gerontol.* (in press).

CHAPTER 6

1. *Environmental Nutrition*, May 1998, p.7.

2. M. Paolini et al., *Nature* 398:760, 1999.

3. M.E. Shils et al., *Modern Nutrition in Health and Disease*, 9th edition. Baltimore: Williams & Wilkins, 1999.

4. I.D. Podmore et al., *Nature* 392:559, 1998.

5. R. Weindruch and R.L. Walford, *The Retardation of Aging and Disease by Dietary Restriction*. Springfield, IL: Charles C. Thomas, 1988.

6. Interview with Sir Peter Medawar in *Omni*, January 1984, p. 63.

7. G. Kolata, *Science* 223:1161, 1984.

8. In 1983, Dr. John Holloszy, one of the best exercise physiologists in the country, wrote, "… scientific evidence that strenuous exercise has long-term health benefits or slows aging is meager and unconvincing." J. 0. Holloszy, *Med. Sci. Sports Exerc.* 15:1, 1983. (I might add that the health benefits are by now established, but there is still no evidence that exercise actually retards aging.)

9. It was not until 1984 that the American Cancer Society officially acknowledged the probable role of diet in promoting or preventing cancer.

10. L. Alhadeff et al., *Nutrition Reviews* 42:33, 1984.

11. Shils et al., op. cit.

12. Both an increase and a decrease in cholesterol have been attributed to intake of vitamin C, but in none of the studies in humans was the effect statistically significant (Klevay, 1976). Very large doses of ascorbic acid given over a six-month period have not been toxic in laboratory mice (Deschner et al., 1983). One short article reported that vitamin C given to pregnant rats in dosages equivalent to 20 grams per day in humans may cause kidney damage (Lavender, 1978). However, at least a few humans have taken doses of vitamin C up to 15 grams per day without known ill effects (White, 1981). Convincing evidence of severe vitamin C toxicity has been found in guinea pigs. When kept on an unfortified wheat diet and given large doses of vitamin C, the guinea pigs experienced a high death rate within 25 days (Nandi et al., 1973). But when milk casein was added to the wheat diet, thus supplying the essential amino acid lysine, no toxicity at all was seen. Thus, large doses of vitamin C might be harmful to a person on a meatless, amino acid imbalanced diet. But this is reductio ad absurdum. There seems to be reasonable evidence that vitamin C may interfere with the absorption of copper, an essential trace element, from the gastrointestinal tract (Finley, 1983; Shils et al., op. cit.). Vitamin C may also increase intestinal iron absorption, and the iron-vitamin C complex may have pro-oxidant activity (Shils et al., op. cit.). So don't take vitamin C with meals. L. Klevay, *Proceedings of the Society for Experimental Biology and Medicine* 151:579, 1976. D. Deschner, *Nutrition and Cancer* 4:241, 1983. L. M. Lavender, *Federation Proceedings* 37:321, 1978. J. D. White, *New Eng. J. Med.* 304:1491, 1981. B. K. Nandi et al., *J. Nutr.* 103:1688, 1973.

    E. B. Finley, *Am. J. Clin. Nutr.* 37:553, 1983.

13. H. J. Roberts, *J. Am. Med. Assn.* 246:129, 1981.

14. Bieri et al., *New Eng. J. Med.* 308:1063, 1983.

15. The Federal Register of 1979, a publication of the Food and Drug Administration stated that the maximum safe dose of vitamin E is certainly greater than 400 International Units, and that doses up to 3,000 units for up to 11 years had had no detrimental effect.

16. R. Vieth et al., *Am. J. Clinical Nutrition* 69:842, 1999.

17. Nutrient-balance studies have forced an increase in RDAs for calcium from the previous 800 milligrams per day up to 1,200 milligrams per day. At the lower figure, 30 to 40 percent of men were found to be in negative calcium balance.

18. H. Kamin, *Am. J. Clin. Nutr.* 41:165, 1985.

19. *Nutrition Reviews* 57:210, 1999.

20. Only a single and limited study has addressed this problem. While mice fed half of RDA levels of (all) vitamins lived 12 percent less long than controls, there was no difference in survival between mice fed regular RDA and those fed four times the RDA amounts of (all) vitamins (Kokkonen and Barrows, 1985). Of course four-times-RDA amounts of vitamin E, for example, would still be quite small in terms of an antioxidant effect. C. C. Kokkonen and C. H. Barrows, *AGE* 8:13, 1985.

21. R. Anderson et al., *Am. J. Clin. Nutr.* 33:71, 1980.

22. I. M. Corwin and R. K. Gordon, *Annals of N.Y. Acad. Sci.* 393:437, 1982.

23. B.N. Ames, *Science* 221:1256-64, 1983.

24. They need to be paired because in addition to swirling around the central nucleus, each electron spins on its own axis; and to maintain stability in the universe, for reasons known best to the high priests of physics, every electron spinning to the right must be balanced by one spinning to the left. Atmospheric oxygen is a rare exception to this rule, having two unpaired electrons, a phenomenon exploited by all aerobic (oxygen-using) organisms.

25. R.S. Sohol and R. Weindruch, *Science* 274:59, 1996.

26. K.B. Beckman and B.N. Ames, *Physiological Reviews* 78:574, 1998.

27. Many antioxidants, or "scavengers," are enzymes that change the free radicals into stable compounds. Superoxide dismutase, catalase, and glutathione peroxidase are examples of free radical scavengers, and they guard against the superoxide anion radical, against hydrogen peroxide, and against the hydroxyl radical, respectively. Some vitamins (E and C) also have antioxidant properties.

28. J. Marx, *Science* 219:158, 1983. B.N. Ames, op. cit.

29. The relationship holds for superoxide dismutase, uric acid, the carotenes, and vitamin E (Cutler, 1983; Cutler, 1984). However, a number of other free radical scavengers do not show such a relationship: vitamin C, glutathione, and glutathione peroxidase (the enzyme that requires selenium). And if some free radical scavengers do and just as many do not correlate with maximum life span, one could interpret the data in either of

two ways. Dr. Richard Cutler of the National Institute of Aging tends to dismiss the noncorrelating antioxidants as not being important in aging. Whether the cart is before the horse is difficult to say because they are going in a circle. R. G. Cutler, in *Intervention in the Aging Process. Part B: Basic Research and Preclinical Screening*, ed. W. Regelson and F. M. Sinex. New York: Alan R. Liss, 1983, p. 69. R. G. Cutler, *Proceedings Natl. Acad. Sci. U.S.A.* 81:7627, 1984.

30. More fully, the pigment is a degradation product resulting from the reactions of a cross-linking agent (malondialdehyde) with cell membranes. And malondialdehyde comes from free radical processes involving lipid peroxidation. It has been shown that the peroxide levels in serum and brain bear a roughly inverse relation to maximum life span in mammals, right on up from mouse to monkey to man (Cutler, 1983). But again we have a paradox: certain drugs will greatly slow down or inhibit the development of the pigment in mammals, but exert little or no effect on maximum life span. So what is the real relevance of the pigment? R. Cutler, in *Intervention in the Aging Process*, op. cit.

31. Sohol and Weindruch, op. cit.

32. Beckman and Ames, op. cit.

33. A. Tappel et al., *J. Gerontology* 28:415, 1973. D. G. Hafeman and W. G. Hoekstra, *J. Nutrition* 107:656, 1977. R. D. Lippman, *Review of Biological Research in Aging*, ed. M. Rothstein. New York: Alan R. Liss, 1982, p. 315.

34. Antioxidants such as vitamin E or the chemical agent Santoquin were reported to improve the immune response of mice (Harman et al., 1977). The height of the response was greater in antioxidant-treated animals. That sounds like a favorable result. However, examination of the data reveals that the time at which the immune response peaked was later in the treated mice. If aging were really being retarded, the peak should come sooner, as that would represent reversal of what is seen in normal aging. When rich and not-so-rich antioxidant mixtures were fed to mice, the former but not the latter inhibited the buildup of age pigment; but only the latter improved the biomarkers represented by treadmill performance and kidney function, and neither antioxidant mixture improved survival (Tappel et al., 1973). Thus a clear picture does not emerge. D. H. Harman et al., *J. Am. Geriatrics Soc.* 25:400,1977. A. Tappel et al., op. cit.

35. Some extension of species maximum life span may have been achieved by antioxidant therapy in invertebrate species such as fruit flies. (See also Sohol and Weindruch, op. cit.)

36. E. L. Schneider and J. D. Reed, *New Eng. J. Med.* 312:1159, 1985.

37. Below are reproduced, adjusted to the same scale, the seven "best" survival-curve studies using antioxidants that I can find in the biological literature. Even where some differences were detected between antioxidant-fed and normally fed animals (chart F in the figure), neither population exceeded the maximal life spans for the species. Compare these curves with those of Figure 3.1 from CRON diet studies in naturally long-lived mouse strains. The difference is striking.

NOTE 37 FIGURE (*see next page*) Survival curves of long-lived strains of mice and rats given various antioxidants throughout part or all of their lives

A and B: In male mice (A), treatment by injection with large doses of cysteine or folcysteind (folic acid plus thiazolidincarboxylic acid) on alternate days for 42 days led to increased survival; but in female rats (B) no effect at all was seen (adapted from S. Oeriu and E. Vochitsu, *J. Gerontology* 20:4127, 1965.)

C and D: Survival curves of male (C) and female (D) rats fed either a normal diet or a diet supplemented with selenium (as selenate). We see mild increases in mean life spans in the supplemented animals, but no significant differences in maximum life spans (adapted from N.A. Schroeder and M. Mitchner, *J. Nutrition* 101:1531, 1971.)

E: Survival curves of mice fed normally or given a cocktail containing moderate amounts of vitamin E, BHT, methionine, and selenium, or large amounts of these same compounds. Either there was no effect, or the antioxidants slightly decreased survival (adapted from A. Tappel et al., *J. Gerontology* 2:415, 1973.)

F: Survival of mice fed a diet supplemented with 2-ME (2-mercaptoethanol), compared to that of nonsupplemented mice. A mild (three-month) effect on both mean and maximum life spans was obtained, and the strain is fairly long-lived; but species-specific maximum life span still not exceeded (adapted from M. J. Heidrick et al., *Mech. Ageing and Develop.* 27:341, 1984.)

G: Survival of mice fed the commercial antioxidant Ethoxyquin. Increase in maximum survival, but clearly not a long-lived strain (adapted from A. Comfort, *Nature* 229:254, 1971.)

38. S.W.J. Lamberts et al., *Science* 278:419, 1997.

39. D. Rudman et al., *New England J. Med.* 323:1, 1990.

40. Lamberts et al., op. cit.

41. M. A. Papadakis et al., *Ann. Internal Med.* 124:708, 1996.

42. D.N. Khansari and T. Gustad, *Mech. Ageing and Develop.* 57:87, 1991.

43. D. N. Kalu et al., *J. Gerontol.* 53A:B452, 1998.

44. J.H. Morrison and P.R. Hof, *Science* 278:412, 1997. S.S.C. Yen et al., *Ann. N. Y. Acad. Sci.* 774:128, 1995.

45. Ibid.

46. J. F. Nelson et al., *Neurobiology of Aging* 16: 837, 1995.

47. S. Nemecek, *Scientific American*, September 1997, p. 38.

48. Ibid.

49. E. Hemminki et al., *British Med. J.* 315:149, 1997. S. Hulley et al., *J. Am. Med. Assn.* 280:605, 1998.

50. Morrison and Hof, op. cit.

51. The CRON diet prevents the age-related decline in growth hormone signal transduction (how messages get from the exterior into the cell), so it's possible that growth hormone is decreased because less is needed to evoke the same response. S. Su and W. E. Sponntag, *J. Gerontol.* 51A:B167, 1996.

52. H.M. Brown-Borg et al., *Nature* 384:33, 1996.

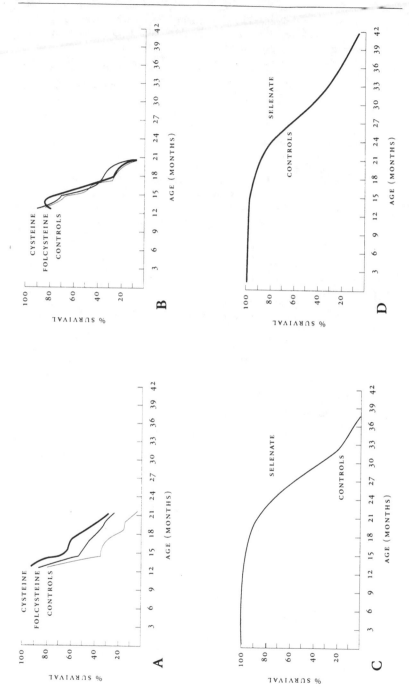

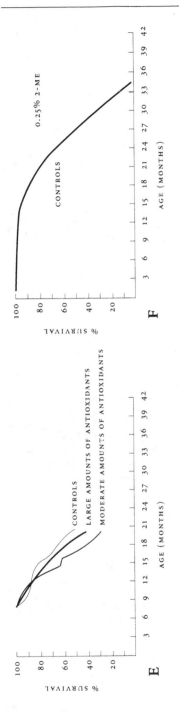

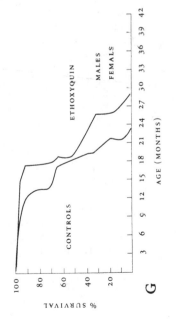

53. J. F. Nelson et al., *Neurobiol. of Aging* 16:837, 1995.

54. Walford et al., *J. Gerontol.* (in press).

55. *Environmental Nutrition*, April 1998, p. 6.

56. *Environmental Nutrition*, March 1999, p. 6.

57. *Environmental Nutrition*, July 1997, p. 6.

58. J. Marx, *Science* 273:51, 1996.

CHAPTER 7

1. W. Empson, *Faustus and the Censor*. Oxford, U.K.: Basil Blackwell Ltd., 1987.

2. Ibid.

3. C. E. Finch, *Longevity, Senescence and the Genome*. Chicago: University of Chicago Press, 1990.

4. D. DellaPenna, *Science* 285:375, 1999.

5. D. S. Michaud et al., *J. Natl. Cancer Inst.* 91:605, 1999.

6. I.E. Dreosti, *Nutrition Reviews* 54 :S51, 1996

7. J. A. Joseph et al., *J. Neuroscience* 19:8114, 1999.

8. Ibid.

9. L. Packard, *Sci. Am. Sci. Med.* 1:54, 1994.

10. Vitamin E works mainly on the cell membranes, where it protects polyunsaturated fatty acids against free radical attacks (Lippman, 1983). It may also to some degree protect the DNA of cells against radiation-induced damage, mutation, and chemically induced cancer (Ames, 1983). And it has been reported to markedly increase the endurance of rats during exercise sufficiently strenuous to cause extensive free radical damage to tissues (Davies et al., 1982). R. D. Lippman, in *Rev. Biol. Research in Aging*, ed. M. Rothstein. New York: Alan R. Liss, 1983, p. 315. B. N. Ames, *Science* 221:1256, 1983. K. J. A. Davies et al., *Biochemical Biophysical Research Communications* 107:1198, 1982.

11. J. Epstein and D. Gershon, *Mechanisms of Ageing and Development* 1:257, 1972. J. E. Fleming and L. S. Yengoyan, *AGE* 4:132, 1981. M. Sawada and H. E. Enesco, *Experimental Gerontology* 19:179, 1984.

12. In the worm *C. briggsae*, the maximum normal life span of 56 days was incrased to 69 days by vitamin E (Epstein and Gershon, 1972). However—and now we must look at the evidence critically—in this and a similar experiment with another worm, *Turbatrix aceti* (Kahn and Enesco, 1981), the effect was obtained only if vitamin E was present very early in life. If it was present for the first six days and then withdrawn, a big effect was obtained; but very little benefit accrued if the vitamin was added after ten days and kept in the diet for the rest of the life of the worms. An effect limited to an early phase of development does not suggest simple protection against free radicals, which of course are generated throughout life. J. Epstein and D. Gershon, op. cit. M. Kahn and H. E. Enesco, *AGE* 4:109, 1981.

13. D. Harman, *The Gerontologist* 8:13, 1968. A. Tappel et al., *J. Gerontology* 28:415, 1973. A. D. Blackett and D. A. Hall, *J. Gerontology* 36:529, 1981.

14. B. M. Zuckerman and M. A. Geist, in *Age Pigments*, ed. R. S. Sohal. North Holland: Elsevier, 1981, p. 283.

15. Age pigment is the insoluble end product of free radical damage to certain components of the cell, which have been further digested, degraded, and stored in vacuoles within the cell. The rate of accumulation of this pigment in dog hearts is 5.5 times as fast as in human hearts and humans live about 5.5 times as long as dogs. The same relationship holds, albeit less proportionately, with other animal species. (See note 28, Chapter 6.)

16. R. P. Tengerdy in *Vitamin E: A Comprehensive Treatise*, ed. L. J. Machlin. New York: Marcel Dekker, 1980, pp. 429–44. L. M. Corwin and R. K. Gordon, *Annals of N.Y. Acad. Sci.* 393:437, 1982. W. R. Beisel, *Am. Clin. Nutr.* 35 (Suppl. 2): 417, 1982.

17. J.G. Bien et al., *New Eng. J. Med.* 308:1063, 1983.

18. T. Yasanaga et al., *Nutrition* 112:1075, 1982.

19. Almost every aspect of the immune system, including resistance to infection, specific antibody responses, responses to mitogens, and "clearance" of particles from the blood, has been shown to be enhanced by moderate increases in vitamin E intake (Stinnett, 1983).

    J. D. Stinnett, ed., *Nutrition and the Immune Response*. Boca Raton, FL: CRC Press, 1983.

20. P. A. Cerutti, *Science* 227:375, 1985.

21. There are two stages in cancer promotion. Vitamin E is a stage one inhibitor.

22. E.B. Rimm et al., *New Eng. J. Med.* 328:1450, 1993.

23. W.J. Blot et al., *J. Natl. Cancer Inst.* 85: 1483, 1993.

24. O. P. Heinonen, *J. Natl. Cancer Inst.* 90:416,440, 1998.

25. L. Packer, in *Vitamin E in Health and Disease*, ed. L. Packer et al. New York: Marcel Dekker, 1993, p. 977.

26. C. E. Melton, *Aviation, Space, and Environ. Med.* 53:105, 1982. R. J. Stephens et al., *Chest* 5:375, 1983.

27. K. Node et al., *Science* 285:1276, 1999.

28. *Nutrition Reviews* 55:376, 1997.

29. M.E. Shils et al., *Modern Nutrition in Health and Disease*, 9th edition. Baltimore: Williams and Wilkins, 1999.

30. Ibid.

31. E. Niki et al., *Am. J. Clin. Nutr.* 62 (Suppl.):1322S, 1995.

32. The frequency of aberrations in the DNA of coal-tar workers dropped from an initial value of 5 percent to a near-normal value of 1.8 percent after three months' daily intake of 1 gram of vitamin C. R. J. Sr'am et al., *Mutation Research* 120:181, 1983.

33. P. J. Hornsby and J. F. Crevello, *Molecular and Cellular Endocrinology* 30:1, 1983.

34. L. H. Chen, *Am. J. Clin. Nutr.* 34:1036,1981, 25

35. J. A. Simon, *J. Am. Coll. Nutr.* 11:107, 1992.

36. The addition of 0.25 to 1 percent sodium ascorbate to their diet reduced the number of rats developing colon cancer in response to a chemical carcinogenic agent from 26 percent all the way down to zero. B. S. Reddy et al., *Advances in Cancer Research* 32:237, 1980.

37. Shils et al., op. cit.

38. Simon, op. cit.

39. J. E. Enstrom et al., *Epidemiology* 3:192, 1992

40. C.J. Fuller et al., *Athersclerosis* 119:139, 1996.

41. B. Kennes et al., *Gerontology* 29:305, 1983.

42. Ibid.

43. R. Anderson et al., *Am. J. Clin. Nutr.* 33:71, 1980.

44. J. E. W. Davies et al., *Experimental Gerontology* 12:215, 1977.

45. H. R. Massie et al., *Experimental Gerontology* 11:37, 1976.

46. H. R. Massie et al., *Gerontology* 30:371, 1984.

47. T.M. Hagen et al., *FASEB J.* 13:411, 1999.

48. E.D. Schleicher et al., *J. Clin Invest.* 99:457, 1997.

49. B.N. Ames, *Toxicol. Lett.* 28:102–5, 1998.

50. S. Jacob et al., *Arzneimittelforschung* 45:872,1995.

51. Some flavonoids antagonize the mutagenic activities of polycyclic hydrocarbons (PHC), including the metabolites produced by p-450 enzymes acting upon these hydrocarbons (Huang et al., 1983). The flavonoid "rutin" has strong activity in this regard. Another flavonoid, "quercetrin," inhibits development of experimental cataracts in a species of rodent from the Andes prone to develop cataracts (Varma et al., 1977). But quercetrin may also be mutagenic (Stauric, 1984). We don't know much about the possible role of bioflavonoids in nutrition in part because there are so many different kinds—more than 500 (Havsteen, 1983). M. Huang et al., *Carcinogenesis* 4:1631, 1983. S. D. Varma et al., *Science* 195:205, 1977. B. Stauric, *Federation Proceedings* 43:2454, 1984. B. Havsteen, *Biochem. Pharmacol.* 32:1141, 1983.

52. Shils et al., op. cit.

53. D. DellaPenna, *Science* 285:375, 1999.

54. *Environmental Nutr.* December 1998, p. 4.

55. *Science News*, September 18, 1999, p. 180.

56. A. Cassidy et al., *Brit. J. Nutr.* 74:587, 1995.

57. DellaPenna, op. cit.

58. M.S. Kursur and X. Xu, *Annual Rev. Nutrition* 17:353, 1997.

59. N. K. Edens, *Nutrition Today* 34:152, 1999.

60. Shils et al., op. cit.

61. R.K. Severson et al., *Cancer Res.* 49:1857, 1989.

62. L. White et al., *Neuropbiol. of Aging* 17 (Suppl. 4):S121, 1996; *J. Am. Med. Assn.* 276:955, 1996

63. *Science News*, October 11, 1997, p. 230.

64. S. Hecht, *J. Cell Biochem* 22 (Suppl.):195, 1995.

65. J. W. Fahey et al., *Proc. Nat. Acad. Sci.* 94:10367, 1997.

66. Edens, op. cit.

67. J.A. Milner, *Nutrition Reviews* 54:S82, 1996.

68. K. Imai et al., *Prev. Medicine* 26:769, 1997.

69. Ibid.

70. K. Imai and K. Nakachi, *Brit. Med. Journal* 310:6981, 1995.

71. Y. Cao and R. Cao, *Nature* 398:381, 1999.

72. Dreost, op. cit.

73. Ziegler et al., *Cancer Causes and Control* 7:157, 1996.

74. G. W. Burton and K. U. Ingold, *Science* 224:569, 1984.

75. H. J. Thompson et al., *Cancer Res.* 44:2803, 1984.

76. Ibid.

77. A. Forman, *Environmental Nutrition*, August, 1997, p. 4.

78. W. C. Willett and M. MacMahon, *New Eng. J. Med.* 310:633, 1984.

79. Peto et al., op cit.

80. D.A. Cooper et al., *Nutrition Rev.* 57:201, 1999.

81. DellaPenna, op. cit.

82. Cooper, op. cit.

83. Shils et al., op. cit.

84. Ziegler et al., *Cancer Causes Control* 7:151, 1996.

85. J.W. Erdman Jr. et al., *Nutrition Rev.* 54:185, 1996.

86. C.W. Hennekens et al., *New. Eng. J. Med.* 334:1145, 1996.

87. Forman, op. cit.

88. Willet and MacMahon, op. cit.

89. E. Giovannucci, *J. Nat. Cancer Inst.* 91:317, 1999.

90. J.S. Bertram, *Nutrition Rev.* 57:182, 1999.

91. R. G. Cutler, *Proceedings Natl. Acad. Sci.* 81:7627, 1984.

92. Cooper, op. cit.

93. Glutathione peroxidase breaks down lipid (and other) peroxides, and also hydrogen peroxide, both of which are among the damaging free radicals generated by normal metabolism. And acting together, the enzymes glutathione peroxidase and superoxide dismutase may prevent the formation of perhaps the most dangerous of all free radicals, the superoxide radical (Sunde and Hoekstra, 1980). Increasing selenium intake in the diet will increase the level of glutathione peroxidase in both rats (Scott et al., 1977) and humans (Thomson et al., 1982). Organically bound selenium gives a greater response in humans than the inorganic form

(Thomson et al., 1982). R. A. Sunde and W. G. Hoekstra, *Nutrition Reviews* 38:265, 1980. D. L. Scott et al., *Acta Biochemica Biophysica* 497:218, 1977. C.D.Thomson et al., *Am. J. Clin. Nutr.* 36:24,1982.

94. A. Griffin and S. Clark, *Advances in Cancer Research* 29:419, 1979.

95. But the "p-450" system is like a two-edged sword. The enzymes sometimes "activate" the simple organic chemicals into forms that are carcinogenic. Selenium may help decrease those p-450 activities that play a role in this activation. Griffin and Clark, op. cit.

96. H. A. Schroeder and M. Mitchner, *J. Nutrition* 101: 1531, 1971.

97. A small bit of additional experimental evidence and one curious piece of anecdotal evidence can be added. An experimental study showed that adding selenium to the drinking water of mice not only decreased their frequency of spontaneous breast cancer but shifted the peak incidence of the cancer to a later age (Schrauzer and Ishmael, 1974). The age-specific peak incidence of cancer is a rather good biomarker of aging, so the shift might suggest an age-retarding effect. For the anecdotal evidence: when Representative Claude Pepper asked a number of centenarians about their health habits, the only common trait was that many of them ate lots of onions. Interestingly enough, we see from the "rich soil" column of Table 7.2 that of the plants we do eat, onions are the best selenium accumulators. G. Schrauzer and D. Ishmael, *Annals of Clinical and Laboratory Science* 4:441, 1974.

98. Griffin and Clark, op. cit. J. A. Milner and G. A. Greeder, *Science* 209:825, 1980. R. A. Passwater, *Selenium as Food and Medicine.* New Canaan, CT: Keats Publishing Co., 1980. Schrauzer and Ishmael, op. cit. L. W. Wattenberg, *Adv. Cancer Res.* 26:197, 1970. H. J. Thompson et al., *Cancer Res.* 44:2803, 1984.

99. Y. Kise et al., *Int. J. Cancer* 46:95, 1990.

100. L.C. Clark et al., *J. Am. Med. Assn.* 276:1957, 1996.

101. A study from the Harvard School of Public Health conducted in 1982 examined the effect of selenium levels in the blood on future cancer risk (Willett et al., 1983). Frozen blood samples were available from participants in a blood-pressure study done back in 1973. One hundred eleven of the participants in the study had died of cancer. Comparing the levels of their blood selenium with levels of 210 persons from the same study who had remained healthy, the investigators found that most of those who developed cancer had low selenium levels even before the onset of the cancer. W. C. Willett et al., *Lancet* 2:130, 1983.

102. B. Liebman, *Nutrition Action*, December 1983, p. 5.

103. R. A. Passwater, *Selenium as Food and Medicine.* New Canaan, CT: Keats Publishing Co., 1980. K. Jaakkola et al., *Scandinavian J. Clin. Lab. Med.* 43: 473, 1983.

104. Schroeder and Mitchner, op. cit.

105. Thompson, op. cit.

106. Organic selenium is usually manufactured by inclusion of selenium in the food fed to yeasts, which then incorporate it during their growth cycles.

But some manufacturers simply mix brewer's yeast with inorganic selenium salts and press the mixture into tablets. Read the label to make sure this is not what you are getting. If it says "organically bound," that's okay. If it says "added to" or "fortified," that's not what you want.

107. L. Aladaheff et al., *Nutrition Reviews* 42:33, 1984.

108. R. B. Pelton and R. J. Williams, *Proceedings Soc. Exper. Biol. Medicine* 99:632, 1958.

109. K. E. Cheney et al., *Exper. Gerontol.* 15:237, 1980.

110. E. P. Ralli and M. E. Dunn, *Vitamin and Hormones* 11:133, 1953.

111. Ibid.

112. J. Selhub et al., *New Eng. J. Med.* 332:286, 1995.

113. Colloquium: homocysteine, vitamins, and arterial occlusive disease. *J. Nutr.* 126 (Suppl 45):1235S, 1996.

114. E. B. Rimm et al., *J. Am. Med. Assn.* 279:359, 1998.

115. M. L. Fonda et al., *Exper. Geront.* 15:473, 1980. C. S. Rose et al., *Am. J. Clin. Nutr.* 29:847, 1976.

116. K. Lindseth and J. Miquel, *AGE* 4:133, 1981. K. Lindseth et al., *12th Ann. Meeting, Am. Aging Assn.*, September 23–29, 1982, p. 18.

117. H. Schaumburg et al., *New Eng. J. Med.* 309:445, 1983.

118. L. Ernster and B. D. Nelson, in *Biomedical and Clinical Aspects of Coenzyme Q*, Vol. 3. Amsterdam: Elsevier, 1981, p. 159.

119. K. Linnrot, *Coenzyme Q10, Its Bioavailability and Effects on Survival and the Cardiovascular System*. Doctoral Thesis, Univesity of Tampere, Finland, 1999. K. Linnrot et al., *Gerontology* 41 (Suppl. 2):10-9, 1995. K. Linnrot et al., *Biochem. Mol. Biology Internal.* 44:727, 1998. K. Linnrot et al., *Brit. J. Pharmacol.* 124:500, 1998.

120. E. G. Bliznakov, in *Biomedical and Clinical Aspects of Coenzyme Q*, Vol. 3. Amsterdam: Elsevier, 1981, p. 311.

121. Linnrot, op. cit.

122. It should be mentioned that—in possible contrast to oral administration—intraperitoneal or intramuscular administration increases the CoQ10 levels in the heart and elsewhere. Bliznakov's method was by injection.

123. Linnrot, op. cit.

124. M.F. Beal, *Biofactors* 9:261, 1999. R. T. Matthews et al., *Proc. Natl. Acad. Sci.* 95:8892, 1998

125. G. Paradies et al., *FEBS Lett.* 454:207, 1999.

126. T. M. Hagen et al., *Ann. N. Y. Acad. Sci.* 854:214, 1998.

127. T. M. Hagen et al., *Proc. Natl. Acad. Sci.* 95:9562, 1998.

128. T. M. Hagen et al., *FASET J.* 13:411, 1999.

129. Y. Suzuki et al., in *Carnitine Biosynthesis, Metabolism, and Function*, ed. R. A. Frenkel and J. D. McGarry. New York: Academic Press, 1980, p. 341.

130. Fanelli, *Life Sciences* 23:2563, 1978.

131. C. Cavazza, *Chem. Abstracts* 100:203597f, 1984.

132. W.E. Lands, *FASEB J.* 6:2530, 1992.

133. W.E. Connor, *Ann. Int. Med.* 123:950, 1995.

134. R. Uauy-Dagach and A. Vakebzuela, *Nutrition Reviews* 54:S102, 1996.

135. G. Fernandes and C.A. Jolly, *Nutrition Reviews* 56:S161, 1998.

136. J. Bezard et al., *Reprod. Nutr. Develop.* 34:539, 1994.

137. R. A. Gibson et al., *J. Pediatrics* 125 (Suppl.):48S, 1994

138. Uauy-Dagach and Vakebzuela, op. cit.

139. See note 63 above.

140. J.P. Tissen et al., *Nutrition Reviews* 57:167, 1999.

141. A. Bartke et al., *Experimental Gerontol.* 33:675, 1998.

142. A. Schwartz et al., in *Intervention in the Aging Process*, ed. W. Regelson and F.M. Sinex. New York: Alan R. Liss, 1983, p. 267.

143. Among the several effects attributed to DHEA (Schneider and Reed, 1985), one is that it may inhibit weight gain by increasing the metabolic rate and by directing energy into a "futile cycle," thereby increasing oxygen consumption and increasing the generation of heat within fatty tissues. These combined processes could be labeled "calorie wasting." If such is the case, one would expect DHEA to increase the generation of free radicals, in which case it might not decelerate aging but the reverse. E. L. Schneider and J. D. Reed, Jr., *New Eng. J. Med.* 312:1159, 1985.

144. T.D. Pugh et al., *Cancer Res.* 59:1642, 1999.

145. A. M. Brzezinski, *New. Eng. J. Med.* 336:186, 1997.

CHAPTER 8

1. J. O. Holloszy, *J. Applied Physiol.* 82:399, 1997.

2. I've been actively involved in sports all my life: Southwest A. A. U. gymnastic champion (on the rings) my last year in high school; captain of the wrestling team at the University of Chicago for two years; scuba diver since the very beginning of the sport in the late 1940s. Even now I spend three 20-minute periods a week at aerobic exercise with my heart rate at 75 percent of maximum, and do about three hours of isometric bodybuilding weekly. My criticism, such as it is, of the exercise mania is not that of a sedentary person trying to justify his laziness.

3. S. Port et al., *New Eng. J. Med.* 303:1133, 1980.

4. R. Leibel. interview at http://www.sciam.com/interview/089leibel.html!

5. C. Bissell and T. Samorajski, *AGE* 6:134, 1983.

6. J. W. Starnes et al., *Am. J. Physiol.* 245:H560, 1983. E. Steinhagen-Thiessen et al., *AGE* 6:143, 1983. A. Z. Reznick et al., *Biochem. Med.* 28:347, 1982. J. A. Chesky et al., *J. Applied Physiol.* 55:1349, 1983.

7. In another study, mice 6, 19, and 27 months old were forced to exercise on a

motor-driven wheel for 30 minutes per day for ten weeks, after which their leg muscles were examined by electron microscopy. In the 27-month-old but not in the younger mice, the exercise actually accelerated the regressive muscle changes normally seen with aging. R. Ludatscher et al., *Exper. Geront.* 18:113, 1983.

8. R. Coleman et al., *Biology of the Cell* 46:207, 1982.

9. A. B. K. Basson et al., *Comparative Biochemistry and Physiology* 71A:369. 1982.

10. Studies in monkeys kept on high-cholesterol diets that have either exercised (one hour three times per week on a treadmill) or not have shown rather convincingly that exercise protects against the development of arteriosclerosis. D. M. Kramsch, *New Eng. J. Med.* 305:1483, 1981.

11. A Hartmann et al., *Mutation Research* 346:195, 1995.

12. E. Hietanen, ed., *Regulation of Serum Lipids by Physical Exercise*. Boca Raton, FL: CRC Press, 1982.

13. L. W. Gibbons et al., *Circulation* 67:977, 1983.

14. C. C. Johnson et al., *J. Am. Diet. Assn.* 81:695, 1982.

15. Losing weight along with the exercise maximizes the beneficial effects on the blood fats. Z. V. Tran and A. Weltman, *J. Am. Med. Assn.* 254:914, 1985.

16. S. Port et al., *New Eng. J. Med.* 303:1133, 1980. M. Rosenthal et al., *Diabetes* 32:408, 1983.

17. S. N. Blair et al., *J. Am. Med. Assn.* 252:487, 1984.

18. J. L. Kilgore et al., *Canadian J. Applied Physiol.* 23:245, 1998.

19. B. Liebman, *Nutr. Action*, November 1981, p. 9.

20. M. Elsayad et al., *J. Gerontology* 35:383, 1980.

21. W. W. Spirduso, *J. Gerontology* 35:850, 1980.

22. A. F. Kramer et al., *Nature* 400:417, 1999.

23. R. A. Bruce, *Med. and Sci. in Sports and Exercise* 16:8, 1984.

24. Treadmill time to exhaustion is equally good. L. W. Gibbons et al., *J. Am. Diet. Assn.* 81:695, 1982.

25. The age-related decline in maximum oxygen consumption may be different in longitudinal than in cross-sectional studies. Thus, for a contrary view to what I have said about the rates of decline when sedentary are compared with athletic individuals. (Bruce, op. cit.)

26. R. L. Paffenbarger et al., *J. Am. Med. Assn.* 252:491, 1984.

27. A. A. Hakin et al., *Circulation* 100:9, 1999.

28. R. J. Barnard, M. R. Massey, et al., *Diabetes Care* 6:268, 1983. R. J. Barnard, P. M. Guzy, et al., *J. Cardiac Rehab.* 3:183, 1982. J. A. Hall et al., *The Physician and Sports Med.* 10:90, 1982.

29. Holloszy, op. cit.

30. I. Wickelgren, *Science* 280:1364, 1998.

31. E. J. Brierley et al., *Quart. J. Med.* 89:251, 1996.

32. D.L. Ballor et al., *Am. J. Clin. Nutr.* 47:19, 1988.

33. Port et al., op. cit. 0. Segerberg, Jr., *Living to Be 100*, New York: Scribner, 1982.

34. M. Moffat and S. Vickery, *The American Physical Therapy Association Book of Body Maintenance and Repair*. New York: Henry Holt and Co., 1999.

35. Georg Feurstein, *Yoga International*, June/July 1999, p. 39

36. Herbert Benson, *The Relaxation Response*. New York: Avon Books, 1975.

37. P.W. Lemon, *Int.J.Sport Nutr*.8:426, 1998. *Nurt. Rev*.54, part 2:S169, 1996.

CHAPTER 9

1. W. J. Broad, *Science* 204:1060, 1979.

2. *Los Angeles Times*, September 25, 1983, part I, p. 4.

3. R. M. Sapolsky, *Neurobiol. Aging* 16:849, 1995.

4. D. Ornish, *Stress, Diet, and Your Heart*. New York: Holt, Rinehart and Winston, 1982.

5. A. Parachini, cited by *Los Angeles Times*, September 4, 1984, part V, p. 1.

6. R. L. Walford, *Maximum Life Span*. New York: W. W. Norton, 1983.

7. R. L. Walford, *Los Angeles Times*, June 5, 1983, travel section.

8. I don't mean to indicate that an author's mere possession of orthodox "credentials" necessarily means his advice is sound. Dr. Berger's *The Immune Power Diet* is, in my opinion as both an immunologist and a nutritionist, merely one long clinical anecdote, and close to being fantasy—even though Dr. Berger is a medical doctor. And one of the most scientifically nonsensical diet books ever written, the recent *Eat 4 Your Type*, is by a medical doctor.

9. If body fat in women falls below 10 to 14 percent as sometimes happens in heavy-duty exercisers, they may stop menstruating. As long as the quality of the diet is high, this apparently does no harm, and they can start menstruating again by gaining a little weight. But if you are either pregnant or attempting to become pregnant, you should not be on a rigorous dietary program unless that is prescribed by your doctor.

10. K. Cheney et al., *Exper. Gerontol.* 15:237, 1980. R. Weindruch et al., *AGE* 5:111, 1982.

11. P. Verhoef et al., *Am. J. Epidemiology* 143:845, 1996.

12. B. Best, *Life Extension*, June 1998, p. 29

13. *Environmental Nutrition*, December 1998, p. 4

14. H.E. Sours et al., *Am. J. Clin. Nutr.* 34:453, 1981.

15. B. J. Rolls and J. O. Hill, *Carbohydrates and Weight Management*. Washington, D.C.: ISLI Press, 1998.

16. K.B. Beckman and B. N. Ames, *Physiol. Rev.* 78:547, 1998.

17. *Environmental Nutrition*, April 1999, p. 4

18. H. N. Munro, in *Mammalian Protein Metabolism*, ed. H. N. Munro and J. B. Allison, Vol. 2. New York: Academic Press, 1964, p. 3.

19. *Nutrition Action*, September 1984.

20. *New Scientist*, June 5, 1999.

21. P. A. Crapo et al., *Diabetes* 26:1178, 1977. P. A. Crapo, *Nutrition Today* 19:6, 1984.

22. I. Brown, *Nutrition Reviews* 54:S115, 1996.

23. D. A. Jenkins et al., *Am. J. Clin. Nutr.* 34:362, 1981.

24. The fact is that most people have so many amyloses (enzymes that break down carbohydrates) in their gut that complex carbohydrates are broken down to simple ones almost immediately.

25. Dietary fiber is quite different from "crude fiber"—an older, narrower term that designates the part of the cell wall that is left after severe acid and base extraction. Crude fiber values appear in many food tables but are of little value. True dietary fiber may be four to five times as plentiful as crude fiber.

26. M. M. Baig et al., *Drug Nutrient Interactions* 3:109, 1985.

27. The food substance queuosine (found in certain transfer RNAs) may be an example. Experiments suggest that mice cannot synthesize it and must get it from their diet (Nishimura, 1983), but it is not yet recognized as an "essential" nutrient. Sufficient amounts are found in common plant and animal food products such as wheat germ, tomatoes, and yogurt, but might not be present in a junk food diet supplemented with merely the RDA list of essential nutrients. S. Nishimura, *Progress in Nucleic Acid Research* 28:50, 1983.

28. U. Verkhoshansky, *Soviet Sports Review* 17:41, 1982.

29. C. C. Johnson et al., *J. Am. Dietetic Assn.* 81:695, 1982.

30. B. F. Hurley et al., *J. Am. Med. Assn.* 252:507, 1984. L. Goldberg et al., *J. Am. Med. Assn.* 252:504, 1984.

CHAPTER 10

1. Ohaus #720 Triple Beam platform balance: available from (for example) Sargent-Welch Scientific Co., 7300 North Linden Ave., P.O. Box 1026, Skokie 60077.

2. *Nutrition Action*, October 1984, p. 12.

3. *Consumer Reports*, February 1981, p. 68.

4. Ibid.

5. G. R. Beecher, *Nutrition Reviews* 57:S3, 1999. This brief but comprehensive paper contains excellent updated material on the phytonutrients' role in metabolism and effects on resistance to disease and degenerative processes.

6. R. L. Walford, *Maximum Life Span*. New York: W. W. Norton, 1983.

7. I. M. Buzzard et al., *Am. J. Clin. Nutr.* 36:94, 1982.

8. M. Liebman and T. L. Bazzarre, *Am. J. Clin. Nutr.* 38:6127, 1983.

9. *Science News* 127:278, 1985.

10. F.B. Hu et al., *J. Am. Med. Assn.* 281:1387, 1999.

11. *Nutrition Reviews* 42:374, 1984.

12. J. Slavin et al., *Nutr. Cancer* 27:14, 1997.

13. *Science News*, August 18, 1990, p. 109.

14. K. H. Duncan et al., *Am. J. Clin. Nutr.* 37:763, 1983.

15. See note 13 above.

16. S. Belman, *Carcinogenesis* 4:1063, 1983.

17. B. H. S. Lau et al., *Nutrition Research* 3:119, 1983.

18. *Science News*, September 8, 1990, p. 157

19. Garlic also has antithrombotic effects. However, these probably cannot be gained from garlic pills, oils, extracts, or other commercial preparations because most manufacturing processes begin with steam distillation. Fresh garlic is best. Unfortunately, garlic and onions provide a lingering reminder of their ingestion because the sulfur compounds from garlic and onions, when absorbed from the intestines into the blood, find their way into expired air and sweat.

20. K. Kondo et al., *Lancet* 348:1514, 1996.

21. B. Fuhrman et al., *Am. J. Clin. Nutr.* 61:549, 1995.

22. K. Mcnutt, *Nutrition Today* 30:218, 1995.

23. *Sierra Club Bulletin*, July/August 1984.

24. A. Trichopoulou and P. Lagiou, *Nutrition Reviews* 55:383, 1997.

25. *Nutrition Reviews* 57:253, 1999.

26. C. Rainey and L. Nyquist, *Nutrition Today* 32:157, 1997.

27. G. Pascal, *Nutrition Reviews* 54:S24, 1996.

28. F. H. Mattson, in *Dietary Fats and Health*, ed. E. G. Perkins and W. J. Visek. AOCS Monograph 10, Am. Oil Chemists Society, 1983, p. 679.

29. *Environmental Nutrition*, February 1999, p. 1.

30. Ibid.

31. *Science News*, May 15, 1999, p. 319.

32. J. W. Fahey et al., *Proc. Nat. Acad. Sci.* 94:10367, 1997

33. D. Shapcott, in *Nutrition and Killer Diseases*, ed. J. Rose. Park Ridge, NJ: Noyes Publishing, 1982, p. 30.

34. G. L. Feder, in *Aging and the Geochemical Environment*. Washington, D.C.: National Academy Press, 1987, p. 92.

35. Shapcott, op. cit.

36. *East West Journal*, June 1990, p. 51.

INDEX